CANNIBALS, COWS & THE CJD CATASTROPHE

JENNIFER COOKE

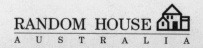

RANDOM HOUSE
AUSTRALIA

Jennifer Cooke is an award-winning senior journalist with the *Sydney Morning Herald* and has reported extensively on the CJD legacy of the use of human hormone drugs in Australia. She researched this book over five years of travelling to the United States, Britain, Canada and South Africa. A former chief reporter with South China Morning Post, she has also written for British newspapers and medical and legal journals.

Published by
Random House Australia Pty Ltd
20 Alfred Street, Milsons Point, NSW 2061
http://www.randomhouse.com.au

Sydney   New York   Toronto
London   Auckland   Johannesburg
and agencies throughout the world

First published 1998

National Library of Australia
Cataloguing-in-Publication Data

Cooke, Jennifer
Cannibals, cows and the CJD catastrophe: tracing the shocking
legacy of a 20th century disease.
ISBN 0 09 183691 3.
1. Creutzfeldt-Jacob disease. I. Title.
616.83

Editorial management by Black Dog Books
Text and picture section designed by Josie Semmler
Printed by Griffin Press Pty Ltd

10 9 8 7 6 5 4 3 2 1

Contents

To My parents John and Margaret
and to all those who have lost their lives prematurely
to Creutzfeldt-Jakob Disease

Preface

THIS IS A STORY of cannibalism and its legacies. It's about the cannibalism recognised for centuries — humans eating other humans. And it's about new-age cannibalism — feeding an animal species back to itself for recycling, for added protein, for profit. It's also about high-tech cannibalism — transplantation of organs, of tissue, of blood or other bodily parts into members of the same species or another species.

And it's about the warnings that should be heeded if the tragedies of accidental transmission of lethal diseases are to be avoided in future.

Transmissible spongiform encephalopathies (TSEs) or prion diseases are rare. But they do appear to be increasing in incidence, largely due to better awareness of them by doctors, better diagnostic criteria and the continuing and alarming spread of the terrible Bovine Spongiform Encephalopathy — Mad Cow disease — to humans in Britain and France so far.

The spread of BSE is but the newest form of accidental TSE transmission. There are lesser-known routes including neurosurgery and human biological transplants such as corneal grafts, brain lining implants and human hormone extracts. The jury is still out on whether blood transfusions and bone grafts pose more than a theoretical risk.

I first stumbled across this amazing story at 4.30 p.m. on November 26, 1992 when I received a telephone call about a bioethics paper to be presented at a conference in Sydney the next day. The paper warned of the potential risk of human hormone drug recipients passing on their risk of contracting Creutzfeldt-Jakob disease to others through blood, tissue and organ donations. Thereafter, as the then medical writer for the *Sydney Morning Herald,* I wrote a series of stories on the legacy of accidental medical transmission of CJD through human hormone injections to treat infertility and short stature in children.

What had begun as an interesting medical story has led to tracks in many directions – neuropathology, gynaecology, endocrinology, virology, pathology, veterinary science, family tragedy and cannibals.

The tireless research that has led to what is already known about these science-fiction TSEs – diseases that defy all known biology and seem to be caused by an "agent" that appears to be driven by non-living protein – is elite stuff. Already it has spawned two Nobel Prizes in medicine. It is an area of science that to date has attracted relatively few pharmaceutical dollars because the rareness of these diseases had rendered commercial viability a virtually zero.

TSEs, including Creutzfeldt-Jakob disease, are some of the most diabolical diseases known to science. Their attack is stealthy, invisible and relentless. The outcome is always fatal. There is no treatment or cure — or hope. A genetic lottery also appears to play a part in the unfortunate circumstance of a CJD death, from whatever source.

This book began as the germ of an idea to chart the tragic legacy of a fertility drug taken from dead bodies to give life to childless couples. It was also to provide information comprehensible to the lay person, desperately sought by families facing the threat of CJD from human hormone drugs in Australia, which was not generally available in the early 1990s. But as time passed, as inquiries were set up and shocking truths were revealed in several countries, the story broadened to include other modes of accidental transmission.

Still an obscure disease with little public recognition, except perhaps in Britain, CJD became a household acronym, almost, from 3 p.m. GMT on March 20, 1996 when the House of Commons was told that the deaths of 10 young Britons from CJD was linked to the BSE epidemic. This was a link the Government had denied for a decade.

This book, which was to have concentrated merely on human hormone drugs, became drastically altered. Many stories have been left out, each as tragic in their own way, as those that follow.

Since the announcement of the link between CJD and BSE-contaminated beef products there has been an explosion of developments that have increased knowledge in all areas relating directly and peripherally to CJD and related diseases.

All the average person ever wanted to know about these diseases, some of the people it affected, and a little bit more, awaits the turned page.

Jennifer Cooke
January 1998

Acknowledgments

THIS BOOK would not have been possible without enormous help. Thanks, in particular, must go to the families with members who died of CJD and who co-operated in the lengthy research of this book and — Ted Allender and Noel Halford, Lee and Kate Allender, Margaret Knight, Stephen and Muriel Cummings, Noel and Janet Baldwin, Ashraf and Parveen Khan.

Papua New Guinea: Dr Michael Alpers for his time and patience.

France: Jean-Bernard Mathieu, Maitre Giselle Mor, Pauline Jadas, Katharine Reynolds and Martin Morrissey at the Paris office of the Herbert Smith law firm, Maitre Monique Pelletier, Cecily Miner, Charles Humblet and Jean Thiessard.

America: Lewis Saul, Simon Beck, Dr Paul Brown who reviewed parts of the manuscript, Barbara Friedland, Candace Sutton and Gary Wilson.

Canada: Dr Michelle Brill-Edwards, Frank and Wendy Murray, Al Hébert, Eric Hébert and André Picard.

South Africa: Chantal and James Taylor, Dr Wolf Katz, Emlyn Hitchings, Professor François Bonnici and Emeritus Professor Lionel Smith.

Britain: Dr Alan Dickinson, David Body, Dr Robert Will, Professor John Collinge and Dr James Ironside, all of whom reviewed parts of the manuscript. Thanks also to Tam Fry, Peter Llewellyn, Caitlyn Delaney, Delyth Jones, Pauline Roberts, Dean Nelson, David Connett, Linda Tsang, Robert Neill, Professor Norman Solkoff, Ken Sutherland and Gaynor Fennessy at the John Fairfax London office.

New Zealand: Donelle Clarke, Anita McNaught, Michael Okkerse and Maureen Macdairmid.

Australia: The Australian Medical Writers' Association for its inaugural grant and group encouragement and enthusiasm, Diane Armstrong for her initial help and belief in the project and to Aileen Berry and Amanda Wilson for their invaluable first draft attention to detail. Geraldine Brodrick gave generously of her time and home hospitality. The John Fairfax editorial library staff members were extremely helpful and senior colleagues at the *Sydney Morning Herald* were outstandingly accommodating in allowing me work around research and writing commitments.

Professor Colin Masters from the Department of Pathology at the University of Melbourne, Dr Ian Humphery-Smith from the Department of Microbiology and Professor Clive Harper from the Department of Neuropathology at the University of Sydney, Dr Andrew Collins from the School of Microbiology and Immunology at the University of New South Wales and Dr Bob Ashcroft of Certain Cell Sorting Pty Ltd who provided reviews and other help for the scientific sections of the manuscript.

Professor John Hilton and Dr Jack Reisanen from the NSW Institute of Forensic Medicine and Dr Steven Collins from the Australian Creutzfeldt-Jakob Disease Registry were helpful on brains. Thanks is also due to Sean Millard, Michael Glen, Margaret Cooke, Helen Plumridge, Brad Norington, Bob Beale, Leigh Dayton, Melissa Sweet, June Giles, Helen Signy, Rhonda Hoysted, Sue Byrne, Suzanne Solvyns, Carol Wilson, Susan Andrews, Frank Peters, Laurie Bell, Lee Strauss, Karen Svensen, Karen Weeks, Joel Griffin, Jerome O'Shaughnessy, Coral O'Connor, Geoff Ross, Bill Smith, Keith Austin, Stuart Gordon and Jo Marshall of the Walter and Eliza Hall Institute of Medical Research. Major thanks must go to Dr Lynette Dumble for her unbridled enthusiasm, encouragement and unceasing help, as well as for rescuing a very large volume of Gajdusek and CJD scientific articles headed directly for the paper recycler.

Thank also to Andrew Kelly, who produced the book in record time and publisher Deb Callaghan, who took the punt when no-one else would.

List of abbreviations
This list shows common abbreviations used in the text.

ACTH	adrenocorticotrophic hormone
AHPHP	Australian Human Pituitary Hormone Program
BSE	bovine spongiform encephalopathy
CJD	Creutzfeldt-Jakob disease
CSL	Commonwealth Serum Laboratories
FFI	Fatal Familial Insomnia
FSH	follicle stimulating hormone
GAGS	glycosaminoglycans
GSS	Gerstmann-Straüssler-Scheinker syndrome
hCG	human chorionic gonadotrophin
hGH	human growth hormone
hMG	human menopausal gonadotrophin
HPAC	Human Pituitary Advisory Committee
hPG	human pituitary gonadotrophin
LH	luteinising hormone
nvCJD	new variant CJD
PMS	pregnant mare serum
prion	proteinaceous infectious particle
PRNP	prion protein
SAFs	scrapie-associated fibrils
TME	transmissible mink encephalopathy
TSE	transmissible spongiform encephalopathy
TSH	thyroid-stimulating hormone

CHAPTER 1

Kuru:
The shivering sickness

THE KEROSENE LANTERNS flicker erratically as the gale howls outside. The grass hut is made of kunai grass, weather-proof and tough enough to slash the arms and legs of unwary visitors to the mountainous interior of the island of Papua New Guinea. The wind's eerie song as it whispers through the grass roof and walls of the hut is like a ghastly dirge for the boy who lies within. Lantern light casts weird shadows on the walls of the hut as a tall, lean white man leans over the table. He is young, not quite 30, and his normal dark crew cut has grown long.

The boy on the table is Kinao. He is no more than eight years old. It is 2 a.m. this cold mid-May morning in 1957 and Kinao has been dead less than an hour. It is perfect timing for the man, who is carrying out a grisly harvest. He opens up Kinao's skull, cuts the optic and outer cranial nerves, and then the spinal cord. The little boy's brain literally falls into his hands.

Kinao's body was carried to this place by his family through driving rain and wind from the "hospital", a long, low structure and the newest building in the village of Okapa.[1] In it 22 children, adolescents and adult women lie stricken. Many have been carried there from their own villages, unable to speak, to walk or swallow even tiny sips of liquid. They cannot appreciate the magnificent view down the valley.

Their relatives, sleeping nearby in small circular houses segregated into men-only and female-only groups, have come with a mixture of suspicion, hope and resignation. Suspicion about what the white doctors are jabbing into their loved ones with their needles and pills and strange foods. Hope that, by trying the western medicine, the evil sorcery that has made their wives and children sick will be miraculously lifted. But mostly they are resigned to the fact that there will be many more deaths, as there have been before, as far back as most can remember.

The village of Okapa is one of some 160 that dot the valleys of the Eastern Highlands of PNG, wedged between the Lamari and Yani rivers to the south and west and the Kratke Mountains north-east of the Fore area. Everyone who lives there knows about kuru sorcery. Historical perspective reveals that it probably started in neighbouring Keiagana and the southern part of the north Fore area in the early 1900s. Slowly it moved south and north, in line with the movement of the locals, killing hundreds. Kuru is one of the key features of life in this part of the Highlands and its mystery has set these people apart from others. Like Kinao, the 22 patients at Okapa hospital are dying of kuru, the local native word for shivering or trembling. Their last months have taken the usual course of this dreadful illness — the staggering, jerking, degenerative symptoms that mean certain death.

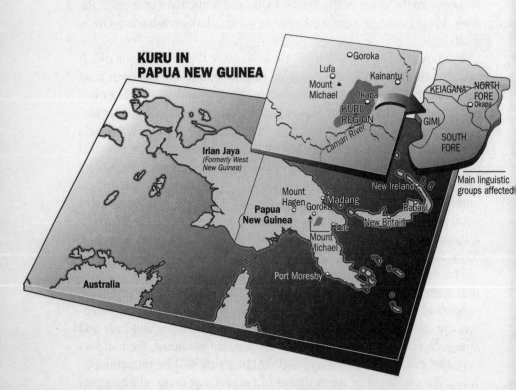

The man, who would later to write of his autopsy on Kinao as a "dastardly" deed, is Dr Daniel Carleton Gajdusek, known to everyone as Carleton. He is trying to work a little of his own Western medical magic on the scourge that threatens to wipe out much of the human life within miles of Okapa. Gajdusek is one of only two westerners in the immediate vicinity and among only a dozen white men seen by the major race of inhabitants of the region — a culturally and linguistically distinct group known as the Fore (pronounced For-ay) people. They practise polygamy and cannibalism, and are war-like in nature, fighting each other with bows and arrows. Hunting and the subsistence farming of small plots of land, clawed back from jungles that dominate mountains up to 3,000 metres, support hundreds and hundreds of tribes, each with its own language.

In 1957 the Fore believe kuru is the result of magic spells by malevolent sorcerers — human enemies. Each year kuru kills about 200 of the 35,000 inhabitants of the Eastern Highlands region, and the 12,000-odd Fore, in particular, are desperate for help. What concerns them most is that kuru kills mostly women and children, and at a rate far outstripping any other disease or accident.

Gajdusek, a paediatrician and virologist, knows there is a logical explanation — medical, environmental or inheritable — for kuru's relentless advance. Already he has found an apparent sharp demarcation circling the Fore people and several other nearby linguistic groups that have intermarried with the Fore. As he works on Kinao's body, still warm in the hour since his death, and works against time to collect the precious organ and tissue samples vital to his search for an answer, Gajdusek's mind is racing: sorting accumulated facts and pondering the elusive cause of kuru. The scientist knows only that nothing of a medical, drug or dietary nature he has tried in the eight weeks he has been at Okapa has stopped or even slowed kuru's relentless pursuit of death. He hopes that expert analysis of the child's cerebellum, the area of the brain that controls balance and motor function, might hold the clue.

Built from native materials and thatched in the traditional kunai grass, Gajdusek's new laboratory hut is doubling as a treatment and autopsy room away from curious local eyes. The crude autopsy — "butchery" as Gajdusek's characteristic candour allows him to admit — is completed using a hand saw, one of the few implements available to open a skull in this jungle setting.[2] And while neuropathologists prefer to use an inflexible long-bladed, round-ended brain knife to cut slices from the jelly-like texture of warm brain, Gajdusek has only a carving knife. He is right in fearing that the serrated edges of the knife make it a sloppy job, but at least pathologists will have brain tissue to study.

Around 2 a.m., as the storm continues to buffet the hut, sending clouds of chaff raining down on the occupants, Gajdusek and a native *dokta boi* helper harvest other organs and tissues from Kinao's frail body in the hope some might yield more clues. The slices of brain are placed in a container filled with a 10 per cent formaldehyde-saline solution, one of several combination chemical agents used for processing brain material. It will help to preserve, or fix, the chemical structure of the brain so that little is altered in the time it takes to travel by jeep and plane to pathologists at the Walter and Eliza Hall Institute of Medical Research (WEHI) in Melbourne, Australia, and the National Institutes of Health (NIH) in Bethesda, Maryland, USA. Also sent for analysis are the whole pituitary gland, a pea-sized organ that sits on a stalk at the base of the brain, and little pieces of Kinao's organs — including the liver, lung, pancreas, kidney, aortic wall and spleen.

By dawn Kinao has been collected by his grieving mother, who is rewarded for her contribution to medical science with salt, axes and a *laplap* sarong. She never discovers the role her small son has played in one of the world's greatest medical discoveries.

Gajdusek was born in Yonkers, New York in 1923 to Czechoslovakian migrant parents. He was a bright child who won all available prizes at his high school graduation. He had been fascinated by science from an early age when his *Tante* Irene, his mother's sister, an entomologist with a PhD from Cornell University, taught him how to dissect a host of insects and helped him design experiments in Petri dishes with larvae, leaves and insecticides. Gajdusek was a quick and early learner with an apparently amazing aptitude for languages. At Rochester University he gained a biophysics degree, then spent three short years at Harvard Medical School earning another degree in paediatrics.

By 1955, when Gajdusek arrived at WEHI in Melbourne, his "hobby" — later described in the subtitle of one of his books as "studies of child growth and development and disease patterns in primitive cultures" — had taken him to the top of Cape York Peninsula. There he charted the presence of measles antibodies in Australian Aboriginal children following a devastating epidemic in 1943. He also visited New Guinea and New Britain to set up child studies on disease screening and genetics aimed at long-term follow up in Melanesians. He had earlier studied and filmed the deadly effects of the rabies virus in the Middle East. He worked at WEHI for about 18 months as a visiting investigator, ostensibly probing influenza-virus genetics and the infectious hepatitis virus with Sir Frank Macfarlane Burnet, who went on to win the 1960 Nobel Prize for medicine. But Gajdusek's work during that time centred on his discovery of the auto-antibodies found in chronic hepatitis, lupus and multiple myeloma patients.[3]

March 13, 1957 marked the beginning of Gajdusek's life-long involvement with kuru. That was the day he arrived unannounced at the home of Dr Vincent Zigas, the recently appointed the district medical officer at Kainantu, a tiny outpost of civilisation with its own basic hospital. Gajdusek had been on his way back to an undefined role within the NIH in America, and had stopped in PNG to further his pilot studies on child growth. He also planned to visit Sir Mac's son, Ian, who was then the patrol officer at Lufa near Mount Michael, north west of the kuru region. But soon after he landed in Port Moresby, a courtesy meeting with a public health official set Gajdusek on the trail of a strange "new" disease in the Highlands. He decided to detour via Kainantu, north-east of the kuru region for a closer look.

Most people retain a distinct first impression of Carleton Gajdusek. Zigas was intrigued by this eccentric and fascinating American visitor who "machine-gunned" him with questions.[4]

> He was tall and lean, and one of those people whose age was difficult to guess, looking boyish with a soot-black crew-cut unevenly trimmed, as if done by himself … He was a well-built man, with a remarkably shaped head, curiously piercing eyes, and ears that stood out from his head … Even standing still, he seemed to be on the move, with top tilted forward, in the breathless posture of someone who never had time enough to get where he had to be.[5]

Gajdusek stayed the night and was infected by Zigas' fascination with kuru — his first taste of "the disease people caught from studying kuru". Those involved would later joke that this was more interesting than the disease itself.[6,7]

> I am in one of the most remote, recently opened regions of New Guinea
> (in the Eastern Highlands) in the centre of tribal groups of cannibals, only
> contacted in the last ten years and controlled for five years — still spear-
> ing each other as of a few days ago, and cooking and feeding the children
> the body of a kuru case, the disease I am studying — only a few weeks
> ago …

Gajdusek wrote excitedly to Dr Joseph Smadel, the research director
and his former boss at the NIH, on March 15, 1957.[8]

Others were less excited at the American's excessive work ethic and
what was seen to be Gajdusek's blatant takeover of a problem on what
was then Australian territorial soil.[9] By the time of Kinao's death,
"Dokta America" or "Coutan", as the local children had begun calling
him, had been in New Guinea for just on eight weeks and controversy
had already erupted around him. Gajdusek's frenzied activity in the
"kuru region" was in part of the "uncontrolled areas" of the country
which were not derestricted until late 1958. This meant that early kuru
investigations needed special government permission — something
Gajdusek did not have. Nor did he have an official permit to stay in the
country, as he was ostensibly there merely to visit Ian Burnet. Zigas,
however, did have official sanction and provided vital medical support
to Gajdusek, who had promptly settled in, happy to sleep on the floor
and work with gusto to solve the riddle of kuru.

Despite protest from WEHI (which had not yet sent its own virologist to investigate the kuru phenomenon) and also polite requests for
him to leave by administrators in the capital, Port Moresby, Gajdusek
refused to leave PNG. And because he was in such a remote part of the
country, no-one was prepared to go and drag him out. A person less
stubborn and with less confidence in his ability to eradicate kuru would
have left.

Gajdusek wrote copious letters trying to smooth out the trouble over
his presence. He worked from dawn until midnight taking specimens,
and laboured for hours at a time compiling family histories via interpreters to identify kuru cases in near and distant relatives. All Fore
adults who were asked admitted to cannibalism, readily telling Gajdusek with pride of their ritual display of love and respect for their dead
relative by eating them. He marvelled in his letters at the accuracy of
local diagnoses of the early signs of kuru. It could hardly be mistaken
in its latter stages.

During this time, the much-respected "Sir Mac" Burnet wrote to an official in the New Guinea administration in April 1957 to provide him with background following Gajdusek's "rather extraordinary intrusion into New Guinea".[10] Describing Gajdusek's auto-immune work at WEHI as "first rate" he said:

> My own summing up was that he had an intelligence quotient up in the 180s and the emotional immaturity of a 15-year-old. He is quite maniacally energetic when his enthusiasm is roused … He is completely self-centred, thick-skinned and inconsiderate, but equally won't let danger, physical difficulty, or other people's feelings interfere in the least with what he wants to do. He apparently has no interest in women but an almost obsessional interest in children, none whatever in clothes and cleanliness; and he can live cheerfully in a slum or a grass hut.[11]

While the discord swirled between Port Moresby and Melbourne, Gajdusek, intent on his work, dismissed it in one of his letters to Smadel. On his faithful Olympic typewriter, carbon paper between the sheets for necessary copies, he described it as "a bit of a spat in the mails with Sir Mac, which is concerned mostly with Australian fears of having 'foreign' (i.e. American) workers studying such an exciting problem in their Territory, and their claim that we are 'stealing' a problem from them."[12]

On April 3, 1957, having returned from his first patrol to map the southern-most extent of kuru in the Highlands, Gajdusek wrote to Smadel requesting any type of funding that could support him for a few months longer studying the epidemic: "I tell you Joe, this is no wild goose-chase, but a really big thing; everything in my medical training makes me confident … I stake my entire medical reputation on this matter."[13]

Self-described in later published correspondence as "a recalcitrant and unpredictable subordinate", Gajdusek's presence developed into a sometimes bitter parochial political issue from which the Australians never fully recovered. However, it is certainly acknowledged among those who came to study kuru after him, that no-one sent from Australia could ever have matched Gajdusek's zeal, command of languages, experience in child health or fanaticism. In a May 1957 letter to Smadel, sent with samples of Kinao's tissue, Gajdusek described kuru as "perhaps the most important epidemiological problem in the world at the moment ... Kuru is a most difficult thing to abandon; it is too good a problem".[14]

The challenge of an apparently new disease drove Gajdusek to work well into each night, sitting on an upturned galvanised iron patrol box, writing letters, documenting dietary habits, drug dosages and progression of symptoms, and collating and classifying the data he collected daily. He and Zigas, who drove his jeep to Okapa from Kainantu as often as possible, doggedly collected urine and blood samples from the hospital patients in the hope that analysis in Australia would provide an answer.

Over the following months, Gajdusek and the local Okapa patrol officer, Jack Baker, crisscrossed Eastern Highlands villages and repeatedly asked the same questions of thousands of villagers, hoping to track kuru cases and chart medical histories. What they found were hundreds of Fore people — as well as a handful from neighbouring areas — dying of kuru. It had become such an epidemic that it threatened the survival of an entire race. Victims included boys and girls aged from five, through to their late teens. Women of all ages were badly affected. Curiously, adult men were rarely touched by kuru.

Gajdusek soon realised that victims were diagnosed often by others in the village. A fine tremor of the body was the first subtle indication, so faint that only a seasoned observer would notice it as they sat in a group around a fire. Weeks later, the victim, no matter how reluctantly, would have to acknowledge trouble walking normally. Regular tropical downpours made immediate mud of the mountain tracks and the villagers were accustomed to maintaining good balance in slippery conditions. Children and adult victims alike would begin to stumble and gradually adopt the peculiar gait that doctors recognise as ataxia but a layperson would describe as drunken staggering.

Soon a sufferer's arms and legs would jerk spasmodically. Walking without a stick became impossible. Some women tending crops of taro and sweet potatoes in their hillside gardens would need a villager on either side to help them return to their huts as dusk fell. Eventually, Gajdusek noted, their speech would become slurred and their eyes might move involuntarily or cross. The tremors would become almost continuous, making the victims appear to be shivering on the hottest of days. Standing up could lead to foot stamping. To maintain some balance while upright, the victim's toes would often claw at the ground.[15]

After several months, sufferers would experience involuntary muscle spasms, jerks brought on by bright lights or sudden loud noise. Women particularly, might burst into tears without warning or, when in groups, would often burst into peals of contagious laughter for no apparent reason. This gave rise to the misnomer of "laughing death" when the term "trembling death" would have been more accurate. Young boys became depressed and sometimes belligerent among relatives. Common to all sufferers was mental deterioration. Dementia, though, was conspicuous by its absence.[16]

Within months of his arrival, and having seen several hundred cases, Gajdusek noted that the terminal stage of kuru arrived six months to a year after the onset of the shivering and staggering symptoms. All bodily functions shut down and when a victim could no longer swallow, he or she would then starve to death. Often as kuru victims lay by the fire, or in shade outdoors during daylight while tended by family members, they developed large ulcers or bed sores on their legs which led to fatal septicaemia. Pneumonia, mercifully, claimed some victims before they could waste away from kuru. Some unfortunate victims died from burns after falling unnoticed into the fires that were the centrepiece of the sleeping huts.

The epidemic was so serious that the polygamous New Guinea Highlanders found it hard to find one wife — let alone more. Many men turned to child marriage for a wife who could tend a vegetable garden and bear his children while he hunted.

On May 27, 1957, soon after Kinao's premature death, Gajdusek performed a second autopsy, five hours after the death of a 50-year-old woman called Yabaiotu. Her brain, however, was left whole and spared the destructive edges of Gajdusek's carving knife. But instead of going again to WEHI in Melbourne, it was sent to the NIH in Bethesda, where Smadel would later provide Gajdusek with his own laboratory to continue this ground-breaking research.

The Australian authorities were not aware that Kinao's tissues had been sent to the NIH until later in 1957. This discovery exacerbated the political issues, which for a time had died down after a decision was taken around April — the easiest at the time — to allow Gajdusek to stay in Okapa. However, the knowledge gained from Kinao and Yabaiotu, whose brains were among a dozen analysed in that first adventurous year of research, laid the foundations for the recognition of a new group of diseases, which would become known as spongiform encephalopathies or literally spongy brain degenerations.

Kuru became the major cause of death for girls in the Fore linguistic group and the biggest cause of death, beyond infancy, after tribal war wounds. The locals were terrified — and not without reason. Kuru would go on to kill at least 3,000 in the decades that followed, most of them adult women.[17,18,19] But the fatal effects of kuru were not restricted to victims of the disease. Pregnancy seemed to hasten the end for women with kuru. Babies born to a kuru victim often died of starvation, despite desperate attempts by fathers to nourish their infants by spitting masticated sugar cane into their tiny mouths. Nursing mothers fed their own children first, so orphans fared worst.

Belief in sorcery was intrinsic to the culture of these people of the Highlands, and a very strict taboo surrounded any mention of the actual operation of kuru sorcery. As a result, the pipe-smoking and bespectacled Zigas — who, with his Baltic features and fair wavy hair, could have doubled for the American actor Danny Kaye — had found it difficult to communicate with villagers during his early patrols through the region. Later, between 1961 and 1963, anthropologists Shirley Lindenbaum and Robert Glasse studied the social effects of sorcery and kuru while based in the largest village of the southern Fore area, Wanitabe. They eventually categorised sixteen different forms of sorcery that the people of the Eastern Highlands believed were responsible for a range of recognised illnesses. Kuru sorcery was one of the worst because the victims always died.

Any male member of a community was believed to be able to inflict kuru. But usually the accused sorcerer was someone who had had a hostile or rival encounter with a male relative of the kuru victim. A kuru sorcerer bent on revenge supposedly took something intimate belonging to the intended victim — like excrement, hair, bits of clothing or discarded food. This was added to a magic bundle made from bark, sweet potato leaves, grass, a twig and a sorcery stone tied up with cane and some vines. The bundle was named and beaten with a stick then placed in a watery, muddy area while a spell was recited. The idea was that as the bundle deteriorated, so did the health of the victim. At intervals the sorcerer returned to beat the bundle, coinciding with the worsening kuru symptoms. As the bundle disintegrated and maggots appeared, the victim's limbs were racked with tremors and death followed.

Zigas performed the first kuru autopsy in early 1957 after gaining permission from the victim's husband to explore his wife's "brain box". But the analysis at WEHI of that brain plus blood samples from 20 live kuru sufferers produced no enlightening result. No virus had been isolated. Nothing abnormal was found at all. Months later Zigas and Gajdusek were no nearer an explanation.

Although both doctors thought kuru was probably an infectious disease, a genetic basis could not be ruled out. It was obvious from their earliest observations that up to four kuru deaths could occur in siblings from one family. These could be years apart. Gajdusek, who with the aid of local interpreters acquired the basics not only of the Fore language but that of the neighbouring Keiagana people, stumbled on an important clue after exhaustive patrols and interviews. Kuru affected not only the Fore cultural and linguistic groups but other linguistic groups, including the Keiagana, Kanite, Auiana (later Auyana) and Kimi (later Gimi) in neighbouring regions where intermarriage with the Fore occurred. But it was years before this apparent random connection made sense.

By June 1957 Zigas and Gajdusek were working assiduously, if dispiritedly due to slow progress, at their "Kuru Centre" — the hospital and native hut "laboratory" containing a microscope, an ophthalmoscope, tuning forks, lab reagents and equipment. Due to the growing workload of experiments, another new house was added to relieve the dining table at the patrol officer's house. For months the table had functioned simultaneously as a desk, a laboratory, a lumbar puncture table and an autopsy bench awash with specimen containers, bottles of rum and lime cordial. Before each meal it all had to be cleared away. Despite a gut instinct by both Zigas and Gajdusek that it was infectious, no thought was given to potential contamination by kuru.

Unimpressed locals told the doctors they were no match for the power of kuru sorcery, but doggedly they continued. The pair took countless urine and blood samples, performed lumbar punctures and other physical and neurological examinations. The medical solutions at hand were tried — long-term doses of vitamin B complex, ascorbic acid, high doses of broad-spectrum antibiotics such as aureomycin and chloramphenicol, which is used against staphylococcus, typhoid and typhus. Folic acid supplements and improved diets including fish oil were tried unsuccessfully. Even phenobarbital, with its anticonvulsant properties was useless against kuru. More drugs were sent via Port Moresby, but there were no reactions either to antihistamines, low doses of adrenocorticotrophic hormone (ACTH), iron therapy, anti-bacterial sulfonamides, or drugs used to treat Parkinson's disease in which symptoms include tremors.

From the 1950s onwards scientists believed all viruses produced fever, antibodies or some sign that the body had recognised a foreign invader. Kuru had none of these. Nor was there an indication of any acute illness before the initial staggering symptoms emerged. There was absolutely no evidence to back an infectious disease theory. In fact kuru appeared to have a strong hereditary component. It could often be traced back over more than three generations: mothers, sisters, aunts, siblings and sometimes male relatives of kuru victims all tended to suc-cumb to the disease. Females were predominantly affected — at a rate of 30 to one in adults, and two to one in children.

Complicating the epidemiological study was the fact that the hamlets in which kuru cases occurred were scattered among almost impene-trable jungle paths. To carry out his work, Gajdusek travelled willingly through leech-infested rivers and up and down thousands of metres of dense mountainside vegetation. He was pursued by wild bees, flies, malaria-carrying mosquitoes and inevitably finished the day with bleeding feet. At night a grass hut floor was the most luxurious accom-modation that welcomed him.

By September 1957 dietary studies on the potential toxicity of native products, plants, minerals and herbs had drawn a blank. Drug therapy — which also included British anti-lewisite, used against heavy metal poisoning — had neither helped nor halted the disease's progression. Blood samples from kuru victims continued to be stockpiled at both WEHI and the NIH.

By this time Gajdusek and Zigas had seen at least 200 active kuru patients and had performed a dozen autopsies, usually within an hour of death. The duo often worked as a team sawing, cutting and sewing up the body and scalp again with "big stitches, dressings, and bands of leucoplast".[20] Three brains from kuru victims who had died since

Kinao and Yabaiotu were sent to a Melbourne University neurologist Graeme Robertson, and the rest went to Joe Smadel at the NIH who assigned a senior neuropathologist, Igor Klatzo, to examine them.

When reports on these brains came back, Gajdusek was as excited as a schoolboy. Robertson had found "surprisingly slight"[21] neuropathological changes to account for the devastating neurological symptoms, and these were mostly in the cerebellum. Klatzo, on the other hand, remarked on striking changes in the cerebellum. In a later paper on studies of the first 12 brains sent to the NIH for inspection, Klatzo made "an interesting finding" in the brain of Yani, the youngest kuru victim who was aged only five when he died in 1957. In Yani's and five of the other brains he inspected, "was the presence of remarkable plaque-like structures".[22] Substantial brain damage was apparent under the microscope, although not to the naked eye. The disease, although apparently genetic, wrote Klatzo, "appears to be closest in resemblance" to a very rare brain disease that few doctors had ever seen — Creutzfeldt–Jakob disease (CJD). CJD was also familial. Individuals in four generations of one family had died by the late 1950s.[23] This observation by Klatzo was a prophetic clue. However it said nothing about the actual cause of kuru. Little was known about the cause of CJD either.

Gajdusek had begun to keep a proper journal, forsaking the scraps of paper and odd notebooks that he had filled for the past 18 months. It was a habit that eventually produced hundreds of thousands of pages documenting his travels, patrols and disease explorations in emerging cultures. It provided a unique insight into his and other scientists' thinking at the times he first encountered various maladies. Gajdusek's journal was also the basis of the first published reports on kuru. Manuscripts drafted and laboriously rewritten by kerosene lamp at Okapa appeared finally in the *New England Journal of Medicine* and the *Medical Journal of Australia* in November 1957, and in the German *Klinische Wochenschrift* in May 1958.

Ten months after his impromptu arrival, Gajdusek left for America. Petty squabbles erupted over priorities for funding. Australian scientists argued the hypothesis that kuru was a wholly genetic disease. But the cause of kuru remained a mystery and the epidemic continued.

From Zigas' formal notification to authorities of the disease on Boxing Day 1956 — "a form of encephalitis amongst the Okapa people" — there was probably not a time when someone hadn't speculated that kuru was linked to cannibalism. Most westerners, including missionaries, miners and government workers living in the Eastern Highlands, knew that many villagers had practised cannibalism. By the late 1950s government campaigns to discourage (including by means of imprisonment) and outlaw endocannibalism, the eating of close relatives as a mourning rite, had been largely successful.

Before those campaigns took effect and as part of the practice of endocannibalism, village women usually opened the bodies of their kin with sharp bamboo knives and stone axes. Their children sat around them as they cut open arms and legs, stripped out muscle and slit the chest and abdomen. The women removed the head and fractured the skull to get at the brain. Soft brain tissue was scooped barehanded into cylinders of bamboo for cooking in the ashes of their fires. Blood and tissue undoubtedly splattered onto the children milling about. Without washing, the women wiped themselves clean on their bodies and hair. Many regarded leaving the cadaver tissue on their hands and bodies as another element of their mourning. With their contaminated hands they picked at sores — tropical ulcers or yaws were very common. They also scratched at bites and soothed crying babies by wiping noses and drying eyes. Then they ate the brains, which they cooked with other food.

Though adult men had similar diets to their families, they rarely ate with them. In mortuary feasts, the men shunned brain and other offal in favour of the occasional meal of muscle, which they enjoyed. After the meat was gone and the internal organs and the brain were removed, villagers sucked marrow from the cracked bones. The bones themselves were sometimes heated in fires for several weeks to make them brittle. Once pounded, the pulverised bones were sprinkled over vegetables.[24] In the north Fore region, it was customary to bury the body for a few days, then dig it up and eat it. That way "the maggots could be cooked as a separate delicacy".[25]

Australian anthropologist Shirley Lindenbaum, with her first husband, Robert Glasse, was the first to suggest that the consuming of dead kuru victims helped explain the remarkable sex and age distribution of the disease.[26] But it was Michael Alpers, a tall, bearded Australian doctor who joined Gajdusek in PNG in 1961, who finally nailed cannibalism as the mode of transmission for kuru.

Alpers was hooked on kuru as soon as he read the first lurid headlines in the *Advertiser* newspaper in late 1957 about the "laughing death". And academics at the University of Adelaide, where Alpers was completing his medical studies, were at the forefront of developing a genetic hypothesis to explain kuru. Bored with his studies, Alpers jumped at an offer to work in New Guinea. Five months after his arrival there in October 1961 Alpers met Gajdusek, by then infamous as "the madman who spends his time over with the kukukukus (the tribe now known as Anga), these weird head-hunting homosexual people that everyone was afraid of".[27] The pair clicked and became firm friends. They shared the same goal — to find the cause of kuru — and began what would be a long and successful collaboration. Earlier experiments using mice, rats and even monkeys had lasted only weeks, rather than months, so they decided they would use chimpanzees, inject them with kuru and watch them over periods spanning years. It was already known that similar diseases in animals appeared to be so slow in evolving that it was years between infection and death. They planned to watch the chimps for up to 10 years, after injecting them with sterile samples of kuru-infected tissue taken within an hour of the death of a Fore victim. This method was intended to avoid any later suggestion of a mix-up, or external contamination, or not having allowed for a sufficient incubation period.

Alpers had been hired by the PNG administration as a government medical officer devoted solely to kuru research. His appointment was the only concrete result that emerged from a doomed proposal, announced by the government in May 1960, to quarantine the entire kuru region. After accepting the hypothesis put forward by University of Adelaide researchers that kuru was solely a genetic disease, the administration had planned to turn the 2300 square kilometres of mountain area inhabited by the Fore and neighbouring linguistic tribes into a "vast concentration camp".[28] It was hoped this would prevent men, by now vastly outnumbering women in many villages, spreading the disease as they moved to find work. The proposal was later dumped.

Fascinated by genetics, neurology, paediatrics and anthropology, Alpers conducted vital epidemiological studies as well as half-a-dozen autopsies on kuru victims — some in remote villages — between April 1962 and late 1963. Death for the Fore was a family affair:

> Everyone wanted to be there so we had to get rid of half the people in the house. Usually the closest relative, the father of the child or the father of the woman or the husband of the woman would assist with the actual autopsy … by holding the body.[29]

During his first autopsy, Alpers set the standard he was to follow afterwards by insisting that every participant wore a mask. His two assistants, who held the sterile bottles into which the brain samples were placed with forceps, also wore gloves. In the confined space of the thatched hut, which generally had a radius of only three metres, those precautions were solely for reasons of sterility, rather than fear of infection.

Another autopsy on an 11-year-old girl called Kigea, who died of kuru in Alpers' own village of Waisa, was more harrowing than normal. Alpers knew the girl and her father, also present at the autopsy, very well. Kigea's autopsy was to prove vital in years to come. All the effort involved in putting kuru brains in a bucket of formalin, walking for hours from a patient's village to Okapa, chartering a small plane from a nearby missionary airstrip to Lae and then forwarding the frozen tissue samples to the Commonwealth Serum Laboratories (CSL) in Melbourne, was essential. Further samples were kept at –70ºC until they could be flown to the USA for inoculation into the brain of a chimpanzee at the NIH.

Alpers and Gajdusek, who returned again and again to New Guinea, visited and revisited Fore villages on field patrols. Laborious and diligent cross-checks, interviews and analysis of field data collected from their own records as well as patrol officers and others working in the kuru region between 1957 and 1963 later filled a file created at the NIH on all known patients.

Alpers moved to America to work with Gajdusek. In 1964, towards the end of the first year of the four he was to spend in Gajdusek's laboratory at the NIH, Alpers was stunned to find something new shining out of the thousands of numbers on his dull charts. Apart from the primary epidemiological statistic — that kuru was limited solely to the Fore people and those with whom they had intermarried — another startling fact had emerged from the data gathered on the 1450 documented kuru cases during that eight year period to 1963.

Alpers and an assistant checked and rechecked their maps and their hand-totted figures, comparing the 1957–59 period with the 1960–63 period. There was no mistake. Kuru had disappeared in children under five years of age and had almost gone in those under eight. Why?

In December 1964, the world's first meeting on slow viruses was held in Bethesda. As a result the first monograph on "Slow, latent and temperate virus infections" was published the following year. In this publication the cause of kuru was said to most likely be the super-imposition of an environmental factor on a genetic susceptibility. What-ever this environmental factor was, it had clearly declined in line with the decline of kuru in children.[30] Cannibalism was one of the items in a long list — including sweet potato, maize, the casuarina tree, salt, steel axes, the domestic fowl, new vegetable varieties and twist tobacco — of known environmental changes in the kuru region over the years. But it was too early to make a definite pronouncement.

It wasn't until early 1967 that some of the puzzling pieces surround-ing the spread of kuru clicked into place. Alpers was composing a paper for the fifty-sixth annual meeting of the International Academy of Pathology, held in March that year, in his makeshift office on the porch of his Bethesda bungalow. He pondered the title of his paper, "Kuru: implications of its transmissibility for the interpretation of its changing epidemiological pattern".[31] What, among the many changes that had occurred in the Fore region since it was derestricted by the Australian administration in late 1958, could account for the disappearance of kuru in small children? Alpers stared distractedly at his third child, baby daughter Deryn, as she tottered around the house following older sister Kirsten and brother James. Suddenly the explanation hit him. It had always been there in the background. The end of endocannibalism was the subject of one well-remembered conversation he had had in 1963 with his friends Shirley Lindenbaum and Robert Glasse: "… It was women and children who ate the infective brain and not the men," he realised. Children growing up free of kuru had also grown up in a community now free of endocannibalism. "The practice of endocanni-balism meant only relatives were consumed, which explained why the disease appeared familial in its distribution," he thought. "Fortunately the disease was not transmitted vertically from infected mother to child; and that too was now clear."[32]

While endocannibalism is now the generally accepted hypothesis of kuru transmission, there was much initial scepticism about Alpers' theory, including the proposition that cannibalism had never been a reg-ular custom. But to Alpers, the vital question remained. Where did kuru originate? It has become generally accepted that kuru was an isolated man-made epidemic spread over a half-century by ritual cannibalism — probably from an initial sporadic case of the similar, if not originally identical, Creutzfeldt–Jakob disease. Gajdusek later speculated in a less popular theory that if a sporadic case of CJD (since found in the early 1970s in a 26-year-old Chimbu tribesman from the Central Highlands) did not start the kuru epidemic, a mutation of a well-known virus, through multiple passages of relatives over decades, may have been the culprit.[33]

No-one born since 1959 has developed kuru. Cannibalism is believed to have largely stopped by about 1957 in the affected villages with the odd sporadic practice reportedly occurring up to about 1962. Alpers' continuing epidemiological studies on kuru — he has been the director of the Papua New Guinea Institute of Medical Research since 1977 — have shown that the disease has been almost, but not quite, wiped out. By the late 1960s it was no longer appearing in anyone under 10 years of age. By the late 1980s no-one under 30 had succumbed to the disease. The youngest victim in the 1990s was in his 40s.

In a remarkable feat of monitoring, Alpers and Robert L. Klitzman, an American doctor who spent a year in PNG, sandwiched their studies on malaria and pneumonia with a study of transmission events of 65 kuru patients. These patients had either died or had been diagnosed with kuru between 1977 and 1981.[34] Gajdusek's early and laborious kuru case histories came in handy in this retrospective study, which was published in 1984. The histories included the names and ages of victims, their relationships with others, the names of relatives who had died of kuru and when this had taken place. Also of use were the Fore's own records, in which ages were calculated by size-comparison with village adults and children. The passage of time was marked by such events as the establishment of the Okapa patrol post in 1954, the start of the building of the road to Okapa in 1955 and its extension to Purosa in 1957.

By studying this cluster of 65 patients, the three investigators were able to show that the incubation period of kuru stretched as far as 30 years: some kuru patients had only ever attended one or two feasts, and then only as young children. Some victims who attended the same feast died within weeks or months of one another, showing an almost identical incubation period and further underlining the feast as the infection event.

From Fore records it was established that two brothers who died within six months of one another in late 1976 and mid-1977 had each been taken by their mother to the mortuary feasts of two women who died of kuru. The first feast was for Nonon, a paternal aunt, in 1948, and the second was for Nen, a member of their kinship line, who died in 1953 or 1954.[35] The brothers had identical incubation periods — either 21 years from Nen's feast or 27 years from Nonon's feast. Others who attended those feasts were found to have quite varied incubation periods. They could have been infected at other feasts not investigated or received a different dose of the infective agent by a different route, such as through a wound or a mucous membrane or by ingestion.

Nen's feast, in particular, was fascinating for the reasons as to why some of those who participated did *not* contract kuru. Of the 16 kin in Nen's village of Awande when she died, 15 were present and 14 took part. Twelve of the 14 died of kuru. According to the paper, the one resident who did not participate was the second wife of Nen's husband who followed her own village tradition of not eating the body of another of her husband's wives. Of the two who participated but avoided kuru, one died of another cause and the other, Omb, Nen's daughter-in-law, ate only Nen's hand. It has since been found that the most infectious parts of the body are the brain and the spinal cord, both of which were favoured by the women. Their children, milling about and being tended by their mothers with their kuru-infected hands, were susceptible to infection. Those who only ate the muscle, as the men did, rarely caught kuru.

A key finding of Klitzman's study of those 65 patients was that incubation could be traced and measured, and that the disease could have a uniform rate of progression in different individuals — even when that progression takes more than 20 years. Only 15 of the more than 2500 kuru deaths to 1981 had known incubation periods of five years or less, and these generally occurred because the victims were young children. There was no such certainty in other cases, since the critical transmission event was not known. Remarkably, some much older women, who must have joined in many, many funeral feasts, had escaped kuru until at least 1981, despite many of their children dying of the disease. "… They may subsequently die of the disease and represent the far upper limits of incubation periods," the authors noted.[36]

By the mid-1990s kuru had almost, but not quite, died out. Long incubation times continue. In 1978 there were 25 kuru deaths, 27 in 1979 and 25 in 1980.[37] In 1982 another 12 kuru deaths were recorded.

Kuru continues to occur at a rate of two to three cases each year. In December 1996 two people died within the usual 12-month-odd course of the disease, the younger of whom was in his mid-40s. His death alone has pushed the known incubation period of diseases like kuru over the 40-year mark. Michael Alpers, who once predicted he would document the last case, fears the disease may have an incubation period longer than the average human life span.

In 1957 Zigas and Gajdusek had little idea of the extent of the medical frontiers their work would open up. That initial research has led to decades of challenging work in neurology, neuropathology, microbiology, neuroimmunology, neurovirology, molecular biology and molecular genetics and collaborations with veterinary scientists and pathologists all working towards a common goal: the cause of a range of frightening brain diseases.

Almost 40 years later, ominous echoes of kuru resound. An epidemic sparked by another type of cannibalism that has led to the slaughter of up to two hundred thousand cows in Britain has emerged, frighteningly, in humans. Its full impact is still unknown.

In time Gajdusek's work on this devastating brain disease would propel him to the pinnacle of scientific endeavour — a Nobel Prize. Ironically, it was also his obsession with childhood diseases in emerging Pacific cultures that, 40 years after his arrival in the kuru region, would contribute to his personal and professional downfall.

CHAPTER 2

Creutzfeldt and Jakob: German pathfinders

HANS GERHARD CREUTZFELDT was only 28 when he met the woman from Grunau who would make him a household name across Europe more than 80 years later. By the time Bertha was brought to see him at his neurology clinic in the University of Breslau on June 20, 1913 she needed help to stand up. Her facial muscles made odd fluttering movements, her eyes jerked strangely. She was extremely tense yet sensitive when touched, and would regularly explode into gales of inappropriate laughter. When Bertha answered his questions, Creutzfeldt realised she had no idea where she was or how long she had been there. Whatever she did say had a staccato quality, as if she couldn't manage smooth speech. Only 22 years old, Bertha seemed to be on a rapid slide into dementia.

Although Bertha's trouble with walking began when she was 16, she had not seen a doctor until she was 21. A year earlier, in June 1912 she had arrived at the university's dermatology clinic with what staff called a "hysterical exfoliative dermatitis", which affected first her hands and face, then her groin and both feet. At her first examination in the dermatology clinic she had spasticity, or uncontrolled movement of both legs, generalised tremors including specific tremor-like movements in the kneecaps and ankles. She also had a weak but definite Babinski sign, in which the big toe moves upwards when the sole of the foot is scraped, indicating a brain or spinal cord abnormality. Afterwards Bertha "had a major hysterical attack" followed by the disappearance of the earlier stiffness in her limbs. She appeared to recover but this was later found to be one of several periods of remission.

Bertha's had been a sad life, Creutzfeldt mused as he took her history. Her mother had died in 1904 at the age of 55 from an unidentified disease. But from the age of nine, in 1899, Bertha had lived in the Catholic convent-run Koppernig Orphanage. And although two of her four siblings were mentally disabled and institutionalised, she had seemed quite normal. Bertha did, however, fit an early description of anorexia nervosa: Creutzfeldt noted that "two years before admission to the clinic she refused nourishment for a period of time under the pretext that she wanted to become slender".[1]

After recovering from her dermatitis attack, in May 1913 Bertha began walking unsteadily, her menstruation had become irregular and she had bouts of hallucinations which led to her examination by Creutzfeldt. Not surprisingly, as her bodily functions began to fail, her personal appearance became slovenly and she "assumed peculiar postures, in that she bent over to her left and pressed her hand against her heart", Creutzfeldt noted.

Creutzfeldt also recorded her extreme mood swings — euphoric one minute, unresponsive the next. Muscles in her face, arms and legs twitched very obviously. The jerking of her eyes, a condition called nystagmus, was obvious. Often distracted and incoherent, she made odd grimaces at times, claimed not to be able to read any more, which underlined a general slowing in all her mental faculties, and frequently burst into spontaneous laughter. One possible cause of this untreatable condition was multiple sclerosis, but the jerkings and parrot-like repetition of words and actions seemed to rule that out.

By July 1913, two months after Creutzfeldt's initial examination, she had noticeably worsened. Continual jerks racked her body. She felt pain easily and continued to repeat certain words. Increasing stiffness was apparent in her face, arms and hands, though not her legs. Bertha was soon totally confused and demented. By the time spring brought warmer weather, she was mute and gripped by echopraxia, a condition in which the sufferer involuntarily imitates the actions of others. In early August Bertha began having almost continuous epileptic seizures. Her body twitched uncontrollably, her face became expressionless. Before long she had slipped into a light coma, where she stayed, twitching, jerking and fitting until she died on August 11, 1913.

During her subsequent autopsy, Creutzfeldt found "a peculiar disease picture". Her brain had atrophied — literally shrunk. There was an obvious loss of neurones — the basic building blocks and tiny message transmitters of the brain. There was also pronounced astroglial hypertrophy, a swelling of the glial cells, or astrocytes, which protect the nerve cells. If the glial cells are swollen it means the nerve cells are damaged. Bertha also had degeneration of the corticospinal tracts on each side of her brain, which indicated death of the nerve cells that controlled voluntary movement. And although the tissue was destroyed in the cerebral cortex, the layered grey matter that covers the brain and is where most of the thought processes occur in humans, surprisingly there was no inflammation.

After World War I, Creutzfeldt resumed his peacetime career as a neuropsychiatrist at Alzheimer's clinic at the University of Breslau. In 1920 his paper on Bertha was published in a German neuropsychiatric journal.[2] A year later Alfons Maria Jakob, a neuropsychiatrist working in the University of Hamburg-Friedrichsberg's psychiatric clinic, leapt into print.

The bespectacled Jakob, born the year before Creutzfeldt in 1884, detailed four cases of rapidly progressive fatal dementia that he labelled "spastic pseudo-sclerosis", a term vastly out of date with diagnostic terms today.[3] Using the term "spastic" indicated there was impaired motor function and "pseudo-sclerosis" meant that it "appeared" — although it probably hadn't — that areas of the white matter in the brain, its wiring, had hardened. The white matter hardens in cases of multiple sclerosis.

In the early twentieth century, syphilis was always the prime suspect in neurological illness. In its tertiary or terminal stage, which was often many years after initial infection through direct contact such as sexual intercourse, syphilis caused fatal brain damage. But Jakob knew his cases were not syphilis. His next thought — that all of them could be an atypical form of multiple sclerosis — was quickly discarded. Another look at the brains of his cases clearly showed a disease he had never seen or heard of before that had devastated the cerebral cortex. And whatever this disease was, it was, unusually, non-inflammatory. All four of his patients had had normal urine, blood and spinal fluid tests. Jakob noted a "remote relationship" to a few cases in the literature to that time, which were so odd they had been labelled simply "strange disease". "The only one I should like to consider as identical with my cases is Creutzfeldt's case, published after the completion of my studies ..." he wrote in his paper.

The third of Jakob's cases was Ernst Kahn, a 42-year-old salesman who found himself commissioned into the German army when World War I began. In May 1918, while fighting in Romania, Ernst complained of stomach pains, vertigo and aching legs. Then for a while these symptoms went away. But by the time the armistice was signed in November 1918, Ernst's legs had become weak. He could not walk normally and developed double vision. When he stood with his eyes closed he lost his balance. His handwriting became shockingly illegible. By the time he visited Jakob's psychiatric clinic in January 1919, he had developed dysarthria — slurring or difficulty articulating words. He had obvious facial twitches and when asked to poke out his tongue, he struggled to do so.

By March 1919 Ernst's walk had become a stagger and his memory was worsening. Like Bertha he hallucinated, was often unable to say where he was and before long could no longer walk and speak. Ernst died of pneumonia after a spell of demented stupor nine months after his initial symptoms began. A post-mortem examination of his brain revealed an almost identical pattern of degeneration to Bertha's. The only difference was that Ernst did not have the corticospinal tract degeneration — the easily identifiable erosion of the nerve cells, and the synapses at the nerve cell junctions — which Bertha had.

In 1923, two years after publishing details of his first four cases, Jakob's description of the demise of a German woman named Auguste Hoffmann helped propel him into the elite scientific clique whose members have diseases named after them. Auguste was only 38 when she became confused and forgetful. Her speech was slow and becoming slurred. Within five months she could neither sit nor stand, had lost coordination of her muscles, and her limbs had become rigid. Thirteen months after her symptoms began she died, having become demented and racked by seizures. When Jakob examined Auguste's brain under a microscope he found that the grey matter was devastated by spongy holes. There were far more holes than there were in Ernst Kahn's brain, which probably reflected the fact that she had lived longer after the symptoms began, Jakob thought. Decades later, when Jakob's case slides were reviewed, it was discovered that the holes in Ernst's brain were hard to spot (and so not mentioned in the report) because of inadequate chemical staining techniques at that time.

With Jakob's cases, a new disease was identified. For some time it was called Jakob's disease but later when both Creutzfeldt and Jakob were given the credit, it shuffled between the awkward Jakob-Creutzfeldt syndrome and Creutzfeldt-Jakob disease. Today, controversy surrounds the issue of whether Creutzfeldt has been wrongly credited with discovery of the disease that bears his name. Later reviews of Bertha's case suggest Bertha did not have CJD as it is diagnosed today, but some other degenerative brain condition with overlapping symptoms.

In 1982, the results of a three-year review of Bertha's case paper and most of Jakob's original case reports and slides, which are still kept in the archives of the University of Hamburg's department of neuropathology, were published. An Australian pathologist, Dr Colin Masters, conducted the review while working in Gajdusek's laboratory at the NIH in the late 1970s.

Of Jakob's first five cases, Masters and Gajdusek found only Ernst and Auguste, with their clinical symptoms and obvious spongiform change in the brain, fitted today's CJD profile. Subsequently, case studies by Jakob stuck fairly narrowly to today's concept of CJD. Jakob's first reported case appears with hindsight to have been a form of motor neurone disease with dementia. But by including that case, as well as another two that now appear to have been some form of toxic-metabolic brain infection, confusion followed for years on what constituted a spongiform encephalopathy. It was not until 1968, when CJD was first found to be infectious, that other neurological conditions with overlapping symptoms could be definitely excluded from the CJD definition.[4]

There was no tissue available from Bertha's case. Creutzfeldt had not mentioned any brain holes and there was the hazy issue of her mentally disabled sisters. Was she susceptible to an inherited disorder? Masters and Gajdusek agreed with an earlier review published in 1977, that Bertha was impossible to define as a true CJD case. In fact, it was impossible to define what she had at all — apart from suggesting it might have been an acquired toxic-metabolic brain infection, like that of two of Jakob's first-described patients who did not have CJD.

But long before the review was carried out Jakob had stamped his name on CJD, both with his initial published descriptions and his identification in 1923 of a familial form of CJD. It is now thought that up to 10 per cent of CJD cases are inherited. In strict figures that is not many. An individual stands more chance of winning lotto than dying of familial CJD.

CJD was the first disease to be formally reported in what would soon be realised was a group of diseases to which kuru would shortly be added in the late 1960s.

By 1960 the terminology to describe fatal conditions like CJD and kuru had gone through several name changes. Scientists and doctors regrouped and split diagnostic terms. From the term "slow viruses" they branched into "unconventional viruses".

A new term, "subacute spongiform encephalopathies", was found in the title of a long, fascinating and ultimately very important paper published in the journal *Brain* in December 1960. Dr Sam Nevin headed a group of English neurologists who focused attention on a group of eight patients at the Maida Vale and the Brook Hospitals, both in London, who had symptoms reminiscent of some of Jakob's patients. Nevin and his colleagues recounted the histories and brain pathology of the patients who died between 1952 and 1958 of a collective condition they described as "subacute spongiform encephalopathy".[5] They didn't think these patients fitted Jakob's initial and confusing "pseudo sclerosis" group of cases. Some sort of dysfunction of the blood vessels in the brain was their best guess at the cause of these eight deaths. Some were later found to have died of CJD accidentally transmitted via contaminated neurosurgical equipment.

It was not until 1968, however, more than four decades after Jakob's first crop of cases was reported, and following disagreement over the specific symptoms that constituted CJD, that experimental transmission of the disease to other animals became the definitive sign of the disease. That same year a German doctor, Kirchbaum, produced what was a highly-regarded monograph on CJD in which he suggested spongy change was a secondary phenomenon. By the late 1970s, however, it became accepted that tiny spongy holes, evident in most cases but only visible in brain sections under a microscope, were to be the defining piece of pathology in the brain that stamps the patient a victim of CJD. Subsequently, these diseases have acquired the more logical title of transmissible spongiform encephalopathies (TSEs). This literally means a slowly progressive brain infection that produces spongy-looking holes in the brains of victims, which in turn can be transmitted to other humans and animals who will contract the disease and die.

The 1920s became an historic era in terms of the discovery of spongiform encephalopathies in humans. A group of Austrians are credited with the co-discovery of a definite familial form of this class of disease, which differs from the familial form of CJD identified by Jakob and his students in a 1923 publication.[6] Josef Gerstmann, an Austrian neurologist, was working in the Maria-Theresien-Schlossel Mental Hospital in Vienna when a 26-year-old woman visited his clinic complaining of memory loss, slurred speech, clumsiness and uncontrollable mood swings over the previous 12 months.

When Gerstmann examined the woman he found she could no longer walk without staggering. Her arms would tremble, and she had some intellectual impairment. She slowly worsened over the next couple of years, developing jerking of the eyes and dementia. She died six years after her symptoms began. Her illness was similar to that which had killed her father and some of his relatives in their thirties and forties. Gerstmann's 1928 report mentioned "holes" in several deep cortical layers of the brain and, distinctively, multicentric plaques — later described as deposits of protein.

In 1936, together with Ernst Sträussler and Isaak Scheinker, Gerstmann reported the case that would link their names to the syndrome, which became known as GSS. It is even rarer than CJD and has since been linked to an inherited genetic mutation. Major differences between GSS and familial CJD are: the earlier age of onset of GSS; the rarity or lack of microscopic holes in the brain; the distinct addition of protein deposits; and more than double the usual duration of illness, to an average of more than four years. GSS was first transmitted to laboratory animals in 1981 and has been classed as an inheritable variant of familial CJD.

After the identification of GSS in the 1920s and 1930s, CJD research tapered off, helped by the eruption of World War II. Confusion with other brain diseases continued even after kuru was discovered in 1957. It was due, according to Gajdusek's friend and colleague, epidemiologist Dr Paul Brown, to "the enduring failure of neuropathologists to credit spongiform change as the linchpin of diagnosis, because of an excusable reluctance to attribute significance to holes".[7]

CHAPTER 3

Scrapie:
The trouble with sheep

DECADES OF RESEARCH into an old European sheep disease has provided the groundwork for advances in the understanding of TSEs and their diabolical ability to survive anything that easily kills viruses and bacteria. In English it is known as scrapie — a name which replaces earlier descriptions of "rubbers", "schrewcroft", "goggles", "rickets", "shakers" and the Scottish terms of "scratchie" or "cuddie" trot.[1]

Scrapie has been described repeatedly over the years as an obscure and incurable disease in sheep. It can cause tiny holes in the minuscule brains of its cloven-footed victims. It is the equivalent of CJD and has at least 20 different strains that can be transmitted to experimental animals. Despite this knowledge, gained over more than 60 years of intensive research, the agent of this insidious sheep-killer remains only partially understood. Britain, where most cases of scrapie are reported, has increased its research efforts over the last two decades. This trend has spread worldwide with the recognition that scrapie is the best-known prototype for a completely new disease — bovine spongiform encephalopathy (BSE), otherwise known as mad cow disease.

Most cases of scrapie that have appeared over the past three centuries have been described in Britain. Over this time the British sheep meat industry and its offshoot, fine wool, tied up an important slice of the national economies of some European countries. But scrapie outbreaks have also been recorded in Hungary, Bulgaria, the Netherlands, Iceland, France and Germany over the past 200 years. This century, outbreaks have been reported in Belgium, Italy, Spain, Switzerland, Cyprus and even Japan. Israel reported its first outbreak as recently as 1993, and a small outbreak in imported sheep in Norway in 1996 resulted in the slaughter of 10 per cent of the country's sheep. Imported Suffolk sheep were found to have scrapie once they arrived in Canada in 1938 and in the United States from 1947. In the 1950s the US banned imports of British sheep. New Zealand had a single instance in sheep imported from Britain in the early 1950s.[2] And, during the same era in Colombia, Brazil, South Africa and Kenya during the 1960s and 1970s, British Hampshire Down sheep died of scrapie.[3]

In Australia scrapie made its only appearance in 1952. On a farm outside Melbourne, a group of 10 Suffolk sheep imported from Britain were quarantined for three weeks on arrival. Little more than a year later, they were all slaughtered after four of the nine ewes died of scrapie. To ensure complete eradication of the disease on the property, all the nine locally-bred Suffolk ewes that had been mated with the one imported ram were destroyed, as were the 12 lambs they bore, and another 12 Romney rams grazing in an adjoining paddock. The property was quarantined for 12 months and the paddocks in which those sheep grazed were ploughed and left fallow for that period. When the case was reported six years later, the disease had not flared in any other sheep on the property.[4]

Even today the real incidence of scrapie is not known, despite it being a notifiable disease in the European Community since January 1993. Some reports have estimated that it affects one third of British flocks.[5] Farmers can face ruin with a scrapie attack rate of only 10 per cent due to a loss of confidence in prized breeding flocks. Great pains are often taken to conceal scrapie in a flock in Britain. A sheep thought to have the earliest signs has often been sold for slaughter, even though scrapie may not actually be the cause. And when definite scrapie symptoms are too advanced for sale, an affected sheep is likely to be buried quietly to avoid tricky questions.

Over the centuries shepherds and flock owners have developed a keen awareness for any of the telltale symptoms that spell doom for rams and ewes alike, symptoms usually appearing in the sheep from middle age and also part-way through pregnancy.

Initial clumsy movements lead to stumbling or wobbling. Scrapie-affected sheep develop a fine tremor of the body or the head, or sometimes both and can fall right over if forced to hurry with the rest of the flock. As death looms, despite eating normally, the sheep can lose weight to the point where it appears to be wasting away. It tires easily and appears confused. Sometimes the animal walks — this simple act becoming increasingly difficult — a fair distance to scrape or rub against the nearest tree, fence post or any solid object.

When inevitable death occurs, sometimes after six months or more of symptoms, it is usually at night.

Farmers, sheep breeders and scrapie researchers wondered why Southern Africa, Australia, New Zealand, North and South America were largely unscathed by endemic scrapie, despite their flocks being built up since the early 1800s from western European stock. These stocks included various breeds of sought-after Spanish merinos, some of which were badly affected by scrapie at the time of their export. In the early 1800s, when the disease was already considered to be infectious, crossbreeding increased. Certain new crossbreeds were free of scrapie. Others were not.

In the 1930s strands of evidence emerged from two sources that scrapie was caused by a transmissible agent and might also be transmitted naturally by infection or contact. Two French microbiologists, Cuille and Chelle, in 1936 published the results of experiments in which they successfully transmitted scrapie via injections of infected spinal cord material. Later scrapie was transmitted to goats.

But of great significance, and with more explosive implications, was the louping-ill vaccine accident of 1935. Louping-ill is another fatal ovine illness, the equivalent of yellow fever in humans. Spread by ticks, it is a conventional virus that affects many Scottish sheep and which leads to brain inflammation, lethargy, poor coordination and death within days. Researchers at the Animal Diseases Research Institute at Moredun, a centre originally specialising in sheep diseases, had developed a louping-ill vaccine some years earlier. Infected sheep brains and other tissues from affected sheep were used as a source of the disease. In a common method of preparation the virus, hiding in liquefied sheep brain suspension, was inactivated with very dilute formalin. Formalin is a fixing and preserving chemical solution, which scientists of the time thought killed all viruses and microbes. The louping-ill virus, present but dead in the solution, was still able to cause the production of antibodies to it in the bloodstreams of the vaccinated sheep. It was a success. There was no hint of louping-ill in the lambs treated.

But about 15 months later disaster struck. The first of about 1,200 sheep treated from one contaminated batch of the vaccine, made from infected sheep brain, began to exhibit the first insidious signs of scrapie. The eventual toll was high — about seven per cent of the 18,000 immunised sheep. Two other batches used were not contaminated.[6] An exhaustive series of experiments followed to rule out the possibility that scrapie was caused by some unknown toxic agent. These "serial passage" experiments involved the injection of scrapie-infected brain and other tissues into sheep in a series extending over several years. The infected material was diluted each time it was prepared for injection into the next passage group. In this way, scientists were able to prove that whatever sinister agent caused scrapie, it actually replicated or "grew".[7]

The louping-ill accident and its implications for pooled tissue transmission of diseases remained largely unknown by the wider scientific world. While the scrapie agent's exceptional resistance to inactivation was reported at the 1939 International Microbiology Congress in New York, there are only five (mostly brief) references to the louping-ill accident in veterinary literature between 1940 and 1954.

In 1947 a fresh scare occurred in America. The lethal disease was contracted by farmed mink, which had never been linked to a scrapie-like disease. It happened on a ranch in Wisconsin, best known as America's dairy state. That year it affected only mink over one year of age on a farm in Brown County, but with utter devastation. From November 1947 to March 1948, almost all of the 1,250 adults at the mink ranch died after the onset of behavioural changes. These symptoms included the normally neat and clean mink walking with a jerky stepping action and scattering their feed, eating and swallowing with difficulty, and biting their own tails when the tails were not arched squirrel-like over their backs. After about a month, as death approached, the minks slept for long periods, had the occasional convulsion and, in a bizarre exit, were often found dead "with their teeth firmly fastened to the mesh of the wire cage".[8] Also strange was that, although being fed and housed identically, none of the babies born to any of the dead mothers contracted the disease.

A later study of long incubation diseases in mink found that 125 pregnant mothers sent from that Brown County farm in April 1947 to another farm — this time over the Mississippi River border in Winona County, Minnesota — all died of the same condition. The symptoms appeared as they did in their original herd, in November that year. The two farms had no feed items in common, and again, none of the babies died.[9]

Common to all the dead mink were two injections in June 1946 of a tissue vaccine to prevent distemper, followed by a single booster shot in February 1947 as well as a diet of beef by-products — uncooked meat from dead and sick cattle — cereal, fish, tripe and liver. When six of the brains of the mink were examined later they had obvious neuronal degeneration and some had holes in nerve cells — a basic resemblance to those in scrapie.[10] Scrapie-infected sheep and goat tissues were initially blamed as the most probable culprits.[11] Subsequent blame focused on cattle tissues from broken down cows — particularly because scrapie had not been found in Wisconsin sheep before 1947.

The Brown County outbreak of disease in mink added weight to the idea that scrapie-like diseases could be contagious to other species, particularly when uncooked material was part of the diet. Later outbreaks of what became known as transmissible mink encephalopathy (TME) occurred in America in 1961, twice in 1963 and in 1985. Reports since have linked all of them to mink fed cattle tissue from "downer" cows[12] — cows found dead or dying, for which a diagnosis of the cause of death is not worth the cost. Renderers usually cart them away.

Before scrapie was found to be transmissible, scientists relied on the chemical formalin to kill infectious organisms. Frighteningly, both the distemper vaccine used on the mink in 1947 and that used on the Scottish sheep in the 1935 louping-ill vaccine had been formalinised. Scrapie became the prototype of a new class of replicating infectious agents, known for many years as "unconventional" or "slow viruses". Victims of these diseases showed no inflammation or other responses to indicate infection. Their immune systems did not appear to know they were infected. This distinguished them from conventional viruses. Viruses could be killed relatively easily (either in or out of the host) and shouted their presence in the body by producing antibodies, through inflamed tissues, swelling or dead cells and obvious sickness in their hosts.

But the discovery of the unique and terrifying properties of the scrapie agent — around the time world attention was riveted on the growing influence of American divorcee Wallis Simpson on Edward VIII, Britain's new king — remained locked largely in the world of veterinary science.

Over centuries, various theories about the cause of scrapie have been argued, debated and dismissed as rubbish. They include causes attributed to a skin mite, close inter-breeding of sheep (called in-and-in breeding) and stall feeding in which sheep were housed very close together. Even excessive sexual activity by rams in the early stages of the disease was touted for a while.[13] During the inter-war years, when new vaccines for various livestock diseases were developed, it was expected that a scrapie vaccine would also be formulated. Bacteria and many of the diseases they caused were becoming better understood, but animal disease investigators had to come to terms with an altogether different class of disease agents — viruses. Bacteria were microscopically small independent entities, but viruses were smaller still and dependent on entry to living cells. And so size offered the simplest differential. By using various types of filters with very fine pores or channels, it was possible to exclude bacteria from a finely dispersed suspension of infected tissue. If the solution, lacking bacteria, could pass on a disease, then the agent of that disease must be some organism smaller than the smallest bacterium. Hence the term "filterable virus" came into use.

In the mid-1930s there were two distinct views about the chemical nature of these filterable viruses. One view was that they were made exclusively from a protein. The other opinion — accepted by the end of the 1930s — was that nucleic acids (the building blocks of genetic material) were the essential feature of viruses, and that the protein was simply a protective cladding for the virus. By the late 1950s, viruses were recognisable by characteristic shapes beneath the microscope. As a result, vaccines could be generated. In addition, it was known that viruses could easily be inactivated by formaldehyde,[14] and knocked stone dead by UV radiation.

Like viruses, the entity that caused scrapie was found to be filterable. But the comparisons stopped there. "The agent", as its researchers called it, was unlike any other known infectious organism. No-one could detect, or recognise it under even the best microscope. A conventional vaccine was not — and still isn't — possible. And the agent was extremely resilient — neither the intense gamma radiation, nor heating to a temperature higher than boiling point in an autoclave could inactivate it. This latter failure meant that standard pre-1970 means of sterilisation in operating theatres and research labs were inadequate — the instruments and containers could be contaminated.

As World War II was ending, a British veterinary virologist Dr D. R. Wilson was the subject of much official criticism over his failure to make a vaccine for scrapie. His critics apparently understood little, if anything, of the unique biological properties of the agent that Wilson was encountering. Wilson had made the earliest careful observations on most of the unexpected physical and chemical properties found in scrapie. But he was so affected by his critics that he suffered a nervous breakdown and published little before his retirement from the Moredun Institute in Edinburgh. His most valuable work was included in colleagues' papers published during the late 1950s, after he had left. Discoveries based on livestock often take a long time to be taken seriously by medics engrossed in their research on humans. Even so, these delayed findings should have sounded a warning in other fields of medicine.

In the 1950s funding for scrapie research increased in the United Kingdom, where it was causing serious problems in the Suffolk breed, the most popular source of rams for crossbreeding. Proponents of the different theories about the cause of the disease gradually divided into two main camps. In one camp were those who believed that naturally occurring scrapie was caused solely by an inherited recessive gene. In other words, a sheep inevitably developed scrapie if both parents carried a gene for it. A sheep could not get scrapie from environmental factors because scrapie was not infectious.

Opposing them was a group that maintained scrapie *was* an infectious, transmissible disease (as countless experiments have since shown), but which was under the control of a sheep gene, called "sip" (scrapie incubation period). This gene determined the sheep's response to any scrapie agent that might enter its body, whether the infection became established and, if it did, how quickly it would kill. This infectious view is the one generally accepted by those in agriculture and science today.

During the 1950s an enthusiastic and committed scrapie investigator in Britain was H.B. (James) Parry. His lone but loud voice first prompted the idea that scrapie was a myopathy — a disease of the muscles. Later he substituted that for the hereditary theory of the first camp. Parry was a qualified veterinarian who, in the early 1950s began a 25-year field study on scrapie in a range of sheep breeds. This was done in collaboration with shepherds and flock owners in England, Wales and Scotland. But in 1980, the affable Oxford-based 68-year-old, his research still unfinished, died suddenly from a heart attack. His unfinished research — the staggering volume of information on sheep breeding habits, historical records and his prized epidemiological data on scrapie incidence — lay abandoned.

Ranged against Parry's view of scrapie were most scientists with direct experience of the subject, including his chief opponent, the tall gangling Alan Dickinson, who also worked in Edinburgh but at the Animal Breeding Research Organisation (ABRO), three kilometres away from the Moredun Institute. Parry's genetic-only theory on the cause of naturally occurring scrapie was finally debunked more than three decades later, when the results of a study were published in March 1997.[15] Scrapie-associated genetic variants, present in sheep affected by scrapie in Britain, are also present in Australian and New Zealand sheep but there has been no scrapie in either country since 1952 when infected British imports were destroyed.

Scrapie is believed to be endemic in sheep in Britain and other European countries because maternal transmission of the agent can infect the lamb. This may occur before birth. However, there are better opportunities for infection after the birth when the highly infectious placenta is eaten not only by the ewe but also by other sheep in the flock.

Work by Dickinson's group showed that a fully functioning immune system appeared necessary for any scrapie-type agent infection in an animal — except in the case of experimental injection of infected matter directly into the central nervous system. This unexpected discovery gave a clue about maternal transmission. It would be expected to occur only in those species with a fully functioning immune system at birth. Such an immune system has evolved as a necessity in animals such as sheep, cattle, deer and elk. (Deer and elk were to suffer a new TSE identified in Montana, USA, in 1980 called chronic wasting disease.[16]) To escape potential predators, these ruminants need to be able to struggle to their feet and be mobile as soon as they are born. With mink and mice and man, which have immune systems that are immature at birth but which develop shortly afterwards, maternal transmission would not be expected. Nor has it been reported to date.

Alan Dickinson began his career as a geneticist interested in livestock growth. From 1955, however, his life's work began: the search for the overall biology of scrapie — what caused it and how it developed in animals. This interest developed from his work at ABRO. From then on, until his retirement in 1987, Dickinson built up a team of experienced researchers. They gained Medical Research Council (MRC) support in 1981 as the Neuropathogenesis Unit (NPU), housed in a highly specialised building dedicated to scrapie and related diseases. From 1961, in repeated and complex experiments on sheep and goats in collaboration with John Stamp at the Moredun Institute, and with his colleagues at ABRO, Dickinson discovered a widely differing range of scrapie strains. Tens of thousands of genetically ideal mice and well over 1000 sheep and goats were used in the experiments. Because no scrapie-like diseases occur naturally in lab animals such as mice, there could be no source of confusion or contamination from them.

The first hint of strains occurred in the early 1960s. Ian Pattison, a Scottish veterinary pathologist, began using goats for scrapie research. He used scrapie-infected brain from sheep. These sheep had been similarly injected in a long series of "passages" of the agent, begun years earlier by Wilson, from one group of sheep to the next. Pattison injected crossbred goats with some of the eighteenth passage of scrapie brain tissue left over in a few separate passage lines. What he found eventually was that two lines differed in their main clinical symptoms. In one, the goats became predominantly drowsy, with no scratching. In the other, they remained active but needed to scratch convulsively. By itself this was no proof that different scrapie strains existed. For instance, both lines may have had the same scrapie strain but in one line the goats could have been carrying an innocuous, undetected conventional virus along with the scrapie which altered the symptoms.[17]

Proof was in the package of specially inbred mice. In 1961 Dickinson isolated in mice a single gene with two alternative varieties, or alleles. It was dubbed the "sinc" gene (the mouse version of the scrapie incubation period [sip] gene). These variations in sinc could produce large differences in the length of incubation before infection became obvious. The question of what particular variant lengthened incubation, and which one shortened it, depended on the strain of scrapie.

Effectively, the intensity and distribution of cell damage in the brains of diseased mice was determined by sinc, once two other factors were fixed. The first was the route of infection — whether the infectious agent entered the brain or spinal cord directly, or via some other method. The second was the strain of the agent — scrapie being but the first disease known to be a TSE.

Of great interest decades later were the following Dickinson findings. An injection of scrapie into mice brains gave the shortest range of incubation periods. Injections through more peripheral routes such as muscle, resulted in longer incubation periods and the need for much higher doses of the infective agent to trigger infection. Infection orally was the slowest and needed the highest doses. And for each route, it was found eventually that the higher the infective dose, the less time it took for the disease to kill.

With conventional viruses, the standard method of identification is a quick lab test for significant differences in the protective protein covering. Although made by the infected host's cells, this protein is specified by instructions within the virus's own genetic material. It is against this alien protein that the host's immune system reacts. The antibodies produced by the host can be prepared and used as a standard lab test to detect the virus in others. With TSEs there are no antibodies. The host's immune system does not notice the deadly replication that leads to a brain full of tiny holes because there is no alien protein to give the game away.

Despite decades of research into exactly how scrapie is spread and which routes are the most important, the full structure of the agent — the "thing" that begins the process that results in brain damage beyond repair — is still unknown and contentious.

Advances in scrapie research remained largely out of view of mainstream science and medicine. But the work that identified the different scrapie strains proved invaluable to this audience when BSE emerged in British cattle in the 1980s. The 1935 louping-ill accident — in which pooled sheep tissue used in vaccinations caused scrapie — was a tantalising clue to later disaster. A quarter century later, fledgling experiments on humans, using drugs made from pooled human tissue, forged ahead. Far from sheep, another accident was waiting to happen.

CHAPTER 4

Kuru and scrapie: The breakthrough

IN THE NORTHERN SUMMER of 1959, American veterinary pathologist Dr William Hadlow stamped his name forever on the remarkable history of TSEs. In so doing he added a key piece of the puzzle that showed kuru was the same type of disease as scrapie. For months Hadlow, working at Britain's Agricultural Research Council Field Station (ARCSF) at Compton, had been examining goat brains — a species not naturally afflicted by the disease, but susceptible to experimentally-induced scrapie. Work at Compton was exciting, even though the director was disappointed the Americans had not sent a virologist who would stand out among the comparative army of pathologists.

Hadlow's examination of sliced sections of brain under a microscope showed the holes in the nerve cells that all pathologists relied on at the time when making a diagnosis of scrapie — "indeed it was the fashion", he recalled decades later.[1] What he found most fascinating were the increased numbers of swollen astrocytes, which created a regular pattern of destruction across scrapie-affected brains. After a year of watching live sheep and goats degenerate and noting the changes in their brains after death, the American decided that scrapie was unique.

That view was about to change. On June 28, a colleague from Montana turned up unexpectedly. Over a pleasant dinner he casually mentioned to Hadlow an exhibit he had seen in London the previous day, which had included "a strange brain disease of a primitive people in New Guinea".[2] Intrigued, Hadlow journeyed to London, to the Wellcome Museum of Medical Science. On the first floor, Hadlow was drawn to large colour photographs that told the story of kuru. The display also showed the neurohistologic changes in the brains of kuru victims. It suddenly hit him. The kuru brains had holes in the neurones, just like those in scrapie brains.

Before returning to Compton that day, a fascinated Hadlow went to the Royal Society of Medicine and found several of the kuru references cited at the exhibit. These included an article published earlier that year by Gajdusek and Zigas in the *American Journal of Medicine.* Hadlow mulled over the "uncanny" resemblance between kuru and scrapie.

Two weeks later he sent a letter to the *Lancet,* which appeared in the issue of September 5, 1959. This letter was to become seminal in the annals of research into TSEs.

> I do not suggest that these diseases are identical or even counterparts, but in my opinion their overall resemblance is too impressive to be ignored ... the general ... features of scrapie closely parallel those that characterise kuru ... each disease is endemic in certain confined populations, whether this be flock or tribe, in which the usual incidence is low, about one or two per cent. Sheep, or person, may become clinically affected months after they have been moved from flocks or communities, where the respective disease is endemic.[3]

Hadlow also set out the "remarkably similar" changes found in the brains of kuru and scrapie victims. These followed common clinical symptoms such as ataxia, tremors and behavioural changes. There was no hint of a cause, or indeed of any infection. There was only a strong suggestion of some sort of genetic predisposition. The most telling similarity, Hadlow noted, was the "soap bubble" vacuoles, or holes, in brains affected by both diseases.[4] With evidence of scrapie transmissibility already established between sheep and goats, Hadlow thought it imperative to test transmissibility by injecting primates, such as chimpanzees, with kuru. He concluded his letter with the suggestion.

On July 21, 1959, only days after sending his letter to the *Lancet,* Hadlow, fearing a printers' strike at the time might hold up publication, sent a copy to Gajdusek, the one person he knew would be interested. By this time Gajdusek was back in New Guinea for more field patrols and follow-up work at the Kuru Research Centre in Kainantu. Clearly eager for more information, Gajdusek replied in early August, after his return from a 17-day epidemiological patrol through the most inhospitable conditions the Highlands had to offer. He told Hadlow that the possibility of an infectious cause was still being "pursued extensively", and referred Hadlow to more thorough descriptions of the pathology of kuru that he had just published with senior NIH neuropathologist Igor Klatzo and Zigas.[5] Klatzo's lengthy paper stated that "Creutzfeldt-Jakob disease appears to be the closest in resemblance" to kuru in the 12 kuru brains he had studied.[6] (A *Lancet* editorial also carried Klatzo's observation in October 1959.)

When Hadlow's letter was published it was a shock to everyone working on kuru. Few in medical research had had much interest in sheep, let alone heard of an ancient and rare disease called scrapie. But it was a turning point in the history of research into TSEs. Hadlow and Gajdusek met briefly in November 1959 while Hadlow was touring the US with leaders of two of the rival British scrapie research teams. The group was explaining facts about scrapie to worried farmers who had imported British sheep. Following this meeting, Gajdusek visited Compton, the Moredun Institute in Edinburgh and Icelandic scrapie expert, Pall Pallson, to broaden his knowledge of scrapie. It was a compatriot of Pallson's, Bjorn Sigurdsson, who had first raised the idea in the mid-1950s of "slow virus infections" in animals. Gajdusek returned from that trip convinced that injections of kuru tissue into animals, especially primates, and then long-term observation was a priority.

In July 1961 Hadlow, who had returned to Montana, declined an offer from Gajdusek and Smadel to join a team at the NIH. It was a chance to follow up his own suggestion in the *Lancet* and experiment with kuru on primates. Hadlow thought that anyone who took on such a job would be little more than "an exalted handler of apes". He has since admitted how wrong he was.

The 1950s was the dawn of an exciting era in medical science. In what began as a giant international experiment, miracle drugs made from the pituitary glands of dead bodies were used to alleviate infertility and replace vital growth hormone in tens of thousands of stunted children around the world. It did not work for everyone. Even for those in which it did, these drugs left a fatal legacy — scores of patients would die as a result of this high-tech cannibalism.

Pioneering work on both sides of the world led to the wonder drugs that were useful in two very different kinds of medical problems. The first was stunted growth in children. The second was infertility in men and women. Although these problems originated from different sources, a common net result was the inability of the pituitary gland to secrete enough of its hormones.

In the United States, at the Tufts University School of Medicine in Boston, Maurice Raben developed a method of extracting human growth hormone (hGH) — one of the essential elements necessary for child growth and metabolism. Conditions such as diabetes, pituitary tumours, and radiation therapy directed at the head can halt or affect the secretion of hGH. Children who lack sufficient hGH are called pituitary dwarfs — normal in all respects apart from their growth. Unless treated, they remain abnormally short.[7]

In 1958 Raben reported the successful trial of two milligram doses of hGH two or three times a week over 10 months on a 17-year-old youth with deficient growth hormone output. The patient finally grew 35 centimetres to 163 centimetres tall following seven years of hGH injections.[8]

That same year, in Sweden, a young gynaecologist called Carl Axel Gemzell teamed up with biochemist, Paul Roos, to perfect their chemical "recipe" for the extraction of hGH. By 1958 Gemzell had also used purified gonadotrophin on female patients who had trouble ovulating. Several had become pregnant, two of them with twins. Gonadotrophins had been found in the late 1920s to be the hormones produced by the pituitary gland, which stimulate the ovaries and testes. Infertile women, and men with low sperm counts were then prescribed one of two drugs. One choice was human chorionic gonadotrophin (hCG), a hormone produced by the placenta and excreted into the urine by pregnant women. The other was blood serum from pregnant mares — pregnant mares serum (PMS). PMS became so popular that it was marketed commercially by four companies in Britain before the outbreak of World War II. Results, however, were disappointing.[9] When it was realised that animals could develop immunities to hormones from other species, doctors experimented with combinations of hCG and PMS in the hope that the hCG would overcome the production of antibodies to PMS. But it had too little effect.[10]

In 1954 a small group of European and British scientists interested in follicle stimulating hormone (FSH) formed themselves into the "Gonadotrophin Club" to share information. The hormone had by now been isolated from the urine of menopausal women, as well as from the pituitary glands of healthy women who had died prematurely.[11] The group included Dr J. Brown of Edinburgh (later of Australia), Dr A. Crooke and Dr W. Butt of Birmingham, Dr E. Diczfalusy of Stockholm and Dr B. Lunenfeld of Geneva.

By 1961 the prescribing of high doses of PMS had resulted in 60 cases of hyperstimulation in women — far too many eggs released from the ovaries. This condition had killed two women and resulted in surgical intervention including the removal of both ovaries in others.[12]

Hormone extraction for medical use in humans relied on a rather gruesome source — cadavers. The pituitary gland is about the size of a pea or the tip of the little finger, and sits in a little cavity at the base of the brain. It is known for the hormones it secretes. But it was the front half of the pituitary that was of immediate interest to the Gonadotrophin Club and others interested in producing hGH for short-statured children. This section produced FSH and luteinising hormone (LH) as well as hGH, prolactin (which stimulates the secretion of breast milk), adrenocorticotrophic hormone (ACTH) and thyroid-stimulating hormone (TSH).

Early experiments had shown that growth hormone was species specific. As early as 1956 it was known that growth hormone from fish did not work in rats, that cattle-derived bovine growth hormone was useless in monkeys, and that neither cattle nor monkey growth hormone was the same as that produced by humans.[13] The only way to obtain a hormone from a human gland was to take the whole gland from someone no longer using it. So began the worldwide practice of removing pituitary glands from the dead. In the early days pathologists and morgue attendants were persuaded to help science — sometimes for a small inducement fee for the extra work it entailed — by removing the glands. In the Raben method of extraction, pituitary glands were taken from the bodies and stored in a small jar of acetone, the fluid that, in less scientific circles, removes nail polish. Acetone got into all the tissues of the gland by removing fat and water and made them shrivel like prunes. It was thought likely that acetone deactivated any known bacteria or virus agent. The whole gland was then ground into a paste in fresh acetone with a blender or an electric meat mincer. The mince was then filtered and washed repeatedly with cold acetone. In one of several acetone-stored extraction procedures, modified from Raben's method, the mince was spread out on a tray to dry, and turned at intervals with a spatula to break up lumps.[14] The hGH and other hormones needed were then extracted in a harsh chemical process from this pituitary powder, which could be stored for several years at a low temperature. A batch of

1000 glands would yield about 100 grams of pituitary powder.

In contrast, by 1963, Gemzell and Roos had succeeded in producing, via a totally different method, a purer hormone extract. It started from a different basis: the use of whole glands that were freeze-dried straight after autopsy removal and kept in their own glass vial. The duo also used a thin gel substance called Sephadex, a product that had become available in Sweden in 1958 and which filtered heavy molecular weights like viruses and bacteria from the lighter weights of the hormones. Because it was purer, less than five milligrams of hGH a week was effective in making a child grow.

Raben's method was considered by many to be a "harsh" unsophisticated method of extraction, the product of which was not completely soluble in water, and it was a more expensive method of manufacture.[15] Sometimes the hormone was denatured, or unfolded from its original shape, which meant it could stimulate antibodies in patients that made them immune to the treatment. Because the hormone was not totally pure, batches also gave lower yields and up to 50 milligrams of hGH was needed per week to make a child grow.

In the 1960s reports surfaced of children who had developed allergies from the impurities and other pituitary hormone fractions that sometimes remained in the hGH injections. Lumps or pain at the injection site were reported. It soon became apparent that the younger the child being treated, the better the result.[16] Children with both short stature and hypoglycaemia — low amounts of essential blood sugars — improved on hGH.

About half the children affected by hGH deficiency also have hypothyroidism — a deficiency of hormones produced by the thyroid gland — which hGH therapy can reveal. During the 1960s these children, in addition to hGH, received a drug called thyroxine. Sometimes there was a risk of children developing hypothyroidism as a result of pituitary-derived hGH therapy. Other risks included weight gain or even diabetes if too much hGH was used.

Both hGH and hPG were always in short supply. There were simply too few pituitary glands collected to meet the demand, which grew as more doctors became better at diagnosing hypopituitarism and explaining the benefits of hGH therapy to parents. It would not be until much later that any side-effect worse than antibody production, which rendered the hGH useless in some patients, became clear.

In Sweden in the late 1950s Gemzell had organised an effective pituitary collection procedure in which he asked pathologist colleagues in six hospitals, around Stockholm initially, to remove and immediately freeze the pituitary glands of cadavers. Unlike in other countries, it was ordinary practice in Sweden to remove the brain at every autopsy and he was eager for as many glands as possible. But, recognising the possibility that the dead may have had hepatitis, which was untreatable and potentially fatal, he asked that no glands be taken from anyone who had died of an infectious disease.[17]

"Because of the purity that we had managed to achieve, we were able to get a greater yield of useable hormone from cadaveric pituitaries rather than from menopausal urine," he recalled in a statement for a court case decades later. Gemzell was referring to the "gallons of urine necessary" to extract human menopausal gonadotrophin, hMG.[18] One pituitary gland provided the same amount of gonadotrophin as three litres of post-menopausal urine. Each week, Gemzell — who later continued the practice at hospitals around Uppsala where he was professor of gynaecology at the local university — collected up to 60 pituitary glands. From this he would produce a batch of hGH each month. Each batch was completely used up before another batch was made. "Donors" of human pituitary glands were in short supply, and concerted efforts began in various countries to encourage pathologists to collect glands to be used in extractions of both hPG and hGH.

While Gemzell was improving his hPG therapy, by 1963 the Institute Farmacologico Serono in Rome, part of the Swiss pharmaceutical company, Ares-Serono, had meanwhile extracted gonadotrophins from the hMG found in 80,000 litres of urine from menopausal Italian women. In exchange for small gifts, the urine of Italian nuns and women in small towns and villages was collected at regular intervals by the Serono tanker.[19] Although more expensive to produce, hMG soon overtook hPG use around the world. Except, that is, in Australia. Not only was hMG available commercially, urine was easier to collect in large amounts than pituitary glands. In addition, there appeared to be little difference in the effectiveness of hMG as opposed to hPG.

In the late 1960s Swedish endocrinologists, including Professor Kerstin Hall (who was later to become professor of endocrinology and diabetology at Sweden's prestigious Karolinska Institute) approached Kabi Pharmacia, one of the country's largest pharmaceutical companies, to manufacture much needed hGH on a commercial basis. Kabi had extensive hospital contacts and was already making blood products for haemophiliacs. It was experienced in the purification and exclusion of infection in the manufacture of biological products made from human sources. While there was initial resistance within the company (due to forecasts of poor demand), it was decided that the company would produce hGH in "the national interest".

Doctors prescribing the drug were seeking the safest most effective drug possible. They wanted reassurance that Kabi did not use any animal pituitaries, or glands that had clinging remnants of brain tissue, which occurred if the stalk was not removed properly. They wanted a guarantee that glands used did not come from cadavers that might carry hepatitis, or diseases such as Alzheimer's, Parkinson's and meningitis.[20] Roos, whose process using frozen pituitaries and Sephadex gel filtration had been simplified to the point that "any trained biochemist could apply it", advised Kabi Pharmacia (later called KabiVitrum and Pharmacia & Upjohn) on larger scale production.[21]

The company began selling hGH registered as Crescormon in 1971 to countries where no large-scale production of the hormone was taking place. Kabi requested that pituitaries for the production of hGH be provided by the country requesting it (such as Hong Kong,[22] Japan and other Scandinavian countries) because its own supply of pituitary glands could not keep up with demand. Despite Kabi's initial fears, by 1982 Crescormon was outselling all other Kabi products.[23]

In Norway in 1963, Dr Olav Trygstad, a paediatric endocrinologist at the University Hospital in Oslo, went to Sweden with his biochemist wife, Irene Foss, studied the Roos method of extraction with frozen pituitaries and modified it into the Trygstad method. Norway's National Health Service gave Trygstad his own product licence in 1963. Worried about contamination by viruses such as hepatitis, Trygstad and Foss included in their method, like in the Roos method, use of a Sephadex gel chromatography column to filter molecular particles by size. This was considered "fine tuning" after rapid centrifugation had flung off heavily weighted bacteria and viruses.

These contaminants were large molecules compared with hGH. Heavier weights travelled quickest through the tightly packed Sephadex gel beads to be discarded at the end of the column. What remained at the top or middle of the column after 24 hours were the lighter weight hormones. The column was discarded after every two batches were processed.[24]

By 1974 there were at least 12 different hGH extraction methods in use in countries including America, Britain, Australia, Switzerland, Austria, Norway, Sweden, France, Germany and Finland. Commercial hGH was made by four European and Scandinavian companies — Kabi, Organon, Ares-Serono and Nordisk. Trygstad has since estimated that up to 1.3 million pituitary glands were used to manufacture hGH in Europe — including in Zurich, Vienna, Helsinki and Oslo — from the early 1960s to 1985. That is roughly 40 to 50 glands worth of treatment each year for each child.[25]

Commercial manufacture of hGH meant its production, at least in Scandinavia, was taken out of small research laboratories and given to large pharmaceutical production laboratories. In the latter, safety standards could be maintained or even increased. And with all applications for product licences internationally, preparation methods received close scrutiny. Commercial collection of glands for a fee, however, was conducted worldwide. Nordisk in particular collected glands from Africa and Asia, which it processed in a laboratory separate to that in which pituitaries from Scandinavia, Britain and western Europe were processed.[26] This was due to the fact that both Africa and Asia had a high rate of endemic hepatitis, a transmissible disease.

Meanwhile the fertility hormone hPG, a combination of FSH and LH, was being trialled far from Gemzell's original patients. In Australia it began experimentally in the early 1960s on women who could not ovulate naturally for a variety of reasons — one of them being an emerging social scourge, anorexia nervosa. Between the early 1960s and mid-1970s national programs of manufacture and distribution of hGH — usually government-sponsored and provided free to patients — had sprung up in countries including America, Britain, Australia, France, New Zealand, Israel, Japan and South Africa. Where local hormone supplies failed to meet demand, commercial preparations were bought from the four European suppliers — although these were expensive supplements.

On a much smaller scale, the fertility drug hPG was manufactured for national programs. It was made during the 1960s in Britain, where at least 300 women were treated in at least six hospitals. These figures are probably higher due to hPG's use on some in-vitro fertilisation (IVF) programs as a stimulant for egg production.[27] One of the early trial patients of hPG, before IVF came into existence, was Beryl Friel, who in 1960, at the age of 40, was overjoyed at the birth of her daughter, Jackie. Her gynaecologist, Dr Rowath, had overseen her five treatments with hPG at the Victoria Hospital in Swindon, Wiltshire.[28]

Five healthy examples of what could be achieved with the new fertility wonder drug were the Lawson quins. Born within 24 minutes of each other at New Zealand's Auckland National Hospital for Women on July 27, 1965, they were the first quins in the world to be born after hPG therapy. Although this wasn't the largest of multiple births by then — a set of septuplets was born the previous year in Sweden — the quins survived low birth weights, which other multiple birth babies did not. A set of quins was born in Sweden only three days later to Mrs Karin Olsen of Orda, but none survived. Mrs Olsen had been treated by Gemzell and had previously had one child on the hPG treatment.[29]

The Lawson quins thrived, and became national celebrities and joined an elite club of surviving quins around the world. Overnight the non-identical quins and their parents — 26-year-old Shirley Ann, a statuesque former department-store model and beach carnival surf queen, and 28-year-old Sam, who had recently switched from labouring at a brickworks to running his own fish and chip shop — were front-page news around the world. Offers of gifts, products, cash, furniture and baby products flooded in with bags full of mail.

Shirley Ann Lawson had had no fertility problems until after the birth of her first child, Lee Ann, then aged five. Afterwards she had failed to menstruate and felt lethargic — except when she tried three courses of the anti-oestrogen drug, clomiphene citrate. Due to a hormonal imbalance, she had lactated for the next five years. It was then decided to try hPG, which was successful on the first course of injections. Nineteen days after her first injection Shirley Ann felt ill with morning sickness. Two weeks later, at only seven weeks pregnant, her uterus had grown to the size of a normal 12-week pregnancy. By the time she was 12 weeks pregnant she was the size of a normal 20-week pregnancy. At 18 weeks, Shirley Ann was X-rayed.

The film showed four foetuses and "there was room for another", which shocked the doctors.[30] She was admitted to hospital at 19 weeks and stayed there until the birth, seven weeks premature. Her only complaint, apart from discomfort due to her size during that time, was insomnia. Her wedding ring was sawn off her swollen finger the night before the birth. The babies — named in order of birth Samuel Christian Clayton, Lisa Gay, Deborah Ann, Shirlene Jan and Selina Joy weighed between 3 lb 3 oz and 4 lb 2 oz.

In successive interviews after her record birth, Shirley Ann cheerfully admitted to being the first in a group of five original infertile New Zealand "guinea pigs" to be treated with hPG at the National Hospital for Women.[31] There was a history of twins on both sides of the family and Shirley Ann's mother, Mrs Hilda Menzies, was widely quoted as saying that her new grandchildren were descendants of the *Bounty* mutineer Fletcher Christian, on her husband's side.[32]

The birth was the subject of a four-page article in the *Lancet,* which detailed dosages of the drug and measurements of the babies in the womb.[33] Other women had received the same dosages and conceived single babies, hospital authorities claimed at the time. Mrs Lawson's treating doctors, Dr D. C. Liggins and Dr H. K. Ibbertson, were both senior lecturers in the post-graduate school of obstetrics and endocrinology at the Auckland University professorial unit. They admitted in the *Lancet* article that "future modification of therapy will no doubt diminish the chances of a repetition of this sequence of events" — despite its happy outcome this time.

By this time the drug had been on trial for two years in the Australian states of Victoria, New South Wales (NSW) and South Australia. This trial had a close to 100 per cent success rate and had produced twins in both Sydney and Adelaide, according to Dr James Brown who had made the drug in Melbourne.[34] In Germany three pregnancies were reported in a group of 19 women on hPG by 1964.[35] In America hPG had reportedly been used on 30 women in New York.[36] They were part of what would be a group totalling less than 300, most of them volunteers in short-term physiological studies rather than as a clinical therapy for infertility.[37] While Gemzell treated 572 women up to 1975, by far the largest program involving hPG was in Australia. More than 1,800 women were given hPG either as primary therapy for anovulation, the failure to ovulate, as test doses to check their initial response, or as stimulation on IVF programs. This large hPG use evolved due to several factors including cost, ease of production and the arrival from Edinburgh in the early 1960s of Brown, who joined the endocrine unit of the Royal Women's Hospital in Melbourne.

Brown found that a local colleague, Dr Kevin Catt, was already making hGH at another centre in Melbourne. Competing for scarce pituitary glands made no sense, so Brown and Catt devised a method of production where hPG was extracted first by Brown and hGH from the residue by Catt. It became known as the Brown-Catt method. From 1963, as pressure for a national hormone program in Australia increased, there was little point in doctors buying hMG or going to the trouble of making it. The government intended to provide pituitary-derived hormones free as pharmaceutical benefits.[38]

Refinements of the original extraction methods for both types of hormone followed in the 1960s and 1970s. Glands used were either stored in acetone or frozen, and at least 12 different extraction methods evolved worldwide. No method was perfect. Antibodies continued to affect some hGH preparations. Some children did not grow at all. Others grew, but because they had begun treatment as teenagers, their final height was still shorter than average — although taller than they would have been without treatment.

Some women treated with hPG failed to fall pregnant. Of those who did, some aborted. Others developed polycystic ovaries or abdominal pain. Superovulation, which resulted in many multiple pregnancies, became a distinct problem. The dosages of hPG necessary to induce normal ovulation in one woman might result in hyperstimulation and a multiple pregnancy in another. These wild fluctuations were often blamed on a woman's physical response rather than her doctor's dosage.[39] Few women were warned that hyperstimulation was potentially fatal.

Many patients did not know that the hGH or hPG being used to treat them was made from pituitary glands. If they did, it did not occur to them that the glands had to be sliced from the brains of dead bodies. In America, however, the source of the hormone was well known. Parents of children needing supplementary hGH for a variety of medical conditions went on what became known as pituitary drives — campaigns to convince people to donate their pituitary glands in the event of sudden death — much like present-day organ donation awareness campaigns and drivers' licence arrangements.[40] Some nationalised government-sponsored programs encouraged the removal of pituitary glands during post-mortem examinations, with a payment given to some mortuary attendants and pathologists. The practice began in the United States and Canada in the early 1960s, where pathologists were paid US$2 and C$2 respectively. In Britain, mortuary attendants were paid a shilling per gland, which increased to 20 pence in later years.

In Australia, from 1967, payments of 20 cents per gland were common to mortuary attendants (although some refused payment). Others never received a cent. The bounty rose to 30 cents per gland in 1974 and to 50 cents in 1977. These payments paled beside the comparatively huge amounts offered by commercial companies during the same period. In the United States $10 a gland was offered.[41] And Nordisk paid more than US$15 each for glands from Africa and Asia. Kabi paid a similar amount for glands primarily from the West Indies and South America.[42]

It was not until the 1980s that the highly infectious nature of the CJD agent in human tissue was appreciated by much of medical science. Nor was it known until then just how good acetone was as a preservative: not only did it preserve pituitary glands for months at a time, it preserved the CJD agent as well. No-one involved in the collection of pituitary glands thought to exclude anything remotely like a slow virus when production of these miracle drugs began. This was chiefly because no-one in fields outside veterinary science and neurology had ever heard of them.

But in 1965, as Shirley Ann Lawson prepared for the birth of her quintuplets, on the other side of the world inside a drab cinder-box building at the Patuxent Wildlife Research Center in Laurel, Maryland, a pair of chimpanzees was about to change the course of medical history. The chimps, Daisy and George, would also lay a mantle of scientific respectability on those associated with the brilliant but eccentric Carleton Gajdusek.

Daisy and George were among about 12 chimps in the enclosure, eight of which had a timebomb ticking away in their brains. Those select eight were sharing the sparse interior of their "home" with hundreds of mice. Another 75 monkeys of various types, some of them harbouring their own timebombs, had been bought from "shady primate dealers" in the south of the United States.[43]

Gajdusek's laboratory at the NIH had been extended to include the "study of slow, latent and temperate virus infections". It was the first laboratory of its kind in the world. The laboratory at Patuxent, and the building constructed next door in 1963, which then housed the chimpanzees, monkeys and mice, was run by Joe Gibbs, a former navy man with a wry sense of humour. Gibbs had been a medical microbiologist involved in conventional virus research and had developed a vaccine for the fatal Rift Valley fever. Then in 1961 he agreed to join Gajdusek's exciting new venture investigating "slow viruses" like kuru.

By August 1961 several hundred mice had been injected with scrapie-infected sheep tissue. In the two years that followed more than 10,000 mice and non-human primates were injected with liquefied brain tissue infected with a variety of human brain diseases. These included kuru, amyotrophic lateral sclerosis (ALS), Parkinsonian dementia, Pick's disease, Alzheimer's disease, Schilder's disease and multiple sclerosis. And chimps other than Daisy and George were injected with kuru or other chronic nervous system disorders including schizophrenia, motor neurone disease, multiple sclerosis (MS) and ALS. While the aim was to determine if these other diseases transmitted to laboratory animals, these chimps were also performing the function of controls for the kuru-injected chimps, which were the animals that carried the most promise at that stage.

But it was the early injections of kuru tissue into chimps that made the Gajdusek team famous and set the "mad scientists" on a path of respectable accomplishment in a brand new area of disease work. August 1963 was the start of the kuru transmissions, which Gajdusek and Michael Alpers had agreed in New Guinea to commit themselves to for 10 years if necessary. Gajdusek and Gibbs injected Daisy with a kuru brain solution taken from the 11-year-old Fore girl, Kigea, from Waisa, whose death and autopsy in the presence of her father in March 1963 had so affected Alpers.

The following month, as the political career of US President John F. Kennedy rolled towards its fatal climax in Dallas, liquefied brain from another kuru patient called Eiro was injected into the brain of two-year-old George. Eiro was a 13-year-old boy who died in September 1962. He had been Alpers' first autopsy patient. Both injections were made into the left frontal cortex of the brain. The animals were lightly anaesthetised with ether, but minutes later were sitting on the secretary's desk and walking around Gajdusek's lab.

Such long-term experiments on chimpanzees, rather than on monkeys that were cheaper and easier to house, were unprecedented and considered a long and doubtful shot. This pessimism was shared not only by others inside the National Institute of Neurological Diseases and Blindness that housed Gajdusek's lab, but also outside the NIH. Gajdusek was also considered quite mad in an affectionate sort of way. He was insistent, however, that the more expensive and more difficult chimpanzees should be used over monkeys.

In early 1964 Michael Alpers, by now very familiar with the similarities between kuru and scrapie, arrived to work in Gajdusek's lab. He stayed four years. At the end of 1964 the world's first meeting on slow virus infections was held and from that the first monograph or book on slow virus infections was produced in 1965.[44] For the first time, current knowledge on kuru and other slow virus infections like measles was to be found within two covers. Of note was the inclusion of the first report on a new scrapie-like disease in farmed mink fed on "downer cows". It was called transmissible mink encephalopathy (TME).

Also included in the monograph was an addendum by Gibbs. In it he detailed early signs of progressive ataxia and tremors noticed in George and Daisy since May — 20 and 21 months respectively since they had been injected with brain suspensions from Kigea and Eiro. Gibbs had never seen a kuru patient, nor watched any of the hundreds of feet of cine film the amateur cameraman Gajdusek had taken during his last seven years of patrols in New Guinea. But Michael Alpers certainly had. At Patuxent he examined and photographed the chimpanzees on a regular basis long before they became sick. Once their symptoms had begun, a string of doctors and world-renowned neurologists examined Daisy and George during the last months of their lives. From May 1965 everyone there noted the increasingly abnormal behaviour of George and Daisy.[45]

The chimps, as well as six others that had been injected with kuru between September 1963 and February 1964, had become friends with everyone who dealt with them. It was distressing for all to see Daisy and George change for the worse. They both showed initial signs of apathy. But while Daisy remained apathetic only for several months, George — whom it was soon shown was a girl and was renamed Georgette — showed a more rapid deterioration. The chimp developed a droopy lower lip, lost coordination, staggered around the cage and soon could not eat properly. Unable to pull the skins off her bananas properly, Georgette ate them straight from the floor of the cage in what became known as vacuum-cleaner eating. Daisy, also after several months of apathy and a droopy bottom lip of her own, began showing early signs of disease. By July 1965 she began to walk with a stagger and developed a specific nodding of the head which had also affected Georgette.

One day, while completing clinical notes from more neurological tests on Georgette for reflex, vision, balance and sensory perception, Alpers was jolted by the conclusion he had absently written down. All the signs — the jerking ataxic walk, shaking, truncal tremors and involuntary nodding of the head — added up to only one thing: kuru. It had all been documented, photographed and filmed together with the observations of all those doctors. The chimps had been given superb nursing care, perhaps better than many humans suffering a similar neurological disease would have received.

"Joe," said Alpers when he went to see Gibbs immediately afterwards, "I really think this chimpanzee's got kuru. I think we should get Carleton."[46] Joe didn't disagree, though he had been somewhat sceptical. In any case Gajdusek was on patrol in New Guinea.

After cabling Gajdusek with the condition of the two chimps, Gibbs received the following reply: "Say nothing of this development: we may well have contaminated the animals with scrapie".[47] Gibbs doubted this very much because he had always been scrupulous in separating scrapie-infected animals from others. Gajdusek was persuaded by telegram that despite his doubts he had better come back. He returned immediately to America. If it was kuru, this was what they had all been working towards.

Tired, put out and very sceptical, Gajdusek went straight to Patuxent the morning after his arrival in late July 1965. There Joe Gibbs, the two animal handlers and Mike Alpers watched as Georgette emerged from her cage. "She came out and she was very ataxic, she fell all over the place. She was shaking, she was grimacing, which is a particular feature of kuru in chimpanzees and occasionally does occur in human beings. She also showed dislike of light so she was screwing up her eyes. Then she sort of fell over," Alpers recalled years later.[48] Gajdusek couldn't believe what he was seeing. "I've just come from seeing patients two days ago in the bush out of Okapa and you've dragged me here and now this chimpanzee performs in exactly the same way. It's uncanny," he declared.[49]

July rolled into the heat of August 1965, two years after the injection of kuru tissue into Georgette and Daisy. Agents such as manganese deficiency (thought to produce vague neurological symptoms in primates), trace metal diseases and parasites such as tape worm had to be firmly rejected as even remotely possible causes of the observed symptoms. Over the next few months, as Daisy and Georgette rapidly deteriorated, Gibbs, Alpers and colleagues scoured the scientific literature for anything on primate or chimpanzee neurology. The little to go on did not fit the chimps' symptoms. Soon Georgette was huddled at the bottom of her cage barely able to move.

In October 1965, five months after Georgette first became unwell, she was gently put to death by exsanguination. She was anaesthetised with ether and bled to death from a vein, sparing her further suffering. Bleeding also provided blood samples and in reality meant less mess than with other procedures.

A London-based neuropathologist, Mrs Elisabeth Beck, flew to Washington to oversee the correct handling of the brain and tissues by Joe Gibbs and Michael Alpers. Her work had previously included inspecting scrapie brains with H. B. Parry and examining eight kuru brains sent from New Guinea by Gajdusek. Now she was to be part of the most important aspect of the experiment — confirmation of kuru transmission, if that was what had killed Georgette.

A piece of every part of Georgette was put into separate, sterile vials for later examination during the day-long autopsy. Mrs Beck, Berlin-trained but among those who had fled to Britain from Nazi Germany, was later employed at the Maudsley Hospital in London. During Georgette's autopsy she personally placed the friendly chimp's brain into a bucket filled with a formalin solution and suspended it with some string around the major arteries. As she boarded the plane for London she remarked that a Nobel Prize would result from what she fully expected to be a transmission of kuru.[50]

After four weeks, Georgette's brain, by now solidified sufficiently for slicing, was sent to London. Mrs Beck waited several more weeks — so there would be no question about the brain's structural stability — before cutting it up. Under a microscope, she scanned thin slivers of each part of the brain for telltale spongy holes and deposits of amyloid protein known as plaques. Amyloid plaques were to become a typical, though not uniform, feature of kuru.

Daisy was killed in December 1965. She also had deteriorated to the point of being huddled on a shelf of her cage, with difficulty swallowing and hardly any coordination in her limbs.[51]

In January 1966 Mrs Beck's eagerly anticipated telegram arrived in Gajdusek's lab. "Neuropathology of chimpanzee indistinguishable from human kuru. Stop."[52] Everyone crowded around Gajdusek grinning widely. Joe Gibbs came in from the woods in Maryland and worked into the night composing the paper that would alert the world to their discovery. Michael Alpers wrote the clinical features section, Joe Gibbs added the laboratory work and Gajdusek wrote the beginning and end of the letter.

By this time, a third chimpanzee called Joanne, who had been injected with kuru from a victim called Kabuinampa in February 1964, had developed strikingly similar symptoms to Georgette and Daisy. From August 1965, just after Gajdusek's flying trip from New Guinea to look at Georgette's symptoms, Joanne had become lethargic. Within weeks she had lost much of her coordination and had developed tremors in her limbs. She also developed "a wide-based stamping gait in which she never rose much above her haunches", shivering tremors and would grimace when examined. Joanne's deterioration had been followed — only weeks before Mrs Beck's cable — by a fourth chimp, a male injected in November 1963 with kuru from a patient called Kariwani.[53]

Late on the night they wrote their letter for publication in the prestigious journal *Nature*, Gajdusek and Alpers drove all the way from Bethesda to the general post office in Washington. Having missed the NIH mail that day they wanted to be sure this was sent. Two weeks later, in the February 19, 1966 issue of *Nature* the letter on the transmission of kuru to a chimpanzee was published.[54] It was followed in November that year by an article in the *Lancet*, which fully detailed the pathology of Georgette's brain. It also included the exciting outcome that, excluding Georgette, Daisy and Joanne, three other chimpanzees injected with kuru brain suspension had developed the disease after incubation periods of 18 to 30 months.[55]

Another doctor, Paul Brown, well remembers the jubilation in the lab at Mrs Beck's histopathologic confirmation of Daisy's kuru. A wiry native of New Jersey, with a dry wit and striking pale blue eyes, he had fallen under Gajdusek's "Pied Piper" spell in 1963 and had spent his compulsory army service researching kuru.[56] During his six weeks in New Guinea, Brown continued Alpers' collection of kuru brains under optimal conditions. These were to be used for continuing experiments on chimps via injections of kuru tissue through alternative peripheral routes into the body, rather than just into the brain. Brown's New Guinea research, during his training to be a specialist in internal medicine, included performing an autopsy on a woman who had died of kuru. He placed her brain and other organs in a canister of liquid nitrogen and arranged for payment to her family of several tins of beef stew and a blanket. Brown also collected the specimen from Kabuinampa, which was injected into the chimp Joanne in February 1964. Away from Bethesda while he completed his training during the drama years of 1965 and 1966, when one chimp after another succumbed to kuru, Brown never missed the excitement again. He returned to Gajdusek's lab in 1967 and witnessed the silencing of the sceptics the following year — the first of his next 30 years with Gajdusek.

When Daisy and Georgette developed kuru but all the other primates injected with various other (clearly non-transmissible) neurological diseases remained stubbornly well, Gajdusek decided to inject other chimps with the kuru-like and fatal CJD. But because the disease was so rare, it was difficult to locate tissue from a CJD brain in America. Elisabeth Beck and her boss at the neuropathology department of the Maudsley Hospital, Dr Peter Daniels, provided the first specimen. A piece of brain taken during the biopsy of a woman five months before her death from CJD was given to them by Dr Bryan Matthews, a Derbyshire-based neurologist later to become Professor of Clinical Neurology at the University of Oxford. This brain tissue was injected into the brain of a chimp at Patuxent and the waiting game began again. Almost on cue, 18 months later the chimp developed CJD. The initial letter on this transmission sent to *Science* in August 1968 was greeted with "some incredulity", according to Professor Matthews decades later.[57,58] Another article on the CJD transmissions, published in *Science* in 1969, detailed how a suspension of the biopsy patient's brain, along with brain tissue from other British, Canadian and American CJD patients, was injected into chimpanzees. In addition, infected brain tissue from the first two chimpanzees that contracted CJD was injected, in turn, into several other chimps. This was the serial passaging process that had long been used in scrapie studies in Britain. "Both retransmission and serial passage from chimpanzee to chimpanzee have been successful", the authors of the *Science* article stated. They added that the symptoms differed markedly from experimental kuru, with obvious dementia, jerks, muscle contractions and drowsiness — just like that found in human CJD.[59] Later, when further successful injections of tissue into chimps occurred it became more difficult to distinguish kuru from CJD in those animals.[60]

The transmission of CJD to chimps, which finally proved that it was an infectious disease, was big news in the worlds of neurology, virology and microbiology. In other scientific and medical disciplines it was barely noted. For those who already knew that CJD was a disease that could be inherited, there was profound shock when it was found to be infectious as well. Paul Brown recalls that people initially doubted the veracity of the kuru transmissions. "But when the CJD animals started coming down, that was it."[61]

In hindsight this research was a giant pointer. It should have alerted the science world to the transmissibility of such terrible brain diseases. But kuru was seen merely as an exotic disease affecting a few tribes in one small area of a largely unexplored third-world Pacific island country. And because CJD was so rare — its description to that time found under at least 25 different names in medical literature — most neurologists, let alone family doctors, had never seen a case in their entire career. The penny certainly did not drop that these discoveries could threaten large human populations.

Attempts to transmit other degenerative diseases of the central nervous system (including the brain) — Parkinson's disease, MS, Alzheimer's disease, motor neurone disease, ALS and schizophrenia — all failed. There were, however, two false alarms that caused consternation for a time. One involved a sheep injected with MS that coincidentally developed natural scrapie as well. The other was an apparent transmission of Alzheimer's disease, which was later blamed on a laboratory labelling error.

Eventually other primates, including the spider monkey, the squirrel monkey, the capuchin monkey and the woolly monkey developed experimental kuru. Transmissions also succeeded in several species of Old World monkeys, all of which had much longer incubation periods than chimpanzees — sometimes up to 12 years.[62] Kuru in later years was also successfully transmitted to goats, minks and ferrets. And though neither kuru nor CJD would transmit to sheep, the brain pathology looked just like scrapie.[63]

Later, in 1981, another inheritable disease of the TSE family would prove transmissible — the very rare Gerstmann-Sträussler-Scheinker (GSS) syndrome. And much later, after its discovery in 1986, the aptly named hereditary disease, fatal familial insomnia (FFI), would finally transmit to laboratory mice in 1995. But that was all far into the future.

The transmission of kuru to chimpanzees made it the first human disease to be proved a slow virus infection. This was a breakthrough in the recognition of kuru as one of several chronic, degenerating, non-inflammatory, inheritable diseases that would become known as TSEs. Man might have landed on the moon but as the decade of the 1960s closed, medical science was no nearer to solving the mystery of what it was that actually caused these so-called slow viruses.

CHAPTER 5

And then there were nine

GERALDINE BRODRICK was lying on her side in bed, too sick to move, when the doctor arrived. Her husband Len ushered him into the master bedroom of their semi-colonial sprawling three-bedroom brick home in Hughes, the first suburb in the rapidly expanding Woden Valley area in Australia's capital city, Canberra.

It was mid-December 1970, and the usual hot Christmas was only 10 days away. Geraldine was known around Canberra as a charity worker and hostess of some note, for which roles her effervescent personality and dry wit were perfectly suited. In addition to her normal role as secretary of a local branch of the Red Cross Society, she had taken charge of the decorations for the Red Cross annual ball — a large social affair at which the diplomatic corps, headed by the Swiss Ambassador, were always honoured guests. Hardly able to move all day, Geraldine was worried that her traditional large self-catered Christmas functions for family and friends would not go ahead.

Geraldine's abdomen had swollen to the size of a football. There was something very wrong. Ian Ferguson, her GP, only had to look at her and note the extreme swelling and tenderness to know instantly that she had a large ovarian cyst. His gentle examination also revealed a uterus that was as extended as a three-month pregnancy. "That cyst will have to come out," he told her bluntly. "Sometimes, if they are a certain type, they do subside on their own but this is pretty big. Now, I think you're also pregnant. If you are, there would be a 90% chance of losing the pregnancy."

Geraldine was startled. "If I am," she said disbelievingly, "I couldn't possibly be more than two weeks."

A diminutive 1.5 metre tall, the attractive 28-year-old brunette regularly appeared in the social pages of local newspapers. Her mother had been a well-known Sydney mannequin in the 1940s before her premature death at 39, from cervical cancer. Both her father and her step-father were dead. Perhaps as a result, Geraldine had always wanted a house full of children, and had delivered two daughters within the first two years of her marriage. But this wasn't Geraldine's only reason for wanting to remain pregnant.

Her problems had started nearly four years earlier, after the birth in March 1967 of her second daughter, Jacqueline. Geraldine had noticed that the persistent lethargy, facial acne, gradual weight gain, headaches and depression, all of which had developed while breast feeding, had worsened. She was weepy and short-tempered and not coping with housework. Also, her hairline was receding — a fact her husband had underlined one night when she had piled her long dark brown hair into its customary chignon. "You're going bald," he'd told her. "And so are you," she'd retorted, stung. It was time for action.

Despite a battery of tests, Geraldine's Canberra gynaecologist could find no obvious cause for her problems; the hair thinning was simply attributed to the toll of pregnancy. Geraldine was prescribed a contraceptive pill, which she took every day for 12 weeks after Jacqueline's six-month birthday. Following the caesarean births of both Jacqueline and her older sister Belinda, Geraldine's gynaecologist thought it best that she not conceive again too soon. He also thought that the Pill might stop some of the symptoms annoying her.

But by the time Jacqueline was a year old, the hair loss and other symptoms had worsened. Geraldine was not menstruating either, which meant she was not ovulating. More tests and several courses of the oestrogen blocking synthetic drug, clomiphene citrate, taken to stimulate the pituitary gland's production of hormones necessary for ovulation, had failed to yield anything.

With no improvement by 1968, her gynaecologist referred her to one of the most highly qualified fertility experts in Sydney, Professor Harvey Carey. Carey, who had pioneered the use of tailor-made mini ("traffic light") pills from his hormone clinic at Sydney's Royal Hospital for Women, was often labelled "absent-minded" because of his tendency to lose himself in his research and, in so doing, get locked into his rooms for the night.

"Right," he told Geraldine in Sydney at her first consultation, "we'll have to start from scratch." What followed was a battery of tests even more arduous and prolonged than those she had had in Canberra. But

none of the measurements of hormone levels, blood sugar, basal metabolic rate or oestriol levels, nor the results of X-rays showed a conclusive result. All that was known was that Geraldine was still not ovulating — or menstruating. Technically she was infertile. So Carey put
Geraldine on a mini-Pill, tailored to her as determined by her blood and
other tests. The aim was to raise her hormone levels to the level at which
a pregnancy was possible. This was done in the hope that the pituitary
gland might kick in and take over again. If this happened, there was a
possibility that she would regain her former vitality.

In mid-1968, Geraldine was again put on clomiphene citrate to
induce ovulation. But apart from massive fluid retention and a face of
moon proportions, nothing happened and it was back to another round
of head X-rays, tests on the hypothalamus and hormone levels. Again
they were inconclusive. Carey then suggested the drug of last resort for
women who desperately wanted a baby: pituitary gonadotrophin.
Although Geraldine didn't mind the thought of more children, she was
not desperate. What was desperate was her need to feel better, to rid
herself of the endless headaches, the ever-present depression and the
600-kilometre round trip to Sydney for useless tests and drug monitoring every few months.

Geraldine had been a nurse before her October 1964 marriage to Len
Brodrick, a self-employed meat wholesaler from a large pioneering
family in the Canberra area. She was not averse to asking questions
about drug treatment effects, good or bad. Gonadotrophin, Carey
explained, had a risk of multiple birth, probably higher than the twins
and triplets that had been born after clomiphene treatment. There were
the Lawson quins for a start. And only three years previously the Jones
quads of Melbourne had received national prominence.

And there was one more thing — the possibility of over-stimulation
of the ovaries. Geraldine, whose nursing training had not included
obstetrics, did not pursue the issue. She did not know until much later
that hyperstimulation, as it was called, was painful and potentially life-
threatening. She knew the drug was extracted from human pituitary
glands, unlike other gonadotrophins that were extracted from the urine
of either pregnant or menopausal women. Agreeing in principle with
organ and tissue transplants, a pituitary donation certainly did not put
her off, as long as the family of the donor had agreed.

"I knew gonadotrophin was the last resort," she recalls. "The point was, I was terrified they'd pat me on the head and say 'Go home, you'll be all right.' Because I knew I wasn't going to be. It just wasn't going to right itself, obviously. The worse I felt, the less able I was to do anything and the more depressed I became. I mean I was in my twenties. I was literally in menopause at 25. So the only thing they'd come up with was if I could fall pregnant again then maybe the whole system would just right itself. Now that, to me, made sense."[1]

Between late 1968 and mid-1970 Geraldine had four hPG treatment courses, each of about two weeks duration, for which she stayed in hospital. After the final injection of hPG in each course, following injections on successive days of human chorionic gonadotrophin (hCG), she returned to Canberra. Each morning at home she took her temperature to check for the slight rise that always indicates ovulation. And every day, in a five-litre plastic container, she would deposit every drop of her urine for the next three weeks. The container, in a brown paper bag, went with her everywhere — to kindergarten, to dinner parties, shopping, to friends' homes. At the end of each day she would shake it up and pour a sample into one of 21 test tubes provided for each day of the three-week period. Each tube was marked, labelled and frozen. At the end of the three weeks, an express courier was called and paid for by Geraldine to speed her set of test tubes to Sydney. There, a biochemical laboratory would test the oestriol content that indicated overall oestrogen levels in her body for each day.

All of these four treatments, which began with low doses and gradually increased to higher doses, used hPG manufactured by Dr James Brown at the Endocrine Unit of the Royal Women's Hospital in Melbourne. It was on the labels. Geraldine would feel better over a few days as the hPG worked its magic. But as the hormone levels subsided again, she would be back to dabbing on make-up over acne craters she had filled with thick calamine lotion.

At the end of November 1970, fearful for her continued sanity if she was not made well soon, she practically begged Carey for "one last attempt". He replied: "All right, but this will definitely be the last one". Her fifth and last course began on November 25, 1969, using half the dose of her highest previous course. It stopped with her last injection on December 4, 1970.

Now, 10 days after that last injection, and with her GP by her bedside, the ovarian cyst which had been gradually making its presence felt, had swelled to the point where Geraldine was so sore she could not get out of bed. Len Brodrick, a quiet reserved man approaching his thirty-second birthday, was clearly concerned about his wife.

The GP, Ian Ferguson, took a urine sample for what was a very early pregnancy test but it came back negative the next day, December 15, 1970. He trusted his instincts, though, and was sure Geraldine was pregnant. In fact the pregnancy may have caused the ovarian cyst, which was a common enough occurrence, he thought. He took urine again and a week later, just before Christmas, it came back positive. Geraldine estimated that she was only 17 days pregnant because that was the length of time that had elapsed since her last injection of hPG. She was elated, sick and frightened all at the same time.

Ferguson was unhappy. He thought the cyst might kill her, or at the least threaten her reproductive organs. But Geraldine was determined to keep her pregnancy. She opted to do nothing except rest and hope the cyst would just go away, which it did. While she stayed in bed Len cooked the turkey for the first quiet Christmas in years.

Later, while recalling the hPG injections that led to that pregnancy, Geraldine said her doses were half what they had been on her four earlier courses. "I knew I had no hope of ever being treated again. So I was not going to lose that pregnancy. The children were not the main driving force. I just wanted to feel better again."

Carey wrote a short note to her in January 1971 thanking her for the letter in which she announced her pregnancy and suggesting she travel to Sydney in the next two or three months. "We could carry out an echoscope [the forerunner of today's ultrasound test] examination to see if there is more than one baby present."[2]

Organising and appearing bright and bubbly on February 20 at a large Red Cross charity event, also Len's thirty-second birthday, was a nightmare for Geraldine. It was her last outing for months. She was getting awfully big for only two months pregnant and needed to rest constantly. Standing side-on before the mirror, she knew she looked as big as she did at four months with Belinda.

Then the headaches started. They were severe and unrelenting. After repeated doses of Panadeine failed to take even the edge from the pain, Len packed Geraldine's head in ice. That didn't work either so she was given a pain-killing injection. Afterwards, she began to haemorrhage and was taken by ambulance to Royal Canberra Hospital. After 24 hours in the labour ward, where the bleeding stopped spontaneously, she stayed on at the hospital for two weeks for complete bed rest, and missed Jacqueline's fourth birthday at home. A physician was called about the continuing headaches and told her privately, when she asked, that she was having at least three babies. "I thought it was more than three. I could feel them turning over. It was very weird because I thought if I can feel three and I am only this far along it's got to be more," Geraldine recalled.[3]

After another week of bed rest in a private hospital, Geraldine shocked herself again. Now three months pregnant, she looked at least six months along. Carey wanted her in Sydney for an echoscope as soon as he heard about the possible triplets. The more babies, the more chance of prematurity and death. But he warned that she should not be immobile all the time or she might develop blood clots.

On April 7, 1971, a week after her twenty-ninth birthday, and with the air already crisp in Canberra, Geraldine and Len Brodrick flew to Sydney for her echoscopy. Barely able to zip up the maternity dress she wore to hospital before having Jacqueline, Geraldine and her husband went straight to a city maternity boutique where she bought a size 16 pillar-box red dress for her normally size-10 frame. She felt like a dumpy fire engine. The dress certainly covered what looked like an eight-month pregnancy, but it hung to her ankles and the sleeves had to be rolled up just to hold her handbag.

Ultrasonic echoscopy was then the most advanced method of checking on the developing foetus. Pregnant women, contact gel smeared on their abdomens, had to lean upright into a plastic bladder which bordered a tank of water. Sound waves from a variety of angles in a line around the womb — similar to radar — were used to measure pulses that were emitted from different organs and tissue of the baby. The pulses were converted into dots, which registered on a screen to produce an anatomical cross-section of the mother and babies. This could then be photographed, analysed, and the size and number of babies measured. Standing through the 40-minute procedure was too much for Geraldine, with babies "climbing up under my rib cage and wriggling under my shoulder blades". She fainted several times from the breath-

lessness of standing for such long periods. The echoscope was interrupted and done in two takes, making it difficult to confirm the actual
number without risking double counting.

The two young women conducting the echoscope procedure asked
how many babies she thought she was having.

"I think it's at least three," Geraldine replied.

"One," said one woman operating the machine.

"Two," said the other, after a pause.

"Ah, three," said the second one again. Then there was silence. Geraldine fainted again and had to be revived with another glass of water. She
didn't notice that the counting had stopped.

Later she was ushered into Carey's office, leaving Len, the door ajar,
in the waiting room. The doctor talked at length about the weather and
asked how she had been feeling until now. Finally Geraldine, unable to
take the suspense any longer and wanting confirmation that she was
having triplets but probably quadruplets, blurted out: "Well how many
is it?"

"There are at least six," he replied, looking straight into her eyes.

Geraldine was speechless. Carey's face receded as the blood pounded
in her ears. She heard him say: "We don't really expect you to carry
them. In fact, I don't think you could carry them another week. Your
size — everything's against you. That many babies is just not on. I
really don't think you'll carry the pregnancy to a term where they will
be viable."

Geraldine didn't want to hear this. She'd carried them this long. She
would have to endure a "birth" of some sort, whatever happened, so she
determined that she would take each day as it came and survive the
pregnancy in small stages. "What if I do continue to carry them past
next week?" she asked. "If you do I want you back here in May, and you
will stay here until delivery." He paused. "But you won't. I just want
you to go home and lead a normal life." Hell, thought Geraldine. I
haven't done anything since December. How do I start now?[4]

When Geraldine left Carey she saw Len had heard what had been said
and turned ashen. They travelled in silence by cab back to the Went-
worth Hotel, where they had held their wedding reception, and decided
over dinner to tell the family only that she was expecting triplets. Anything over triplets would have excited immediate unwanted interest in
Geraldine, who was already well enough known in Canberra. The

nation's capital city had never had its own set of quads, let alone sextuplets. They thought triplets a good enough excuse for her to be "resting" and out of circulation for so long. And if they lost the babies, well, noone would need to know any more.

Back in Canberra Geraldine got through one day at a time in her insular world — in bed. It was in bed that she would shell the peas and peel the potatoes for dinner. She couldn't lie on her right side because the babies resting on her stomach would give her heartburn. So, on her left side, pillows tucked around her and a hot water bottle at her back, she lay and knitted, needles in the air, for Belinda and Jacqueline, because there was a fair chance she would miscarry at any time. She ate her Vita-Wheat biscuits with honey and drank her tea — basically her only sustenance for months, because eating was too nauseating and too much effort.

Soon Geraldine could not sleep because the babies continually crawled up under her chest bone. Later the pummelling of tiny limbs became so intense that it cracked a rib and resulted in such severe bruising that it appeared she had varicose veins on her chest. And after every sleepless night Carey's words echoed in her brain: "If you're still around in May, come back". All that Geraldine could hope for was to reach 30 weeks gestation.

By Saturday June 12, 1971, Geraldine was just over 27 weeks pregnant. The skin over her abdomen was stretched so tight it was as thin as tissue paper. A gaggle of the world's media had for days been camped outside the Royal Hospital for Women, then in Sydney's inner-city suburb of Paddington. Word had leaked out of the hospital that Geraldine Brodrick, a former Sydney nurse and mother of two small daughters, was expecting six babies. The first anyone in the hospital knew that the secret was out was when a telegram arrived unexpectedly from a baby formula manufacturer the previous Wednesday, offering milk supplies free for the expected multiple birth.

Two days previously, on Thursday June 10, Associate Professor Leslie Stevens, from the paediatrics department at the University of New South Wales, asked Geraldine if she had made any of what he termed "legal arrangements". "No, why?" She looked at him blankly. He explained, briefly mentioning the media frenzy that had surrounded the birth of quads at nearby Crown Street Women's Hospital several years earlier. He didn't want a similar debacle to ensue. The media had got hold of photographs of the quads, all of whom had subsequently died, and had them published — before the mother had had a chance to see the babies herself.

He also asked if she had had any contractions. "Just those Braxton Hicks ones," she replied breezily, "the ones you get before you go into labour." Professor Stevens hurried off, alarmed, and told her that her husband should come to Sydney that night. Three hours later she was in labour — three months before her due date.

Leaving Belinda, 5, and Jacqueline, 4, in Canberra, Len arrived in Sydney and was immediately engulfed in a war of media offers for the story of the babies. He asked Geraldine, who was distracted by continuous contractions, what she thought about it all. She didn't much care about any offers at that stage, but eventually suggested he accept the one with the most privacy. The offer by John Fairfax and Sons Ltd — publishers of newspapers and magazines, including the *Sydney Morning Herald* and *Woman's Day,* and owner of ATN Channel 7 — was the lowest bid at $6,000. Later it included accommodation and airfares to Honolulu, two dresses and one swimsuit for magazine advertisements — nothing like the "six figure sum" quoted in the press that their friends and family believed they had received.

Geraldine and everyone inside the hospital knew more than the press and public outside. More echoscopes in the past few weeks had confirmed seven babies. It could have been more, the obstetrician Dr Bill Garrett had maintained, after examining the photos. A world authority on the echoscope, which had been developed in Australia during the previous decade, Garrett advised the hospital to be prepared for at least nine, just in case.

While his wife had the most public of labours with at least 36 people present, Len Brodrick was also under the spotlight, busy giving the first of many interviews to which they had been contracted over the next two years.

Seated on a bench in the nearby 662-acre Centennial Park, Len Brodrick told an ATN Channel 7 reporter, smoke curling up his arm from his cigarette, that the sudden and all-consuming media attention of the past few days had "come as a shock to me". He had emerged from several sleepless nights "fairly well", but was not prepared at all for the frenzy of world interest that had ensued when the story leaked out.[5] And it was all rather embarrassing. Len's family and many of their friends knew Geraldine was pregnant, possibly with triplets, but knew nothing abut the fertility drug that had caused it, of which details had been plastered all over the press. Geraldine's extended family knew nothing at all. No-one had expected the pregnancy to last so long.

As the clock in the crowded labour ward ticked past midnight into June 13, the contractions accelerated and the delivery room rapidly filled. Along one wall were nine black strips of tape forming Roman numerals. Underneath were nine humidicribs. Electricians were on stand-by in case of a power failure, and the 39 medical and other staff present jockeyed for position between machines and medical equipment.

Seated beside Geraldine was Sister Mary Clements, a nun training as a midwife. She knew that being present for the Brodrick births and having the honour of baptising them immediately they were born, before they had been handed to their paediatrician, would be one of the greatest experiences of her life. "I can't take much more of this," Geraldine grated out towards the end of her 56-hour labour, desperate for a caesarean birth, drugs — anything — and regretting she had passed on the offered gas. "We'll be right, we'll get there," said Sister Clements calmly, holding Geraldine's hand, clammy despite the chill of winter outside.

Geraldine knew that the fate of her babies was almost out of her hands. Her abdominal skin had stretched to almost breaking point. The doctors were terrified that her two previous caesarean scars could rupture internally. Carey wanted a normal delivery. A caesarean delivery of so many babies was in the realms of the unknown, and any disaster could have happened. Also, with no precedent, doctors were unaware of the effect of a numb mother on such a large birth, so Geraldine did not receive an epidural until 20 minutes before the babies were born. She could not bend over because her belly was so big. Len, the biggest man in the room, had to hold her in as curved a position as she could manage in full labour. Due to their number, the babies were causing contractions that started up under her arms, so 10 minutes later Geraldine was given a top-up epidural in the middle of her spine.

Exhausted after spending the last two days by his wife's side, Len was encouraged to go and have a cup of coffee in Geraldine's private room in the neonatal ward. He fell asleep, expecting to be called in time for the births. He woke bitterly disappointed to be told it was all over.

The nine paediatricians, nine paediatric nurses led by Sister Betty Horner, theatre nurses, a camera crew recording the historic event for the hospital, the medical superintendent of the hospital Dr John Greenwell, Garrett the obstetrician and specialist in echoscopy who had detected the nine babies, the anaesthetist Dr Richard Climie, Carey, Stevens — watched in wonder as without problem, Geraldine and Len Brodrick's third daughter entered the world at 4.53 a.m. on Sunday June 13, 1971. Everyone was stunned when she cried spontaneously. She was christened immediately by Sister Clements. The girl was the biggest, weighing in at two and a half pounds, and was placed in the first humidicrib under the Roman number I.

Geraldine giggled before dozing off under the instant relief the epidural gave her after the unrelenting waves of pain of the previous two days. She and Len had joked that with their luck, if it was septuplets, they would all be girls. "Oh my God, that'll be nine weddings!" she'd gasped.[6]

Two minutes later the second baby, a boy, was born dead. No-one said a word. The silence did not register on the semi-conscious Geraldine, who was by now quite numb from the chest down and greatly relieved that her responsibility was over; it was now up to the experts. Sister Clements baptised him before handing him to the paediatrician in charge of baby number two. His next brother, born a bare three minutes later, was also stillborn, and was christened immediately while everyone looked on in silence.

At 5.04 a.m. a third boy was born, this time alive, and he was placed quickly into the first of six extra humidicribs that had been bought by the hospital especially for the record birth. Geraldine didn't ask the sex of the baby. She knew everyone in the room was "extremely busy".

Six minutes later, another boy, alive, was placed in the next humidicrib and the hopes of those in the room began to rise again. At 5.13 a.m. another girl was delivered and placed in the humidicrib next to her two live brothers. Another girl was born three minutes later, followed by another four minutes later. Finally at 5.25 a.m. — 32 minutes after the first baby was born — the last of the Brodrick nontuplets, another live boy, was born. Richard, as he was to be called, after Climie, the anaesthetist, and also Richard the Lionheart, fitted snugly into the palm of his paediatrician's hand. He weighed only 12 ounces.

The next full recollection Geraldine had was of Len saying: "There were nine and there's seven alive darling." Later, after a quick look revealed that none had apparently inherited his ears, Len told Belinda on the phone, "You have three new brothers and four new sisters."

At a press conference later, and sitting in a row so long it could not be captured in one shot by television cameras, were seven of those involved in the history-making exercise. Lacking in sleep, they fronted the world's media with details of the record-breaking feat.

"Mrs Brodrick was delivered of her first child at 4.53 this morning," the hospital's medical superintendent John Greenwell began. "There were a total of nine babies delivered. Of those nine, seven were living and two were stillborn, and there was evidence that no life had been there for some time."[7] Garrett added that the two stillborn boys had succumbed to a simple "pressure of numbers".

In her new private room, which rapidly filled with flowers from all over Australia and cards and letters from well-wishers from overseas, Geraldine refused any interviews until someone had washed her hair, which had returned during her pregnancy. Stylist, Alfons Bo, owner of the salon where Geraldine had had her long tresses styled before her October 1964 wedding in Elizabeth Bay, arrived to fix the hair of the world's most famous mother.

Then, in what she described years later as a completely scripted series of questions and answers written by the hospital authorities, and read out in turn by the Channel 7 reporter, Geraldine conducted her first world-exclusive interview.

Q: Why did you take the fertility drug?
A: Obviously because I wanted another baby.
Q: Were you warned about the risk of multiple birth?
A: Most definitely and I was quite prepared to take the risk …
Q: Would you take the drug again?
A: Most definitely.

By the time Len Brodrick returned from celebrating with friends to see his rapidly recovering wife that Sunday afternoon, three of his new children had breathing difficulties and that night, the fourth and fifth born boys and the seventh born, a girl, died. Prayers were said in churches around the country for the Roman Catholic couple.

Overnight, telephone calls from as far as South Africa and South America were received, sheaths of telegrams arrived at the hospital reception desk including one from the Australian Prime Minister, William McMahon, and the Premier of New South Wales, Robert Askin. Twice daily bulletins were issued on the condition of the babies.

A Japanese gynaecologist, Professor Shoichi Sakamoto of the Tokyo University's obstetrics and gynaecology department, was widely quoted in newspapers on the chances of giving birth to nontuplets: one in every eightieth power of 80, or 1.677 billion to one. And Shirley Ann Lawson, mother of the New Zealand quins, wrote an open letter to Geraldine warning that the first years would be an ordeal and that her family would be owned by the country due to the public interest and the joy of watching each child develop individually.

When attention shifted to the four survivors, three of whom were in trouble on their second day of life, all hopes were pinned on the biggest girl, the first-born who weighed 2 lb 2 ounces. Obstetricians collectively gave any baby weighing under 2 lbs little hope of survival.[8]

On Monday night a girl weighing 1 lb 2 ozs died, sparking more calls for prayers to be offered nationally. And in the biggest blow of all, at 11.15 a.m. on Tuesday, June 15, the largest baby died. A tiny girl and boy remained alive.

"We knew the chances of them dying were high," Geraldine recalled years later. "But if you were the parents you were not going to give up hope. When that biggest little girl died we thought 'Oh hell, what chance have the others got?' They really thought she would live."[9]

Meanwhile Len vetted all mail, some of it containing crank letters making horrible comments and demanding money. But most of the hundreds of letters and cards were warm, congratulatory and, above all, hopeful. Some letters, of which almost half came from America along with clippings from local newspapers about the nontuplet birth, contained religious medals. One letter included three sachets containing holy wax blessed by Pope Leo XIII, the pope at the turn of the twentieth century, which the sender asked to have taped to the children's incubators. Geraldine went down and taped them on personally and touched the two tiny but perfectly-formed remaining children as they cupped their hands behind their ears and sucked on their lips.[10]

She personally answered all letters Len allowed her to see, but received no phone calls while in hospital. She was forced to move rooms several times — complete with trolley loads of flowers — after unexpected visitors were caught trying to see her, including one intrepid local reporter who climbed a drainpipe and was forced to backtrack by a fierce nurse.

After developing an acute lung infection, the remaining girl, who had been named Victoria, lost her tenuous grip on life on Friday, June 18, 1971. Geraldine was totally depressed and returned with a vengeance to her smoking habit, which she'd given up on learning she was pregnant. Then, a day later, the littlest one, Richard Leslie Michael Harvey Brodrick — Richard "the Lionheart" — died suddenly. And this after his drop by drop blood transfusion to rid him of jaundice, three days earlier, had looked so promising. Geraldine, who "just knew" he had gone before she was told officially, was devastated. She had been expressing milk for him having been told that, if he kept up his progress, Richard would be going home with her in a few months. In the early hours of the Sunday morning, the red-eyed Carey, Garrett and Stevens were present when, with Len, Geraldine was told the news.

Later autopsies on the babies confirmed they had died from the effects of immature lungs and cerebral haemorrhages due to their lack of blood clotting ability.[11] No photographs were ever taken of the babies. Geraldine and Len had agreed. They didn't need photographs to remember. And they didn't want photos or negatives of their babies to fall into the hands of the media.

The nontuplets were buried at Botany Cemetery in Sydney, near Botany Bay. Geraldine Brodrick considers the weekend of June 13 "our weekend" each year. The simple granite headstone reads: "The nine darling babies of Len and Geraldine Brodrick 13.6.71–19.6.71. It is better to have loved a little than never to have loved at all."

Richard and the biggest girl were single babies. The others were a set of identical twins with tiny blonde curls, a set of fraternal twins and a set of non-identical triplets — eight eggs fertilised which made nine babies. The unique, single placenta, which housed this miracle of nature, looked like a flower with a centre surrounded by petals. Along with film of the birth, it remains in a large glass bottle among the exhibits in the museum of the school of obstetrics and gynaecology of the University of New South Wales, located at the Royal Hospital for Women at Randwick.

A quarter of a century later, when a woman in England called Mandy Allwood fell pregnant with eight babies while taking a fertility drug, all the pain and grief Geraldine thought she had successfully buried was forced back. By this time Allwood, divorced and pregnant to a man who lived with another woman, and who had sold her story to the tabloid press for a reported £2 million, was being urged by doctors to consider selective abortion to give at least two of the babies a chance of survival. The media besieged Geraldine, the only woman alive who could know what Ms Allwood was going through.

Geraldine knew what the media wanted her to say and gave only selective interviews. "It would be an extremely difficult decision to make and I feel very sorry for Ms Allwood that she has to make a decision at all," she said in August 1996. "Abortion was not an issue in my day. It's definitely Mandy's decision and her partner's. Absolutely no-one and certainly not me has a right to give advice."

Mandy Allwood lost all eight babies in her nineteenth week of pregnancy in October 1996.

Like Mandy Allwood's 25 years later, the conception of the Brodrick nontuplets, was an unmitigated medical disaster. "A most extraordinary response, almost an accident of nature," was how the conception was described publicly by Dr H. Pincus Taft, chairman of the FSH subcommittee that oversaw gonadotrophin manufacture and distribution under the Federal Government-sponsored Australian Human Pituitary Hormone Program (AHPHP).[12] According to a much later report into the AHPHP:

> The multiple pregnancy caused a controversy in the community, the medical profession and within HPAC (the program's Human Pituitary Advisory Committee) and its subcommittees.

In July 1971 HPAC sent a report on the matter to the Federal Minister for Health and confirmed what Geraldine Brodrick knew about the dosage on her last course of treatment.

> … it would appear from the oestrogen monitoring data available to the committee that appropriate care was taken with administration of the hormone. The peak oestrogen level at which ovulation was induced is one at which from other records from patients treated in Australia, single pregnancy has resulted.[13]

However the HPAC report stated it was likely that the monitoring assays of the treating medical practitioner were unreliable. It stated it was possible that overstimulation had occurred "at an unacceptably high level of oestrogen excretion, greatly increasing the risk of multiple pregnancy".[14]

The Minister for Health was told in the July 1971 report that the screening and selection of patients for hGH treatment was satisfactory. However, "while appropriate care appears to have been taken" in Mrs Brodrick's case, her nontuplet "pregnancy being just an unfortunate and bizarre occurrence, it is also possible that unreliable hormone assays and unrecognised overstimulation were responsible".[15]

Explaining it himself in a 1976 paper published in the *Australian and New Zealand Journal of Obstetrics and Gynaecology*, Carey — who died in 1991 — stated that "a change in batch and thus a change in FSH to LH ratio may explain the excessive follicular development in relation to the total urinary oestrogen levels".[16] Later it was found that Geraldine was not "initially approved for hPG treatment" but was approved at some unspecified time later by the FSH subcommittee. Due to her two previous pregnancies, she did not meet the selection criteria in the AHPHP guidelines, but this was not included in the information forwarded to the FSH subcommittee by Carey, according to the minutes of a meeting of that committee in February 1981.[17]

In 1970, during Geraldine's first treatments with hPG from James Brown's laboratory in Melbourne, the FSH subcommittee had banned Carey from receiving further stocks of hPG from the government-owned Commonwealth Serum Laboratories (CSL). Not only was Carey not sending in all the appropriate treatment forms, he was found to be treating unapproved patients, of whom Geraldine was one when she began. When first approached about the matter in a letter dated April 10, 1970 from the director-general of health, Major-General W. Refshauge, Carey replied that he hadn't realised his recipients were unauthorised as he was having administration problems.[18]

But in August, after *Woman's Day* magazine had flown the Brodrick family to Honolulu for a two-week holiday, at the start of an eight-part biggest-selling series to that date, Carey emerged fighting. He damned the "departmental red tape" involved in hPG therapy and was critical of the varying balance of the FSH and the LH in hPG, which meant patients received different doses of the drug from different batches. He also acknowledged that he had been cut off from supplies of Brown's hPG from Melbourne and had been banned from further stocks of CSL-manufactured hPG until he gave the Federal Department of Health detailed information about his previous treatments. "I will give them the figures at my convenience — not at their demand," he said of a request to provide material needed for a meeting in 36 hours time.[19]

It wasn't until November 1974, more than three years after the Brodrick controversy that Carey was allowed "readmission" by the FSH subcommittee. His stocks of hPG from CSL resumed with the cautionary note that his urine quality control assays be "satisfactory" before the hormone was issued to him.[20]

After all her heartache over the death of her babies, the symptoms that had led Geraldine Brodrick to hPG returned. They could not be put down to her grief, financial problems or the amount she was eating. The real problem was not identified until 1975 after another gynaecologist, Dr Trevor Johnson, to whom Geraldine had been referred, twigged as to why she had tried clomiphene citrate, had not ovulated and had felt dreadful at the same time. She had very high levels of prolactin, another pituitary hormone that causes lactation in women. Geraldine had not thought much about her irregular ability, if her breasts were knocked or pressed, to produce dribbles of milk even though she had weaned both her daughters. She now realised she had been lactating — at a tiny level — for the past seven years. After tests proved an extremely high level of prolactin, a newly available scanning machine called a tomagraph finally showed what X-rays had failed to reveal. Geraldine had a tumour on the side of her pituitary gland.

In November 1975, Carey, who kept in contact, rang Geraldine with bad news. The tumour appeared from its size to have been there since about 1967 and, as it had grown, the pituitary gland's bony casing had come to rest on the left optic nerve. Test revealed she had already lost some sight out of that eye.

"What are my options?" Geraldine asked in her forthright way.

"If you don't do anything, you'll probably die of a cerebral haemorrhage before you go blind anyway in about two years," Carey replied in an equally frank fashion, adding that surgery was an option.

None too hopeful and recalling her theatre training, which had all been with neurosurgical patients she asked "What are my chances?"

"To be honest with you Geraldine, probably a 50 per cent chance of ending up as a vegetable. It's pretty delicate. It's a nasty area. We couldn't promise you would have your sight after it anyway. But it's certainly your best option."[21] Another option was radiotherapy, which Geraldine, remembering her mother's painful experience with similar treatment before her death from cervical cancer, rejected immediately.

In shock, but relieved to know finally why she was feeling so dreadful, Geraldine opted to do nothing, not wishing to be blind or on drugs for the rest of her life without her pituitary gland, or brain damaged and confined to a wheelchair. The diagnosis also reminded her of a conversation in which the nurse who administered her hPG injections, had told her that the brand of Pill she had taken after Jacqueline's birth had since been found to cause pituitary tumours. Although she didn't know it, a high proportion of other women treated for infertility in Sydney at the time also had pituitary tumours, which caused abnormally high secretions of prolactin.

When her gynaecologist rang in January 1976 offering her the chance to be among the first Australians to trial a new fertility drug — bromocriptine, which had shrunk pituitary tumours in trials overseas, Geraldine jumped at what she thought was her last chance at life. Later, in a review of 90 women who had not menstruated for more than 12 months and who were treated at the fertility unit of the University of Sydney's obstetrics and gynaecology department, 39 per cent of patients were found to have an elevated level of prolactin in the blood, an event often caused by a pituitary tumour.[22]

After 18 months on bromocriptine, Geraldine's prolactin levels finally returned to normal. Her old zip and bounce returned — and she fell pregnant. During the pregnancy, Geraldine stopped taking the drug and her tumour regrew. So after her third surviving daughter, Sacha, was born on December 22, 1977, she resumed taking the bromocriptine. Six months later Geraldine was physically ill after leaving a quaint Sydney restaurant, where she had thoroughly enjoyed her dish of garlic calamari. She was pregnant again. She and Len, after her fourth caesarean birth, finally had a son, Benjamin, on March 30, 1979. Three years later their marriage disintegrated.

Geraldine Brodrick, single mother of four, got on with her life. The drug kept her tumour tiny and, apart from biannual trips to an endocrinologist, she began to think her medical problems were under control.

She was wrong.

CHAPTER 6

Lethal gifts from medical science

IN MARCH 1974 one of the world's premier medical journals, in which medical discoveries of note are often revealed for the first time, carried a disturbing letter. Hundreds of thousands of medical professionals since have read those four paragraphs in the *New England Journal of Medicine* from a group of surgeons in New York.

They reported that a 55-year-old woman, "Linda", had died from CJD 26 months after receiving a corneal transplant from a 55-year-old man. Although he died from pneumonia, the man's autopsy later confirmed — long after his corneas had been taken — that the underlying cause of the memory loss, limb jerking and incoordination that had preceded his death was CJD. Due to the rarity of the disease, it was thought unlikely that the cause could be other than what was obvious: that the woman's symptoms appearing 18 months after her transplant from someone infected with CJD was no coincidence.

"Aside from the importance of this report to the transmission of Creutzfeldt-Jakob disease, there are wider implications to be considered in all transplantation programs with relation to the transmission of slow-virus diseases," the concluding paragraph warned.[1]

By 1990 it was known that CJD transmitted easily via injections of either scrapie or CJD-infected tissue into the eyeball of a mouse. In one experiment, mice were injected with what was called the Fujisaki strain of sporadic CJD. Each week some of the injected mice were decapitated and their brains analysed for signs of CJD. It was only in mice killed after 18 weeks that the first signs of holes in the brain were noticed, starting at the point where the optical fibres branch out from the retina. The spread of CJD was tracked along the visual pathways, all those fibres making railway tracks between the retina and the brain. It offered an explanation of why CJD was transmitted via that corneal transplant in 1974.[2]

But in the mid-1970s, the mere fact that CJD could be transmitted from human to human was something not even noticed in the worlds of gynaecology and endocrinology.

In April 1972, as "Linda" began to deteriorate from CJD, an Australian woman called Jan Blight consulted a gynaecologist in Perth about her lack of menstruation for the previous two years. She and her husband, Lyle, had been married for years. Both her younger sisters had babies and Jan, now 33 years old, desperately wanted one of her own.[3]

Like most Australians, Jan would have been aware that Geraldine Brodrick had conceived her nine babies on a fertility drug two years earlier. Details of the name of the drug were recounted on radio and television and in newspaper and magazine articles published world-wide. She may even have been told that she would have the opportunity to use the same drug, though hopefully any multiple pregnancy, an acknowledged side effect, would be less extreme than Mrs Brodrick's disaster.

She would have had the usual range of fertility tests, including X-rays of the pituitary gland and tests of urinary hormones after problems such as anorexia nervosa, obesity, diabetes, thyroid problems or a history of taking the Pill were ruled out as the major cause of non-ovulation.

Clomiphene citrate in tablet form, which stimulated the release of both FSH and LH in a process still largely unknown, was the initial treatment for women who failed to ovulate. Because of clear evidence that it did not work in all cases, during the late 1960s and 1970s combination treatment with both clomiphene and hCG (extracted from the urine of pregnant women) became standard practice before the last resort, hPG, was considered. All the infertility drugs of the time had side effects including enlargement of the ovaries and ovarian cysts, often after prolonged treatments at high dosage.[4]

Sometimes women were given initial stimulation tests to see if they responded to hPG. This not only saved unnecessary injections, but it used less of precious hPG stocks — there were never enough glands collected to meet demand. For these tests, hPG left over from other patients was used. Permission was not sought before test doses from the FSH subcommittee of HPAC, which oversaw the running of the AHPHP. Permission was sought only if the patient responded. This stimulation test, for some women, actually became the first cycle of treatment and was known as a short treatment cycle.[5]

In 1968 the FSH subcommittee decided that all unused stocks of hPG should be returned to the manufacturer, CSL. However, by 1973 the same subcommittee had agreed that overstocks from one patient could be used on another. Out-of-date stocks of hPG, those more than two years old, could also be used as an "experiment" in stimulation tests.[6]

CSL objected to this use of its hPG in an October 1972 letter to HPAC. Dr Peter Schiff, then the head of research at CSL, stated in the letter that doctors using the outdated hPG should be warned that such use was "experimental at this stage" and could not be recommended by the manufacturer "even though in this case we have no reason to believe that long-term storage has had any deleterious effect".[7]

Dr James Evans, a Melbourne gynaecologist and member of the FSH subcommittee, found that an early batch from CSL was still potent four years after it was made. HPAC had already agreed that with no evidence of harm from outdated stock, patients who had already been treated with a particular batch of hPG could be treated again with outdated stocks from the same batch.[8]

So it was that between May 15 and June 9, 1973, full of hope, Jan Blight attended the Royal Perth Hospital for a series of daily injections.[9] The painful jabs of hPG all came from batch 25 of the drug, which was cost free under Section 100 of the National Health Act.[10] Jan Blight was one of 38 women who received injections from batch 25. She had only one treatment cycle of hPG and it did not work.

In September 1974 Gajdusek's laboratory published precautions in conducting autopsies and biopsies on CJD patients. It was recommended that all instruments be steamed at high pressure in an autoclave for at least 30 minutes. All organs from a CJD patient, however they were stored, should be treated as infectious because a high level of the CJD agent had been found in human brains and livers, and therefore it was presumed to be present in other organs.[11]

The published precautions had been prompted by news, revealed at the tenth International Congress of Neurology in Barcelona in September 1973, that a 56-year-old Boston neurosurgeon had died of CJD in association with another rare and lethal condition, Köhlmeier-Degos disease. CJD-infected brain, with which he came into contact, was considered a possible source of transmission during his work.[12]

Gajdusek's autopsy and biopsy precautions were republished in August 1975, after it was realised that pathologists did not want to deal with CJD bodies at all for fear of contracting the disease in the course of their work. Gajdusek and colleagues outlined the procedures adopted in their NIH lab, where hundreds of animals had been deliberately injected with CJD, kuru and scrapie for more than a decade. These procedures included wearing surgical gowns, gloves and masks, and afterwards autoclaving at a temperature of at least 121 degrees Centigrade for between 45 minutes and an hour any instruments and clothing that had come into contact with the patient. Anything disposable was to be incinerated and all surfaces and the saw used to open the skull were to be washed and later flushed with commercial bleach and additives.[13]

In January 1975 a young Australian woman, Jane Allender, and her husband Ted were considering adopting a child from a developing country. After six years of marriage and a history of menstrual problems, Jane had looked forward to starting a family. But tests the previous year had revealed she did not ovulate and therefore would not be able to conceive.

By the end of January 1975 the Allender adoption application papers had been accepted. The snag was the three-year wait. Three days after that news, on February 2, 1975, Jane had an appointment to see Dr Colin Matthews, at the fertility clinic at Queen Elizabeth Hospital in Adelaide. Just like Jan Blight, her pituitary gland area was X-rayed, she had blood tests and other investigations to rule out obvious causes for her non-ovulation. Ted's sperm count was measured and ruled out as the problem. In April Matthews offered Jane the opportunity to try (what she wrote in her diary as) a "new treatment", something called FSH, which helped women who could not ovulate. She became a private patient of the gynaecologist who ran the clinic, Professor Lloyd Cox. On May 1, 1975 she began the tedium of collecting daily urine specimens, which were analysed for oestrogen levels (a measure of ovarian response to FSH).

After six courses of the drug, administered into the buttock from CSL batches 34, 36 and 44 between May 2 and September 8, 1975, Jane became pregnant.[14] Nine months later it was all worth the trouble. Lee Michael Allender was born on May 14, 1976.

Still unable to ovulate naturally, Clomid (clomiphene citrate) tablets were enough to induce ovulation again and Jane and Ted became parents to Kate on New Year's Day 1978. Jane had her family, and life seemed wonderful.

Among the other women treated at the Queen Elizabeth Hospital in 1975 was Vonda Cummings. She and her husband, Stephen, had married the previous year. After an early miscarriage, Vonda grew anxious as the months rolled past and she failed to conceive again quickly. She consulted Dr Harold Lane, a GP who referred her to the fertility clinic at the hospital. There she was told she was not ovulating, and went on to try clomiphene citrate and perhaps hCG before government-sponsored hPG was prescribed for her. (At the time it was estimated that patient management on hPG cost the Federal Government between A$500 and $1000 a month.)[15]

After two courses of the treatment between October 24 and November 17, 1975 — one of which followed tests to rule out sterility on Stephen's part — Vonda failed to conceive. She was one of more than 200 women who had not conceived of the 390 treated with hPG to the end of 1975. To that time, a total of 202 pregnancies had occurred in 179 hPG-treated women recorded on the AHPHP's computerised file.[16] Several women had miscarried multiple pregnancies but had returned for further treatment.

Stephen Cummings, unhappy about the contrived nature of the treatment and embarrassed at the mechanics involved, was inclined to believe that if conception was not going to occur naturally, they should accept being childless. Vonda agreed and they got on with life.[17]

In January 1977 Vonda suddenly became pregnant. In September she gave birth to Gareth, the first grandson on her side of the family. In 1979 Lauren, his sister, was born. In 1981 Stephen moved his family, as he had always wanted, to his birthplace, Albany, on the far south coast of Western Australia. There, Vonda continued her regular blood donations. It was in Albany that friends and family noticed how she began to change.

Alan Dickinson, the tall, gangling scrapie expert, lived in a large rambling two-storey house near Lasswade, a rural area just outside Edinburgh. He had a routine when he went to bed. He would sleep for a few hours then waken in the early morning, his five children asleep in their beds nearby. In those quiet, black hours he devised scrapie experiments.

All his work with the disease involved confidence, lateral thinking and very long-term planning. Nothing could be taken for granted: not the funding, the numbers of experimental animals that would be at his disposal, the space for those animals, nor the stringent aseptic conditions under which he and his team were careful to keep scrapie strains totally separate. The conditions they worked under, said Dickinson in hindsight, were "appalling". Even so, essential experiments were undertaken over the years and the results were added to the growing body of knowledge about TSEs like CJD, scrapie and kuru.

Around midnight on October 5, 1976, when Dickinson's mind had drifted "in a generalist sort of way" onto scrapie accumulation in sheep tissue, a terrible new thought struck him. It was so horrible — and so logical — that he sat bolt upright in bed, almost waking his sleeping wife Helen. Knowing about growth hormone treatment in children from a brief stint working in California in 1961, he suddenly thought of the possibility — almost probability — that hGH extracted from human pituitary glands might well have been contaminated by the slow, unconventional scrapie-like disease he knew was called Creutzfeldt-Jakob disease. The contamination would not necessarily come from people who had died of the disease. It was more likely, he thought, to have come from people incubating the disease — those in whom physical symptoms had not yet begun but who had died from another cause.

Dickinson thought the risk of CJD contamination was more than merely theoretical. He knew it was real and he found it hard getting back to sleep. "Pituitaries are close to the brain. I had done one or two experiments in mice which I hadn't published, which showed that the mouse pituitary was perhaps one tenth as infective as the brain, and still a problem." He explained years later, "The Medical Research Council (MRC) in London was preparing growth hormone from pituitaries and, with the restricted range of older bodies that the pituitaries were available from, it wouldn't be surprising if they were CJD-affected, but not necessarily infected, at that stage and were being included in batches. I just suddenly realised that modern techniques using filtering columns, which were widely used in biochemistry labs then, could well be concentrating the infective agent within them. The opportunities for infection were alarming."[18]

The next morning he rang a contact at the MRC and revealed his fears. He pointed out the reality of the weird TSE agents that caused scrapie and its human counterpart, CJD. The agent travelled easily through normal filtration and it was resistant to all but the most severe and protracted biochemical inactivation processes. Alcohol storage of tissue containing a scrapie-like agent would enclose the infectivity rather than inactivate it. Normal doses of sterilising ionising radiation were useless. The point was that the protocol — the precise production plan for the hormone — could be tested to see whether any CJD agent present in the starting solution could be removed.

After further contact, on October 14, 1976 Dickinson officially agreed to scrutinise the two preparation protocols used in Britain: that of both Dr Anne Stockell Hartree, who used acetone-stored glands at her University of Cambridge laboratory, and Dr Philip Lowry, who used a newer method with frozen glands. Lowry had recently become a second supplier of hGH for Britain's government-sponsored Human Growth Hormone Program (HGHP) from his laboratory based at St Bartholomew's Hospital in London. Soon Dickinson had spoken to both biochemists, but he did not visit their labs. He knew the weakest link in the chain was not the protocol; it was the competence in handling between steps in the protocol, and the ability to avoid cross-contamination. The protocol could be tested but the risk of cross-contamination between the different stages of the extraction could not.

Dickinson recalled the conversation with Hartree when she rang him in November 1976 to discuss the sending of her protocol to him: "I told her the first decision you've got to take is how to discuss this with your other colleagues because the handling of the pituitaries and the first preparative steps represent risks to those staff. She couldn't have been more level-headed, sensible and understanding. She was not alarmist and not remotely defensive. She was entirely balanced and commendable. And later we received her protocol for comment."[19]

On December 13, 1976, after working in his pre-kuru years with no less than three future Nobel laureates — Linus Pauling (who won two; for chemistry in 1954 and for peace in 1962), John Enders (1954 for medicine) and Sir Frank Macfarlane Burnet (1960 for medicine) — Dr Daniel Carleton Gajdusek became one himself.

On the seventy-fifth anniversary of the annual awards instituted by Swedish chemist and philanthropist Alfred Nobel, Gajdusek and fellow American virologist Baruch Blumberg were awarded their cash prize, gold medal and diploma by the king of Sweden. On stage in Stockholm with Gajdusek to accept the ultimate scientific accolade were eight of "his" children. They were some of what would swell to at least 56 children, mainly boys, whom he had "adopted" with the blessing of families in Papua New Guinea and the Pacific islands of Micronesia. The majority were educated in America, although some had their education in PNG paid for by Gajdusek. When he accepted his prize he said he would use the $80,000 prize to send his children to college.[20]

The children lived with him at his rambling house in Maryland, not far from his laboratory at the NIH in Bethesda, where it was not unusual for high brow academics, including Linus Pauling and the anthropologist Margaret Mead, to sit around the kitchen table talking. One day, as Gajdusek recounted to Australian Broadcasting Corporation science journalist and presenter Robin Williams, six Nobel laureates came to lunch. In such a large household they had all helped with the meal preparations and clearing up. When Gajdusek's nine-year-old "daughter" had been asked at school soon after to describe a Nobel Prize winner, she replied: " Nobel Prize winners are nice people who come to our house to sweep the yard and do the washing-up!"[21]

On February 22, 1977 Dickinson wrote to the MRC, having been sent the hGH protocols of both Hartree and Lowry. His tone was guarded. Making "many assumptions", he seemed to think there might be more of a problem with Lowry's frozen gland collection method than Hartree's acetone-stored method. He suggested that the MRC consider subjecting both protocols to high-strength solutions of scrapie-infected mouse brain. This would show whether or not hGH came out at the end of the processing with scrapie. Dickinson also suggested an assessment of the likelihood of a CJD gland being included among pituitary gland collections, given that it was known that even before symptoms appear, the infective agent accumulated in high titres or proportions in central nervous system tissue. "Third", he continued in his letter, " it will probably be prudent to exclude glands from cases with dementia".[22]

The following month at a meeting of the MRC's steering committee for human pituitary collection, Dickinson's letter was noted — as was the fact that there had been no evidence to date of slow virus infections via hGH, and that the matter should be "explored further".[23]

By the time of Dickinson's letter, Jane Allender was at home with her first child, Lee, and Vonda Cummings was surprised to find herself nearly two months pregnant with her son, Gareth. Almost simultaneously, a dire warning about the danger of transplanted tissue was being sounded in the rarefied world of neurology.

Many in the field, just as they did when American president John F. Kennedy was assassinated and Neil Armstrong set the first human foot on the moon, well remember where they were when they heard or read about a letter in the February 26, 1977 issue of the *Lancet*. In it, Swiss neurologists reported the second and third cases of the feared person-to-person transmission of CJD.

Two Swiss epilepsy patients — a 23-year-old woman with a long history of the condition and a 17-year-old boy — had a total of 16 silver depth electrodes implanted in their brains during electroencephalographic (EEG) investigations in, respectively, late November and early December 1974. Within two and a half years they were both dead of CJD. Two of the electrodes used on the woman and two used on the boy had been used previously in September 1974, on a 69-year-old woman who died soon after of CJD.[24]

What was so disturbing was the fact that the electrodes hadn't simply been transferred from the CJD patients to each of the epilepsy patients. They had been sterilised thoroughly in between each treatment. Or so it was thought.

The Swiss neurologists described how the silver electrodes of the time were heat sensitive and could not be autoclaved like metal instruments. Instead, as was common with heat sensitive instruments, the electrodes were cleaned with a solvent called benzine, disinfected with 70% ethanol and sterilised in formaldehyde vapour in pre-autoclaved metal boxes for at least two days. That sort of treatment was enough to kill almost any microbe loitering in an operating theatre. But not in this case.

This was the stuff of horror movies. It led to immediate reconsideration by some neurosurgeons about whether to ever again operate on anyone suspected of having CJD. At the time, it was fairly routine to attempt diagnosis of a CJD case — before death — by performing a brain biopsy to see if the tell-tale spongy holes showed up in a sliver of brain. The trouble was that it was chancy. The person may well have CJD but the spongiosis could be in an area away from the site of the biopsy.

On September 2, 1977 Gajdusek's Nobel Prize-winning lecture was published in *Science* and received wide attention. It raised concerns about CJD and suggested some additional transmission routes apart from the known oral and/or mucosal route of kuru transmission, including:

… kitchen and butchery accidents involving the contamination of skin and eyes … CJD from corneal transplant suggests that other tissue transplantation may also be a source of infection. It is known that the virus is present in peripheral tissue, as well as in the brain.[25]

In November 1977, as part of its further exploration of Dickinson's CJD concerns with pituitary glands, the MRC wrote to two British experts on viruses, both of whom were also members of the Agricultural Research Council's Working Party on Scrapie. They were asked their views on whether the Hartree and Lowry gland processing protocols would eliminate any slow virus such as scrapie or CJD. Both referees thought a study along the lines of that proposed by Dickinson was essential. In the meantime they thought it was suitable for hGH therapy to continue.

Professor Cedric Mims, who headed the department of microbiology at Guy's Hospital Medical School in London, replied immediately on November 29, 1977. Professor Mims stipulated:

Although the risk is theoretically so low, are there likely to be very occasionally, perhaps exceedingly rarely, pituitaries from people with transmissible dementia agents such as the Creutzfeldt-Jakob agent in their central nervous system (CNS)? Yes. So there should be complete exclusion of subjects with chronic CNS disease or dementias.[26]

Professor Mims concluded that with the recent discovery that the gene for growth hormone could be manufactured synthetically in bacteria, pituitary-derived extracts would become defunct.

"These are my thoughts about the Creutzfeldt-Jakob problem and hGH. I do think we have to exercise great discretion in talking about such matters."[27]

The head of pathology at the University of Cambridge, Professor Peter Wildy replied on December 1, 1977.

In the meantime I am sure that the work on GH has to go forward and any clinical use of this hormone must be regarded as a risk, albeit incalculable. We are in the uncomfortable position of suspecting the worst but not knowing how bad the worst is.[28]

The next meeting of the MRC's steering committee for human pituitary collection noted both replies. After lengthy discussion it was agreed that the Health Services' hGH committee, chaired by Professor David Milner, a paediatric endocrinologist at Sheffield, should be told about the "possible risks by slow virus or scrapie infection of pituitary glands so [the committee] could decide whether to notify the clinicians involved in therapy or whether such action would be premature and cause undue alarm".[29]

Dr Milner, a de facto member of the MRC steering committee for human pituitary collection, who had received all the minutes of meetings he could not attend, recalled years later that the Health Services' hGH committee was told of the interest in the risk of possible pituitary gland contamination at its first meeting on July 12, 1977. "The risk appeared to us to be so remote that we took no further action at that time."[30]

The Swiss paper that revealed the deaths of the two epilepsy patients from contaminated electrodes caused such a scare that in December 1977 Gajdusek felt compelled to publish a set of guidelines for use by people dealing with CJD patients and their bodies after they died.[31]

In Britain there was sufficient knowledge of the potential hazards of CJD that its 1972 publication, *Safety in the post-mortem room,* was updated six years later. CJD was included in a list of infectious diseases around which to be extremely careful. The Department of Health and Social Security published its *Code of practice for the prevention of infection in clinical laboratories and post-mortem rooms* in 1978. It warned that sensible precautions should be taken to avoid accidental inoculation of brain or spinal cord from CJD patients that was being "subjected to homogenisation or disruption for biochemical and other research purposes", and classified them B1. This category also included such infectious micro-organisms as salmonella, the plague bacillus, the organism that caused the often lethal Legionnaires' disease and the killer yellow fever, "which offer special hazards to laboratory workers and for which special accommodation and conditions for containment must be provided".[32]

Person-to-person transmission of CJD was now known in the worlds of ophthalmology, neurology and pathology. But the lessons learned by some from those unfortunate patients in America and Switzerland still went unheeded in general and other specialised medical fields, including endocrinology and gynaecology.

On March 21, 1978, the MRC wrote to Dickinson officially asking him to conduct infectivity experiments on mice to test both the Hartree and Lowry protocols because neither lab was suitable. In fact both labs were found not to be suitable for making any biological products for humans at all.[33] And in the following month, five months after Gajdusek's precautions for handling CJD-infected material were published in the *New England Journal of Medicine,* the MRC sought advice from Gajdusek. It wanted advice on "the question of possible infection of pituitary glands by slow viruses and scrapie-like agents, and whether steps should be taken to ensure that the glands collected are free of such agent".[34]

Gajdusek was overseas. In his stead Colin Masters, the Australian pathologist soon to travel to Heidelberg to start on his review of Alfons Jakob's original patients, replied:

> It would be reasonable to expect that the pituitary gland and/or surrounding tissue taken from a case of Creutzfeldt-Jakob disease would be contaminated with the virus. Therefore, it would seem advisable that tissue obtained from any patient with CJD (or any other dementing illness) not be used in preparations for human use.[35]

In May 1978 Dickinson replied to the MRC, quoting an initial fee of £500 for the purchase of disposable equipment for work to be carried out on 350 mice. Starting with a mixture of 80% brain from scrapie-infected mice and 20% human pituitary, Dickinson was to test both protocols — starting with Lowry's. For each protocol, the mixture would be run through and the purity of the end product tested by inoculating the mice. The aim of the infectivity experiment was to show that the Lowry protocol could produce safe hGH; any of the infectivity added to it was to be removed. It was not aimed at inactivating infectivity. What could not be answered in this pilot test was the point at which the filtering columns in the much longer production runs, reused in making the hGH, would become saturated with any TSE agent present in the batch. But it wasn't until early 1980 that Dickinson had room in his Neuropathogenesis Unit laboratories to run his experiments, and it wasn't until several years after that his results were confirmed.

Meanwhile in 1979, Professor Wildy had upgraded his earlier advice on exclusion criteria for glands. He told the MRC that all patients with dementia should be regarded as having CJD and that they should not donate tissues, blood or organs. In the meantime, hGH production continued using both the Hartree acetone-storage method and the Lowry frozen-gland method. More British children were assessed by endocrinologists and started on long courses of hGH injections. The only exclusion criteria in existence at that time dated from the start of the program nearly 21 years earlier. A circular had been sent to morgues recommending the rejection of glands that were "the site of primary disease".[36]

Advice on potential virus contamination of hGH was sought several times by the MRC. In 1959, when the program began, virologist Professor Wilson Smith advised that a virus would not be expected to survive the acetone-storage method of processing that applied then. It was sought again in 1973, five years after Hartree had switched to the more refined Hartree–Wilhelmi method of hGH extraction from the original and very harsh Raben technique.[37]

Dr David Tyrrell, then head of the Clinical Research Centre in Middlesex, replied that acetone "will not inactivate all viruses but it will inactivate a lot of them. I think that freezing would tend to preserve viruses, though the ones which would survive would be the same ones which would resist acetone treatment".[38]

CJD was not considered specifically until Dickinson's phone call in October 1976 and his follow-up letter in February 1977. And even then, despite repeated warnings to exclude glands from demented patients, the advice was ignored for three years — with potentially lethal consequences. The inaction — apparently prompted by fears that the numbers of glands collected would drop and affect the always scarce supply of hGH, together with the lack of any previous known contamination by CJD in the then 18-year history of the program — would later attract global condemnation.

No-one involved with hGH production knew at the time that the insidious CJD had indeed penetrated batch processing. One young man who began and finished his hGH injections between 1977 and 1980 was already doomed. His name was Patrick Baldwin.

CHAPTER 7

What's in a name?

WHEN EMLYN HITCHINGS took over the manufacture of hGH in South Africa in 1979 his only safety precaution, apart from common sense in handling human tissue, was to wear a surgical mask. The mask did not protect his eyes, one of the presumed entry sites for CJD infection, from inadvertent splashes. The pituitary glands collected from eight large morgues around South Africa, bottled in lots of 50 and stored in acetone, were handled with bare hands.

Hitchings now regards those times — indeed the first half of the next decade as well — as "the dark ages" in terms of knowledge about infections that lurked in tissue from human cadavers. Today he wouldn't handle any of it, even with modern laboratory safety containment procedures such as fume cupboards, laminar flow cabinets, UV light hoods that sterilise conventional micro-organisms in the chamber beneath, and perhaps most sensibly, gloves. Now, at least seven different types of hepatitis and the deadly HIV are to be feared when handling human tissues. Still, for a man who was saturated with liquid live rabies virus in a laboratory accident in the early 1970s, the risk of possible contamination of pituitary glands with a slow virus — had he known about it — would have seemed small.

Collecting glands, each little bigger than a pea, in a long, thin plastic container half-filled with acetone, Hitchings spent about 80 per cent of his time from late 1979 to early 1985 manufacturing hGH. His labour reduced the amount of commercial hGH bought by the South African Government, a large saving for a cash-strapped nation crippled by anti-apartheid economic sanctions.

Overseeing the hGH production was the tall, urbane microbiologist, Dr Wolf Katz. Since 1969 he had been running the State Vaccine Institute, housed then in a group of dated government buildings sitting drably behind a steel fence on the main route through suburban Pinelands, Capetown. Katz was also busy directing the production of a

rabies vaccine, the trialling of a tuberculosis vaccine and the manufacture of foetal calf serum, a nutrient medium added to tissue culture for
growing cells. Making vaccines, Katz says today, keeps him humble
because no-one knows what a virus in a vaccine will do the minute you
think it's under control.

The man who was to put the hGH of Hitchings and Katz to work was
Professor François Bonnici. In 1969, as a 30-year-old newly trained
paediatric endocrinologist from Cape Town, he went to Paris to work at
the Hospital for Sick Children. While studying and working there, he
and other doctors began treating growth-retarded children with hGH
made in Switzerland. On his return to Cape Town in 1970 Bonnici
established paediatric endocrinology units at the University of Cape
Town's two teaching hospitals — Groote Schour Hospital, where Dr
Christiaan Barnard had performed the world's first heart transplant in
1968, and the Red Cross Children's Hospital. At both units he treated
growth-retarded children with hGH imported from KabiVitrum in
Sweden.

By 1971 Bonnici had persuaded the South African Minister for
Health of the need for hGH to be sponsored. He became the chairman
of the National Human Growth Hormone Program (NHGHP) that
would, for the next quarter of a century, treat more than 500 black,
white and coloured children with hypopituitarism. The government
provided funds for the importation of hGH from both KabiVitrum and
later Serono, through provincial hospitals. Later, due to growing
demand on the program, the expense, the availability of local pituitaries, and the ever-present threat of anti-apartheid boycotts, which
hovered over most South African imports, it was decided to make the
drug locally as well.

From the early 1970s a biochemist, named Dr S. W. Stroud, became
involved in the NHGHP. In Pretoria he devised his own method of hGH
extraction, one of about a dozen then used around the world.[1] Initially,
glands were donated with the permission of relatives. The first treatment use of the locally produced drug, based on Stroud's extraction
method, was in December 1974.

In 1976, a year after an organised pituitary gland collection was
begun in South Africa, routine production of local hGH was transferred
to the Health Department's National Health Laboratory Service under

the directorship of Professor Lionel Smith. Smith, who until his retirement in 1984 was responsible for all South African pathologists working in state hospitals and laboratories, asked Katz at the State Vaccine Institute to make a regular supply of hGH. Although commercial hGH was used in South Africa from about 1971, "there wasn't enough," Katz explained. "And we weren't on top of Kabi's list of people to get it. So the kids used to get it intermittently, which wasn't good. So they'd stop and grow and stop and grow. It was an interrupted supply."[2]

Kabi in Sweden prepared hGH sold in South Africa from glands collected outside South Africa. It was against export regulations to send glands collected within South Africa to Sweden. Other countries, however, such as Hong Kong, regularly supplied Kabi with glands for drug production to meet the needs of their local patients. Smith recalls that a prime motivation for the production of local hGH was the "vast number of potential donors coming to the police mortuaries from our high violence rate". The brain was always removed for post-mortem examinations. Removing pituitary glands was little extra effort.[3] And there was the added incentive of cost-saving.

In 1979 local hGH cost just five Rand per injection and was fully funded by the South African Government. That year 26 mainly black and coloured children were treated with hGH, according to institute records.[4] Then in 1980 and 1981 the number of children being treated with local hGH increased to 33 and 40 respectively. In both 1982 and 1983, 49 children received the institute's hGH; 1984 saw a decline in patient numbers. Children were often prescribed hGH for a number of years, which is reflected in these figures. And the injections were given mostly to young children, to take advantage of the vital growing years before bone fusion stopped further growth in the late teens.

Hitchings began processing batches of about 1000 pituitaries — double what Stroud had used in his 1973 recipe. The laborious extraction took days. Katz was always amazed that anything at all survived the rough manufacturing treatment, particularly any active growth hormone. Stone-hard prune-like pituitary glands were the raw material. Glands from the big police morgue at Salt River, a southern suburb not far from central Cape Town and its spectacular towering backdrop Table Mountain, were stored in a mini-freezer supplied by the institute. The container sat alone in the freezer at −20 degrees Celsius for what was thought would be total inactivation of any viruses in the pituitaries.

When the container was full, an institute driver was sent the short distance to collect it.

The most hazardous aspect of the extraction process for laboratory personnel was the grinding of the glands in caustic soda, because of the potentially infectious spray. The alkaline caustic soda dissolved the cells in each gland as they were whizzed around in a large blender. This allowed the various hormones and other substances trapped in the cells to be released. The blended liquid that resulted was centrifuged several times and poured on to a molecular sieve in the shape of a plastic column. It was designed to separate small, intermediate and large molecular weight substances such as bacteria and viruses from the relatively lightweight hGH. Gel chromatography, as it was called, often took up to 20 hours to complete because the liquid depended on gravity to wend its way through the column, which was tightly packed with small beads made of Sephadex gel.

Once this purification step was completed, the hGH was freeze-dried, redissolved to ensure its purity, filtered a last time to rid it of any remaining bacteria, then freeze-dried in single dose vials and sealed. "We were reasonably confident that the hepatitis virus would have been knocked out with the treatment of the acetone and the caustic soda," Katz recalls. "And then of course the gel exclusion at the end. The product we were making had a molecular weight of about 25,000 Daltons and hepatitis is many millions of daltons so it would come right out at the beginning of the column." Even when HIV was recognised "we were reasonably confident that anything that had gone through this sort of treatment would have been inactivated", says Katz. "You didn't think of all the things that could happen in those days like you do now," he says reflectively. "We are more aware now. Now everything is suspect, absolutely everything."[5]

The hGH from each batch was tested afterwards for purity and adverse reactions on rats and mice. As a result total production time was often up to four months. Hypophysectomised rats (rats with their pituitary glands deliberately cut out) were injected with the finished hGH. If they put on weight — a sign of growth — then the hormone was considered active. Mice were also injected with a sample of each batch. They were watched for a time for bad reactions like paralysis or death. The mice never died and the rats put on weight. Best of all, once the children received injections of this drug, they grew.

About 4000 pituitary glands per year were collected during

Hitchings' six years of manufacture. They were taken only from people who had been murdered or killed in the plentiful road accidents that occurred each year in South Africa ("the Easter road toll was always good", according to Katz). Only healthy pituitary glands were wanted, from people who had been known to be free of disease but had died prematurely due to accident or violence. And even those glands had to be fresh, removed from the brain within 24 hours of death, for the best hormone yield. No exclusion criteria existed because the glands were assumed to be from young people who were not harbouring transmissible diseases such as hepatitis, which is endemic in Africa.

Mortuaries kept records of the bodies from which glands were taken. No cash incentives were offered, like they were in countries such as Australia, Britain and the United States. So collection rates for glands were initially slow in 1975, but this improved after the passage of the Human Tissue Act of 1980, which dealt with donations of the body. Objections to removing tissue from bodies were most likely to come from particular religious or cultural groups.[6]

Sometimes Bonnici brought the children under treatment to the State Vaccine Institute to show Katz and Hitchings the end result of their hGH production. Both men enjoyed seeing the practical effect of their laboratory work. At its height in the mid-1980s, South Africa's NHGHP was treating up to 175 children at a time;[7] others received a top-up from imported commercial varieties of hGH.[8] The scientists noted that a few children had a quick growth spurt for several years before developing antibodies, particularly those children being treated with locally made hGH. They had to concede that the imported hGH was purer.

Because of the ever-present worry about potential boycotts on hGH, Bonnici made sure most of the imported and far more expensive hormone was given to black children. His rationale was that he would have a potent bargaining chip in the event of a boycott.

Early in 1980, as Emlyn Hitchings began devoting more and more of his time to hGH production, thousands of kilometres to the north, in London, Dr Alan Dickinson was invited to lunch. His host was Professor David Milner, the newly-appointed chairman of Britain's National Health Services' hGH committee. Milner wanted to hear first-hand about agents like CJD and scrapie, while Dickinson was anxious to know whether doctors and scientists responsible for hGH in other countries had been informed of the risk of CJD contamination, which he had raised three years earlier. The chill of the weather outside was not evident in the warm, brown-panelled Victorian dining room of the Royal Medical Society. Dickinson nodded to a colleague at a table across the room and more than once pursued the subject of extending his warning on the potential of CJD to infect pituitary glands.

"Do you know all the people involved internationally in this whole growth hormone area?" Dickinson asked at the start of their 45-minute lunch.

"Oh yes," Milner replied.

"You know the leading figures?" Dickinson stressed.

"Yes."

"Well, as a consequence of my having raised it, it may have been done already, that people have been very quietly told about the ethical issue of how to confidentially inform the international medical community."

Milner looked blankly at him.

"Just in case it hasn't happened," Dickinson said, "I think you ought to think about this issue and if necessary make sure that you have a quiet word, if this is the way to do it, with people using hGH." At one point Dickinson's question was made more specific — whether those in the United States had been alerted. He knew definitely that hGH was being used there. By the end of lunch, Dickinson felt reassured that Milner would check what action had been taken about alerting others.

Dickinson, who admits years later to tip-toeing around the subject as any discreet government civil servant would have, raised the issue to check whether those responsible in Britain had passed on his warning. He felt he could not alert others himself — he didn't even know who to call — as it was a delicate matter and still only a theoretical risk. However, it was a risk that could cause much damage if the media found out. He knew he had placed himself in an increasingly lonely position. Dickinson, a geneticist and microbiologist but not a medical doctor, had warned the MRC by telephone in 1976 and again in writing in February 1977. As far as he was concerned, he had tacitly handed over the ethical responsibility for further action.[9]

Meanwhile, the numbers of patients on both hGH and hPG regimens was increasing. What had begun as trial therapy in some countries had been formalised by the early 1980s, as it had been in Britain, to routine therapy. The discreet warning that Dickinson requested of Milner was never made. The scrapie infectivity tests remained virtually secret, certainly to the doctors prescribing human hormone drugs around the world and to the patients receiving them. But by 1980, when Dickinson's tests on mice with scrapie-spiked hGH were well under way, the word was beginning to leak out.

In February, 1980 Australia's second largest city, Melbourne, hosted the sixth International Congress of Endocrinology. Among those who attended were Dr Leslie Lazarus, the head of Australia's HPAC, and Dr Derek Bangham, head of Britain's National Institute of Biological Standards.

Soon after his February meeting and informal discussion with Bangham, Lazarus wrote to Dr Ken Ferguson, the CSIRO scientist after whom the pituitary extraction method used in Australia at the time was named. Ferguson also headed HPAC's Fractionation subcommittee, which oversaw the national collection and processing of pituitary glands. In his letter, Lazarus asked for an opinion on the possibility of slow virus infections contaminating Australian pituitaries. This was done after relating the news Bangham had given him in Melbourne: British scientists running the latest version of the hGH program at the Centre for Applied Microbiological Research (CAMR) at Porton Down had installed new handling and extraction procedures to protect both staff and product from slow virus infections.

The issue of unconventional or slow viruses, as CJD was then classified, had been raised in 1971 at an HPAC meeting by that body's only pathologist member, Dr Vince McGovern. He had achieved much in encouraging pathologists to collect pituitaries nationally but due to a ministerial restructure of HPAC in 1976, he was not re-appointed to the committee. McGovern had not been prompted specifically by concern about CJD, but rather by the view of some researchers at that time — following the early transmission of kuru and CJD to chimpanzees — that slow viruses might also cause conditions like multiple sclerosis.

After McGovern raised slow viruses, two further opinions were requested from members of the special virology committee of the College of Pathologists. This resulted in the first amendment of the 1966 exclusion criteria for glands in Australia. In 1971 the amendment widened the criteria from "known virus infections, particularly virus hepatitis" to include "neurological disease of the central nervous system".[10]

Nine years later, when the matter resurfaced in 1980, Lazarus apparently forgot McGovern's initial concern, raising Bangham's news as "a new topic for us to consider". Lazarus had headed the AHPHP since its inception in 1967.[11]

In May 1980, three months after Lazarus spoke with Bangham, the Fractionation subcommittee, which Ferguson headed, discussed the possibility of slow virus contamination of FSH and hGH. Members came to a momentous conclusion. "The subcommittee felt as, at present, a slow virus is not positively linked with a disease present in the community and, moreover, as the technology did not now exist to detect a slow virus, acknowledgment of the potential dangers is all that is possible."[12] Recognising that knowledge and expertise in this area of virology would increase, it recommended instead that samples of each batch of FSH and hGH be kept indefinitely by CSL, which manufactured the drug in Australia.

Clearly, the subcommittee was unaware that CJD was reported in Australia in 1965 at the proceedings of the Australian Association of Neurology.[13] At the time of the May 1980 meeting, members of the committee — fractionation process experts, biochemists and CSL representatives, none of whom were experts in the area of slow viruses, pathology or virology — believed that the only slow virus in humans was kuru. Kuru, certainly, was not in the Australian population, limited as it is to the Fore area of the Eastern Highlands in Papua New Guinea.[14]

After his letter to Ferguson, Lazarus had also mailed to Ferguson an editorial from the *New England Journal of Medicine* of 1979 that contained information about slow viruses, including CJD. It is not known whether the article was among the agenda papers of that Fractionation subcommittee meeting of May 19. If it was not, then it was "incredible", a later inquiry found, that neither Lazarus nor Ferguson told the meeting that CJD was a fatal human disease with a lengthy incubation period before symptoms appeared.[15]

The subcommittee did not seek expert advice from a virologist or neuropathologist, once the matter was raised. Nor did it assess the risk of possible slow virus contamination of glands, because it was regarded as merely theoretical. The subcommittee also did not appear to realise, although Lazarus and other HPAC members were aware at this time of Dickinson's continuing work, that the Ferguson method of human hormone extraction could be tested for potential contamination with the closely related scrapie agent.[16]

Obviously no-one on the committee was aware that, in Gajdusek's 1977 Nobel Prize-winning paper, Australia had been included among the countries specifically noted in the worldwide prevalence of CJD. Gajdusek wrote:

> For many large population centers of the United States, Europe, Australia and Asia, we have found a prevalence approaching one per million, with an annual incidence and a mortality of about the same magnitude, as the average duration of the disease is eight to 12 months ...
>
> The unexpectedly high incidence of previous craniotomy in CJD patients noted first by Nevin et al ... raises the possibility of brain surgery either affording a mode of entry for the agent or of precipitating the disease in patients already carrying a latent infection.[17]

If committee members had searched scientific literature for new information they would have found the paper titled "Creutzfeldt-Jakob Disease: patterns of worldwide occurrence and the significance of familial and sporadic clustering". This included Australia on a world map of CJD incidence. The first author of this paper, published in early 1979, was Australian pathologist, Colin Masters. Masters was, at that time, working at Gajdusek's lab at the NIH, where CJD from the brains of two Australians had already been transmitted to primates.[18]

On May 30, 1980 HPAC adopted the recommendations of its Fractionation subcommittee. Both Lazarus and Ferguson were present. The *New England Journal of Medicine* editorial was referred to in the minutes. Therefore, it is assumed, it was read.[19] HPAC now agreed with the Fractionation subcommittee that the risk of CJD in pituitary glands collected in Australia was remote, despite what was contained in the *New England Journal of Medicine*.

In France, where glands processed to treat what would total more than 1700 children were routinely collected from Bulgaria, Hungary and French hospitals in which elderly and demented patients were treated, an ominous and specific warning about CJD and pituitary glands was issued in 1980. This was four years after Dickinson first alerted the British MRC and shortly before the Australians dismissed the risk as irrelevant. Asked for his advice, Professor Luc Montagnier, the French scientist credited with first identifying the AIDS virus, delivered a written warning to colleagues at the Pasteur Institute, the body which manufactured hGH for use on French children:

> The purification technique that was shown to me does not include any step which could inactivate a virus, even of average resistance ... Even if the different cases of cells on the pituitary gland are not infected, extraction can be contaminated by a virus on neighbouring nerves.

Montagnier stressed,

> Particular attention should be given to the dangers of transmission of Creutzfeldt-Jakob disease, a rare disease (one case in at least a million), but for which the patients carrying the infectious agent could be much more numerous. The infectious agent, similar, if not identical, to those of kuru and scrapie in sheep, is extremely resistant to heat, to denaturing agents, to ionising and non-ionising radiation ...[20]

Montagnier's note also referred the reader to Gajdusek's Nobel Prize-winning paper published in *Science* in 1977. By 1980 three reports had been published by Dr Paul Brown, the Gajdusek laboratory's resident neuroscientist, and colleagues, which centred specifically on the epidemiology and multiple case analysis of CJD in France.[21,22,23]

Montagnier's warning followed the horrifying death from rabies of a French recipient of a corneal graft — an example of the pitfalls of unorganised tissue collection. In 1979, the donor, an Egyptian, had died in a coma, the origin of which had not been identified before the corneas were removed. This case had echoes of the original person-to-person transmission of CJD through the American corneal donor reported in 1973.

A letter from Professor Raphael Rappaport, a doctor involved in the French hGH program, was circulated to doctors involved in hGH extraction in Britain, America, the Netherlands and Canada. Dated January 28, 1980, it stated that:

> There is now a big turmoil and much fear about pituitary removal from autopsies ... and the use of extracted growth hormone. Fortunately this debate has not involved the mass media but we feel it is necessary to investigate the risk of viral infections and even cancer transmission through the extracted growth hormone preparations ...[24]

Montagnier's warning was discussed by the main committee of Association France-Hypophyse (the non-profit organisation responsible for the collection of glands and distribution of hGH) and directives to improve exclusion criteria were issued. Despite this, those actually removing the glands (junior morgue attendants who were paid up to FF50 per gland) continued collecting as many as possible without the knowledge of hospital authorities.

Two years after the Australian HPAC had failed to realise the risk of CJD contamination of collected pituitary glands from its own population, a vastly different scenario emerged. In June 1982 probable disaster was averted when a group of 500 pituitary glands was promptly destroyed after an autopsy report revealed that one of the glands, taken from Sydney's main morgue at Glebe, might have been from a CJD sufferer.

At the time, a pathologist working for the NSW Health Commission was inspecting brain sections autopsied at the Glebe morgue, part of the NSW Institute of Forensic Medicine. The patient from whom a gland had been removed had died at Macquarie Hospital, one of the large exclusively psychiatric hospitals in Sydney at the time. The pathologist told this author he knew vaguely that pituitary glands were routinely taken at autopsy for a national program to extract hormones for human use. He rang the director of the Institute of Forensic Medicine, guessing there might be a problem, and told him to discard the pituitary. The director of the institute told the pathologist that the pituitaries were pooled in batches. "Well the whole batch will have to go," the director was told bluntly.[25] Later, when the director asked what should be done to prevent future near-accidents, the possible exclusion criteria that could be applied were discussed, including known cases of CJD, an age limit to avoid very elderly people, and anyone who died in a psychiatric hospital. Glands were also to be kept in individual containers.

The prompt telephone call by the pathologist had a dramatic effect. CSL was told immediately about the suspected CJD gland, by that time part of a pool of 500. The whole pool was destroyed and Lazarus telephoned the Department of Health in Canberra to inform it of the destruction on June 9, 1982.[26] As CSL used 1350 glands per batch, pooled immediately before processing, the autopsy report from the pathologist must have been received soon after the glands were sent to

CSL. Had it been much later, destruction of nearly triple the amount of glands would have resulted, thus adversely affecting already scarce human hormone supplies.

Lazarus sought informal advice from pathologists after the gland destruction incident but found that few of them knew much about CJD.[27] In December 1982 the exclusion criteria for gland collection was redrafted. For the first time glands from people who had suffered from "presenile dementia (Creutzfeldt-Jakob disease)" were excluded, which appeared to indicate that CJD was the only type of dementia to be excluded.

In February 1983, the *Communicable Diseases Intelligence* bulletin of the Department of Health in Canberra included an item on CJD that linked it with scrapie and kuru, and warned of potential transmission to workers. It stated specifically: "Organs and tissues of CJD patients should not be used for transplantations". It also included a footnote about a similar exclusion in Britain of CJD patients being used as tissue donors "for the preparation of ... growth hormone".[28]

"Instructions for Collection, August 1983", which was approved and sent out by HPAC, became the guide for mortuary attendants and pathologists. A final revision, this time including reference for the first time to HIV, occurred in mid-1985. By then, though, it was far too late.

In the early 1980s scientists were no nearer to finding the molecular make-up of the agent that causes TSEs than when Hadlow pointed out the similarity between kuru and scrapie two decades earlier in 1959. They did, however, know a lot more about what TSEs were not. TSEs were not like any other disease. They caused no immune response such as inflammation, swelling, dead cells, elevated protein in cerebrospinal fluid or obvious sickness. These diseases silently multiplied outside the brain for years and eventually entered the brain where they began caus-ing the symptoms that inevitably killed.

All bacteria, viruses and unpleasant microbes that cause disease in humans or animals contain genetic coding in the form of nucleic acids. Different types of sterilising agents will inactivate microbes, allowing the invaded victim to recover or at least improve their health. With TSEs there is never any improvement and no-one ever recovers.

Since publication of the Swiss electrodes transmission of CJD to the two epileptic patients in 1977, TSEs were known to be resistant to normal surgical sterilisation. Gajdusek's laboratory colleagues found that the brain of the man who had donated his corneas in the case reported in 1974 remained infective. This was despite the brain sitting for seven months at room temperature in a preserving and usually virus-deactivating solution of formalin-saline.[29] Later, TSEs were also found to be resistant to the normal duration of pressurised steaming in an autoclave and to temperatures and doses of ultraviolet and ionising radiation that would usually guarantee the destruction of any other microbe. TSEs are "moderately sensitive" to chemicals that disrupt the membranes of cells. Some of these chemicals include strong stuff like phenol, chloroform, ether, urea, periodate, potassium permanganate, alcoholic iodine, acetone, chloroform-butanol and hypochlorite.[30]

These remarkable qualities — first discovered in scrapie and later recognised in kuru and CJD — led to the question posed in *Nature* in 1967 by the British-based radiobiologist, Tikvah Alper: did these agents lack DNA or RNA?[31] No conventional virus could be isolated or recognised under even the newest electron microscope. Whatever the TSE agent was, it had a molecular weight of between 70,000 to 100,000 Daltons. The tiniest known plant virus is about this size.

By the early 1980s one school of thought held that TSEs were caused by a virus that was really a replicating sub-unit, an entity that might contain its genetic information in a small nucleic acid that had become attached to a cell membrane. The cell membrane somehow camouflaged the virus so that the immune system of the TSE-affected human or animal did not attack. In addition to strange properties, TSEs shared some features with conventional viruses. According to Gajdusek's interpretation, they replicated first in the spleen and later in the brain and they adapted to new hosts like chimpanzees, monkeys, mice, hamsters, even domestic cats, with a shortened incubation period. Like other viruses they could be diluted again and again to the point where they no longer caused disease when injected into laboratory animals.[32] TSEs *could* be destroyed, but it took a lot of effort.

The first breakthrough with modern technology in this field occurred in New York. In 1978 a Scottish biochemist, Robert Somerville, was working at what is now known as the Institute for Basic Research and Developmental Disabilities on Staten Island. He had prepared partially purified preparations of blended brains from scrapie-infected mice and had given them to a chemistry graduate called Pat Merz. Merz looked at the preparations under an electron microscope and, like those who had looked before her, found no virus. But she did find something new and very, very small. She found tiny threads, or fibrils, in the mice brains. There were no such fibrils in healthy mice. Two years later, Merz again found the fibrils in other diseased animals but not in healthy animals of the same species. Her discovery of scrapie-associated fibrils or SAFs, as they became known, was published in 1981. Later it was proposed that SAFs may be the elusive scrapie agent. However, the suggestion was among many theories that have been proposed and rejected over the decades.

Two other major theories that remain today were proposed around the same time as SAFs. The first was by Alan Dickinson, the geneticist and founding director of the Neuropathogenesis Unit in Edinburgh, who discovered the sinc gene in mice that controls scrapie incubation. The second, immediately branded as biological heresy, was put forward by California neurologist and biochemist Stanley Prusiner.

Dickinson, having found many strains of scrapie, had been coming to the conclusion that there had to be more than one type of molecule in these robust scrapie agents. The essential molecule would provide the information for strain properties (a very small nucleic acid, or something similar) and another type of molecule hijacked from the host would provide protection (likely to be one or more proteins). Dickinson called the agent a virino. When he first mentioned this name in a lecture he did not define it precisely — much to his regret in hindsight. Instead he set it in a whimsical context by comparing it with the neutrino, one of the most elusive, basic, uncharged particles of matter.[33] Neutrinos need special laboratory techniques to be detected. Dickinson also amplified the idea, discussing different degrees of protection offered by host proteins, at a scientific meeting in Paris in 1981, although the proceedings were not published until 1983.[34]

Years later Dickinson recalled that researchers expected to find a host protein around the infectious agent, whatever it was, which would explain why the infected animal produced no inflammatory response. "A virino," Dickinson maintains today, "is a hypothetical host/agent hybrid structure with PrP robustly protecting a still-unidentified replicable molecule which specifies agent strain properties and which might be a nucleic acid".[35]

In other words, a virino is a small piece of information-carrying material wrapped in protein manufactured by the host, not the invader. This protein is so strong that it resists being degraded by the most aggressive protein-digesting enzyme, protease K. In its smallest common denominator, a virino is, as Dickinson loves to say "very bad news securely wrapped in someone else's protein".

In 1982, just as Argentina invaded the British-colonised Falkland Islands and sparked a short territorial war, bold young American Stanley Prusiner burst onto the select TSE scene. He published a new theory and, with it, a new name for these infectious, lethal entities. What he proposed extended from Tikvah Alper's 1967 postulation that the extreme resistance of scrapie-infected material to radiation might be due to a lack of genetic material.

Prusiner, having concluded that the central nervous system was the "last great frontier of medicine" by the time one of his neurology patients died of CJD,[36] realised that no-one had any clear idea of the exact molecular structure of the CJD agent. After endless nights of reading, particularly about scrapie, he decided that he would discover the make-up of the agent by applying his chemist's training to the purification process.

By 1981 Prusiner claimed to have achieved 100-fold purification of the scrapie agent. In simple terms he'd produced a sample that contained all the infectivity of a diseased brain but with 99 per cent of the extra material gone. To that he added enzymes which would digest, or gradually destroy, almost all types of protein. He found that what was left in the test tube remained infective. And when he threw in enzymes that usually inactivate unprotected nucleic acids, the experimental hamsters he had been using continued to die of scrapie. The agent had not been killed. He used various techniques to test these outcomes. The protein was always present in the infected preparation but nucleic acid could not be found. Prusiner concluded that a protein must have a lot to do with the disease agent. Or it could be the actual disease agent itself.

This was unheard of. If this were true it would turn all that was known about biology on its ear. According to conventional scientific dogma, to replicate an organism like a virus, genetic material — either DNA or RNA — was required. Prusiner publicly postulated that TSEs did not contain either DNA or RNA. He claimed that the agent was nothing more than a protein — a protein found normally in humans and animals. It didn't replicate like a conventional virus. It converted the existing protein to a different configuration, flipped it into an abnormal shape and made everything around it change too, Prusiner claimed later.

By 1982, when the scientific world sat up and took notice of the tall, imposing 39-year-old with the unmistakable mop of grey curls, Prusiner had thought of a simple word to describe what he claimed was a major — if not *the* — factor in the cause of all the TSEs. He'd observed that in brains of the diseased hamsters, there was an accumulation of *pro*tease-resistant protein (PrP) that he called a *pri*on. The word was a twisted acronym for proteinaceous infectious particle, which, he suggested confidently, should replace other terminology including "unconventional virus" or "unusual slow virus-like agent".[37]

The word (pronounced "pree on") officially entered the scientific lexicon in April 1982, when it leapt off the pages of the leading scientific journal, *Science*, under Prusiner's name. This followed the publication one month earlier of a front-page article on the prion subject in the *San Francisco Chronicle*. Under the heading, "Tiny new life form found", the details of Prusiner's discovery were blurted first to the mainstream media, a move frowned upon by the scientific establishment. The accepted procedure for revealing breakthroughs is for scientific literature to lead the way. And Prusiner's catchy prion tag, backed by nationwide publicity, stuck. A snappy buzz word, it was far easier to remember and pronounce than "spongiform encephalopathy" or "slow virus-like agent", and certainly simpler than "infectious cerebral amyloidosis". But for most established workers in the TSE field "infectious agent" was still the preferable name.

When he proposed his theory, Prusiner did not know why the converted protein behaved the way it did, or when. But he suggested that this normal cellular prion protein — known as PrP^c — at some stage came into contact with an abnormal or what became known as "rogue" or "renegade" type of PrP. Colloquially the abnormal protein, which is produced in nerve cells, has been dubbed the "evil twin".[38] To distinguish it from normal PrP^c the rogue protein was dubbed PrP^{sc}, which stands for scrapie-infected prion protein. Once the rogue PrP^{sc} touched the normal PrP^c, it caused the normal PrP to convert to an abnormal shape, the mechanism of which remains unknown. The conversion from normal PrP^c into the evil and fatal PrP^{sc} becomes an unstoppable chain reaction. The result is brain damage, untreatable, incurable and always fatal. The body's immune system does not detect this damage as it occurs. If it did a cavalry of infection-fighting white cells would be sent into battle against the intruder.

Prusiner's guess was that prion proteins were folded in such a way that they were resistant to destruction by protein-eating enzymes. As a result the PrP^{sc} cluttered brain cells with indigestible protein or plaque. Plaque would then build up to the point where it interfered with vital nerve centres and got in the way of cells repairing themselves. Once the plaque deposits accumulated, the body could not respond normally because the accumulated protein blocked the transmission of messages from the infected brain to other parts of the body.

Prusiner's new idea was immediately tagged as "biological heresy". Others dismissed his alleged prion hypothesis as simply "a fairy tale". His many detractors at the time labelled Prusiner, and his heresy, as "the P words". But the "heretical" name stuck. He had created a new scientific word to fit a scientific entity that was still unknown. And for that he attracted a lot of publicity — a third "P" word which resulted in grant money.

At first, Prusiner's detractors included almost everyone involved in scrapie or TSE research. Soon after Prusiner's *Science* article was published in 1982, Richard Kimberlin, then a senior member of the Neuropathogenesis Unit in Edinburgh, first touted the virino theory in mainstream scientific literature in an editorial in *Nature*.[39] Soon after that, and unnamed as the author, Dickinson stated in an editorial in the *Lancet* that in the 1930s, conventional viruses had been wrongly thought by various experts to be essentially protein. As far as TSE agents went, Dickinson said that the existence of many strains of scrapie was the hardest to explain in protein-only terms.[40]

Some scientists sneered at the time that if the word prion were a true acronym, it would have been a *pro*in. They were horrified that this young scientist had not only put forward what he himself admitted was a heretical hypothesis, Prusiner had proposed it as something that ought to be accepted from that time on. He did not even add the words "hypothesis" or "theory" to show that it had not been proved, his critics fumed. In addition, Prusiner's theory evolved over time to cover possibilities ranging from a protein-only agent to a protein-plus-other-molecules agent. This effectively meant that his theory could extend from bacteria to all micro-organisms, which violated one of the core guiding principles of scientific investigation: that a theory or hypothesis had to be so worded that it could be disproved.

A widely held view among some experienced researchers remains that the protein-only hypothesis is "biology's equivalent of cold fusion". Cold fusion was the fantasy theory, initially accepted amid great publicity in the late 1980s when proposed by two American scientists, that energy could be created by fusing hydrogen atoms from water at room temperature — far cooler than the temperature of the sun. It was later found that this was not possible.

The cold fusion analogy has been attributed to Dr Robert G. Rohwer, the bearded and bespectacled director of the molecular neurovirology unit at the Veterans Affairs Medical Center in Baltimore. A former member of Gajdusek's laboratory, he has dismissed as "outrageous" Prusiner's claims that a prion protein could cause disease, and points to all the data on TSEs being consistent with virus causation. Rohwer and other scientists ask this question: How is it possible that there are so many types of TSE if everything is controlled by the host gene and not the infectious agent? Whatever causes TSEs is very hardy and robust, according to Rohwer — just like other viruses.[41]

Despite this alleged flaw and the fact that the quantity of PrP^{sc} does not correlate well with infectivity, many eminent scientists are comfortable with the prion idea, describing it as the most likely candidate in a lacklustre field of equally unproven theories. They included a virus, a tiny virus-like particle, a plant viroid-like naked nucleic acid, the provirus scrapie theory of H. B. Parry, nucleic acid surrounded by a polysaccharide coat, DNA bound to a membrane and, a few years later, a retrovirus.[42]

Like its source appeared to do, the prion tag replicated. Slightly different terms were loaded onto the PrP designation, which have come to be accepted names by many. These include PrP^{sc}, PrP^{cjd} and PrP^{gss}. The detractors remain, though.

Prominent among them is Alan Dickinson who for a while wickedly papered the noticeboard in his office, before his retirement in 1986, with collages of newspaper headlines including "Stanley: Tiny new life form found", which made him chuckle quietly. He repeats with obvious enjoyment, pronouncing prion with English-sounding vowels, a little ditty penned in 1985 by his friend, the late Peter Wildy, professor of pathology at the University of Cambridge (one of the experts from when advice was sought about the potential for CJD infectivity in hGH).

> The chemical state of the prion
> Is the latest genetical try on
> It's flaccid and placid
> No nucleic acid
> Just protein it has to rely on.

Prusiner, meanwhile, has kept very busy, attempting to confirm a version of his theory. After a bruising magazine portrait in 1986, he refused to speak directly to the media. Although still not proved, his prion hypothesis has gained acceptance and in time has become the simplest word to describe TSEs.

As the first shock waves from the prion protein-only theory settled down, another potential reservoir of the disease was uncovered. Two doctors in Houston, Texas reported the cases histories of four Americans who had died of apparent or confirmed CJD after years of eating wild goat or squirrel brains.[43]

The doctors described the demise of a 45-year-old man whose annual treat was to visit Italy and eat wild goat brain cooked and served at a particular restaurant in Padua. This man showed some of the signs of CJD from about three months after his last foray in his home country, in mid-1975. A year later a brain biopsy revealed spongiform encephalopathy. The man died four years after the onset of his symptoms. Samples of his brain later transmitted CJD to animals in Gajdusek's lab.

The second patient was a 47-year-old east-Texan engineer who had hunted small game, including squirrels. This man loved his squirrel brains, a local delicacy, and often added them as dumplings to his soup. In May 1980 he began staggering and his hands jerked noticeably. An electroencephalogram reading revealed slowing and irregular brain wave peaks, which often signal CJD to neurologists. He died nine months after his symptoms began, but no autopsy was performed and CJD could not be confirmed.

The third patient described in this paper was a 62-year-old from west Louisiana who often ate squirrel brains, although the rest of his family preferred the squirrel meat. He was admitted to hospital with a five-month history of progressive staggering, dizziness, periods of confusion, impaired judgment and a hazy memory. While hospitalised, myoclonic jerks set in, his mental faculties deteriorated and within three months he was dead. Again, no autopsy was performed.

Lastly, the authors included a 68-year-old woman who had eaten cooked squirrel brains her whole life. She showed all the signs of an atypical form of CJD with clumsy hands, slurred speech, staggering, myoclonic jerks and seizures.

Some reservoir of infection in humans or animals seemed probable, the authors concluded. The histories of eating wild animal brains in their four patients, who died of definite or probable CJD — other Americans would also succumb in coming years — supported the hypothesis "that ingestion of the infective agent may be one natural mode of acquisition of Creutzfeldt-Jakob disease".

CHAPTER 8

Hormones: The first victims

JOE RODRIGUEZ WAS looking forward to the holiday break and trip with his parents to Maine, American's pine-tree state on the northeast coast, to see his grandparents. It was not only a welcome break from his studies in San Francisco. Maine in spring brought with it childhood memories of boating on the lake, one of his favourite pastimes.

It was May 1984. As the thin young man stood up from the waiting room seat to change planes in Atlanta he complained of feeling dizzy. It soon passed and before long he was happily ensconced in his grandparents' home. But several days later when his grandfather offered to take him for a spin on the lake he declined, frowning. He didn't need to go for a spin because he was "already dizzy".[1]

His mother took sharp note. Always happy, optimistic and talkative as a youngster, despite his medical problems, it was unusual for him not to try any activity on offer. She remembered the endless visits to the doctor and the piles of medical reports which accumulated first at the Los Angeles Children's Hospital and later, when they moved to Palo Alto, south of San Francisco, at Stanford University. Her son was regarded as a stoic pioneer of a new treatment regimen for growth hormone, which involved thousands of injections. At 15 months old he had been diagnosed with thyroid hormone deficiency. From 29 months he received daily insulin shots after the onset of diabetes mellitus. And in September 1966, when he was not yet three years old, his obvious growth deficiency was treated with injections of hGH.[2]

From then on, for nearly 13 years until April 1980, Joe Rodriguez received thousands of shots of hGH. Because of his diabetes, the hGH injections were given daily rather than two or three times a week, which was standard worldwide at that time. This was to prevent insulin swings in the absence of hGH. His initial source of the drug was from the laboratory of Dr Alfred Wilhelmi at Emory University in Atlanta, and thanks to those unusually large early doses of the drug he grew to be just over 165 centimetres tall.[3,4]

When he returned to school after the trip to Maine, Joe's dizziness continued and his speech began to slur. Dr Raymond Hintz, his former paediatric endocrinologist with whom his parents were still in touch, remembers receiving a phone call on Sunday, June 17, 1984 and meeting Joe's parents at the Stanford emergency room. Joe, now 20, had trouble speaking clearly, had jerky eye movements and mild ataxia, a staggering kind of walk that indicates a problem with the brain.[5]

With worsening and puzzling symptoms, Joe was put under the care of neurologist Dr Richard Gravina, who became alarmed at his patient's mental deterioration, the jerks in his limbs and muscular rigidity. Dr Gravina arranged for Joe to be admitted to the paediatric neurology service at the University of California in San Francisco. There, Joe appeared apathetic, had mild drooling and severely slurred speech. He stood in a stooped position, was very unsteady on his feet and his eyes and limbs jerked. A series of test results were normal, apart from strange peaks recording his brain activity on an EEG.[6]

Hintz was kept informed of developments. Joe, becoming increasingly demented, was presented at a paediatric EEG conference. It was there, for the first time since Joe's troubles began, that Dr Michael Aminoff suggested a diagnosis of possible CJD. However, because CJD was noted as being a disease that mainly afflicted elderly people, it was decided that Joe was too young to be considered a CJD sufferer. He was discharged with no agreement on his condition.

On a wintry November day, six months after his first attack of dizziness, Joe died at another hospital. When his brain was examined after an autopsy at the University, it showed the typical changes of spongiform encephalopathy — infection with patches of microscopic holes in his brain. Aminoff had been right.

The snow surrounding Buffalo in upstate New York in that winter of 1984 was the last that would be seen by a 23-year-old man who had also received countless hGH injections. He had been diagnosed as growth deficient when he was seven years old. It wasn't hard to notice. His fraternal twin was much taller.[7] From June 1969 to October 1977 when he was 15, this young man was injected with hGH several times a week, from about three different batches each year. He grew to be 166 centimetres tall, but at nearly 17 years old had no facial hair and abnormally small genitalia. So he was given additional FSH and testosterone. He joined the Navy in 1979 and after four years was discharged.[8] That was when his problems started.

Walking along a street one day in the autumn of 1983, he felt a bit weak and could not control a propensity to veer to the right. Nor could he explain the increasing difficulty he had in maintaining his balance in the weeks that followed. "Funny" sensations in his head and periodic double vision also plagued him.[9] He became apathetic and careless, his family noticed — a marked change from his usual enthusiastic and conscientious self.

The first doctor he consulted, an ear, nose and throat specialist, thought he was a malingerer. A visit in January 1984 to the Buffalo General Hospital resulted in a 39-day stay and a course of ACTH, another pituitary hormone, which did nothing to halt a severe deterioration in his balance. It reached the point where he could no longer walk or sit without help. A diagnosis of severe cerebellar syndrome was made, and was attributed to probable demyelisation or destruction of the protective covering of nerves.

Soon afterwards, in March 1984 he was back in hospital with head tremors, dementia, slurred speech and jerks in his arms. He was too young to die in a nursing home — mute, bedridden and tube-fed — from the symptoms of the CJD that killed him. It was April 1985, 18 months after his physical symptoms began.

Around the same time as Joe Rodriguez and the man from Buffalo began to deteriorate, 34-year-old Wayne Tatlock had his own problems half a country away in Dallas, Texas. In early March 1984 he began to stagger slightly while walking. And although he was not dizzy, his hand trembled as he attempted to drink tea.

Despite a normal ECG and normal results from tests for inner ear problems and changes in blood pressure, Wayne's condition worsened. At work, where he managed the video department within a music store, he hung onto rails, walls and the service counter to keep his balance. Several times he fell for no apparent reason. And on several visits to his parents' home, Wayne staggered around and was intermittently drowsy and unable to concentrate. A brain scan in late April came back normal.

It was only when his workplace insisted that Wayne take leave of absence for medical reasons that he saw a specialist neurologist, Dr Ron Tintner, at the Southwestern Medical School and Parkland Hospital. A customer at the video store who was also a doctor had noted his balance problems and recommended Tintner. Wayne was tested for inner ear problems and anything like a lesion or patch of disease in his brain that could account for his puzzling symptoms. Nothing abnormal showed up.

When his mother visited him in late May 1984 — he was by now on leave of absence from his job again — she found him "not eating properly and not even leaving his apartment".[10] He was not making decisions and his affairs were going unattended. She took her son home with her to Jacksboro, 150 kilometres north west of Dallas.

When Wayne was three years old his parents, the Reverend Lloyd and Janice Tatlock, were told their son had retarded physical development. After brief trials of thyroid hormone and anabolic steroids during his younger years, Wayne began hGH therapy when he was 12. Without it he would have remained a pituitary dwarf. Throughout his three courses of hGH — February to November 1963, May 1964 to September 1965, and March 1966 to April 1969 — he was also periodically treated with testosterone, cortisone and thyroid hormone.

But on June 18, 1984, when he was admitted to Parkland Hospital for more extensive tests, no-one considered his childhood hGH treatment. All test results came back normal despite the fact that by now he could only walk by leaning on someone else. Wayne also had a slight difficulty recalling current events and was not able to put his finger to his nose — what doctors term the "finger-nose-finger manoeuvre".

Tintner discharged Wayne with a diagnosis of cerebellar ataxia of unknown cause.

In mid-July Wayne accompanied his parents to Jamaica for the World Convention of Christian Churches. On their return, his parents closed his Dallas apartment. While finalising his bills, they discovered that for the previous few months he had been regularly overdrawn and had paid bank penalties, despite an income that was enough for his needs. And he hadn't paid his electricity bill, which meant he had spent his nights throughout May with no lighting.

By early September Wayne became wheelchair-bound, unable to

negotiate the distance from his bedroom to the sitting room by himself. Incontinence and feeding problems followed and his father and brothers had to help him in the shower and later in the bath.

In November Wayne developed a head tremor and his attention span fluctuated. All interest in current events and family news disappeared, short-term memory deteriorated and he also denied that he was sick. However, long-term memory remained good and he liked playing Trivial Pursuit, especially the entertainment questions on which he was usually correct. He spent most of his time watching television. Most noticeable, as the weather became colder approaching Christmas, was his lack of interest in music despite his extensive record collection.

By December Wayne was transferred between a specially installed hospital bed and his wheelchair via a rented hydraulic lift.

Swallowing and opening his mouth soon became a problem and his speech became slurred. Occasionally he choked on even processed food so his parents bought a suction machine. By the New Year, he was totally bedridden, was apparently unaware of any bodily functions and could not control the jerks that racked his arms and legs. Getting a cup to his mouth was impossible. By mid-February he could no longer talk, although he still recognised and understood all around him.

Just after 10 p.m. on February 26, 1985, Wayne died. No-one had really considered that he might have been suffering from the fatal but rare CJD. Not until he was exhumed.

If Wayne Tatlock and Alison Lay, a 22-year-old bank typist from Winchester in England, had ever met they might have compared the fact that they both began staggering for no apparent reason in March 1984. Like Wayne, Alison's childhood had been peppered with medical intervention. When she was two years old she had a pituitary tumour removed. Afterwards her diabetes was difficult to control, indicating a problem with her pituitary gland output of anti-diuretic hormone. She received intermittent doses of cortisone and thyroxine for other hormone deficiencies and grew normally until she was eight years old. It was then that growth deficiency was detected.

From July 1972 until July 1976 she received twice-weekly injections of hGH manufactured at the University of Cambridge via the Raben and modified Hartree–Wilhelmi methods. The drug helped her grow 16 centimetres to a height of 139 centimetres. After leaving school she worked as a bank typist, and at 18 developed symptoms of depression that improved but recurred again two years later after a broken engagement.[11]

In May 1984 Alison became clumsy with her hands, unsteady on her feet, and one evening returned home from work and told her mother she had walked into office furniture. By July a slight paralysis of her legs had been detected and she became increasingly childish and demanding, talking continually and making high-pitched screams to gain attention. Eye tests showed a motor function problem, her speech became slurred and her IQ fell to 80.

By September she could no longer work and her personality had changed, according to her mother, Mavis.[12] Although doctors speculated that her condition might be psychological or a regrowth of her pituitary tumour, Alison's parents otherwise had no idea what was wrong with her. Eventually Alison was unable to stand without support. A brain scan in October 1984 showed no tumour but mild atrophy of the cerebellum. MS was ruled out but an EEG test was abnormal.

Alison's health declined rapidly. By Christmas she could no longer talk or respond. Shocked by her condition, her neurologist admitted her to the neurological unit at Southampton Hospital. From there she was taken to the National Hospital for Nervous Diseases at Queen's Square in London and from there to a psychiatric unit at Basingstoke, where she was visited every day by her parents. The last words she uttered to her parents were "I want to die".

"At length Professor Newsom-Davis (a treating doctor) said that nothing more could be done for Alison at the National Hospital. He explained to us that Alison was dying from a rare brain disease. No mention was made of Creutzfeldt-Jakob disease, even though we believe that this was strongly in the minds of the treating doctors," Mavis Lay said a decade later.[13]

She told a television documentary: "They just treated us like morons, I think, not being able to comprehend what was going on. They were very evasive. They told us as little as possible and we very much wanted to know everything. And so did Alison quite early on in her illness. She was very distressed with all these awful symptoms and nobody had any answers."[14]

Alison Lay died in the Royal Hampshire County Hospital in Winchester in February 1985 — the same month as Wayne Tatlock. A post-mortem examination revealed the unmistakable spongy holes associated with CJD. A paper on the autopsy findings published the following year confirmed Mavis Lay's suspicion — doctors had indeed considered CJD to be the most likely cause of her daughter's deterioration.[15]

The deaths of those four young people changed forever the lives of thousands around the world. They represented a statistically significant cluster of deaths in a short period of time from a disease so rare that a general practitioner might never see one case in an entire career. All four had had pituitary gland problems. All four had received hGH as children. All the American patients and their parents knew hGH was extracted from human pituitary glands taken from dead bodies.

Unlike the families of the three American CJD victims, Mavis Lay was not told of the suspected connection between her daughter's death from CJD and her previous growth hormone treatment. It was only later in 1985, when she was sent a draft of an article for the Lancet, that she first realised they had suspected CJD all along.[16,17]

As the news of the CJD deaths spread beyond the world of endocrinology, Gajdusek discussed the first case with his friend and colleague, Paul Brown, on a plane between Geneva and Istanbul. "Very exciting," Gajdusek kept saying. "Very exciting that case of growth hormone."[18] Brown was quite ignorant about hGH at the time and had never heard of the fact that it was derived from ground-up pituitary glands. "Well it's just Carleton being excited by something," Brown thought dismissively. "It certainly doesn't mean anything. So what! It's just a coincidence."

"So I was as dumb as everybody else," Brown admits now. "Carleton was smart. And Raymond Hintz was the smartest of all. Then bang, bang, two more cases and that was that." [19]

In April 1985 Gajdusek and Brown wagered a dinner on their perceived outcomes of the extent of CJD in the estimated 30,000 growth hormone recipients worldwide. "He [Gajdusek] said it was going to be a major epidemic and I said it was going to be a trivial outbreak," Brown recalls. Both of them were wrong.

On April 25, 1985, the seventieth anniversary of the disastrous landing at Gallipoli of British, French, Australian and New Zealand forces during World War I, the beginning of another disaster was heralded in England. It seemed innocuous enough at the time. One of veterinary surgeon Colin Whitaker's regular clients called from a farm near Ashford, in east Kent, the gateway to England's southern green belt and now a stop on the Channel train to France.

A dairy cow called Daisy, like her namesake chimpanzee exactly 20 years earlier, was behaving oddly. Previously quiet, she had turned unusually aggressive, bashing others in the herd, walking on shaky legs and stumbling, especially on her back legs when shooed away from other cows. Soon Daisy was dead.

Over the next year several more cows in Daisy's herd died of the mysterious ailment. They, like Daisy had been, were sent to the local knackery, rendered down and their remnants made into bonemeal. Other apparently healthy cows in the herd were eventually sent to an abattoir for slaughter and made into steaks and the filling for sausages and pasties. Meat from their spinal columns was mechanically flayed off and used with the brain as filling in meat pies and as flavouring in stock cubes and consommés.

It wasn't long before other farms in the Kent area reported cows with the same puzzling symptoms as Daisy. Over the next 18 months, another 17 cows from Daisy's herd died after showing the same mysterious symptoms. They too were rendered down into bonemeal and fed to animals. Reports filtered back of the sickness on farms in other areas, other counties. No-one could explain it.

The more cases Whitaker saw, the more he thought it looked like scrapie in sheep. He was told not to make that comparison publicly by the Ministry of Agriculture, Fisheries and Food (MAFF). In July 1987, about to address a professional meeting on the condition that had begun killing a few cows in some herds right across England and Wales, Whitaker was asked by a MAFF official not to use the phrase "scrapie-like syndrome". "I actually crossed it out of the slide I was presenting," Whitaker recalls of the thick, black line he drew through the words to make them illegible to the audience. He substituted instead the words "new syndrome".[20]

No-one knew it at the time, but the killer cow disease was set to ruin the British beef industry, poison relations with Europe and eventually, it appeared, cross the species barrier to humans.

CHAPTER 9

Tracking the CJD culprit

W HEN DR RAYMOND HINTZ was told in February 1985 that an autopsy had confirmed that his former patient Joe Rodriguez had died of CJD, he was immediately worried. The verdict brought back recollections of a conference in 1982, sponsored by the Food and Drug Administration (FDA), that had dealt informally with slow viruses and how hard they were to detect in tissue extracts. The accidental transmission of CJD in 1974 via a corneal graft was not forgotten.

Hintz believed that Joe's pituitary hormone extracts, perhaps contaminated with a slow virus, were a probable cause of his death. As a result, Hintz thought it crucial to alert the endocrine community. On February 25, 1985 he wrote to the NIH, the FDA and the NHPP, the overseeing body for the collection and manufacture of pituitary hormones throughout the US:

> Creutzfeldt-Jakob disease is extremely rare in a 20-year-old and it is felt to be transmissible by contact with the infectious agent in the central nervous system of affected patients. This patient (JRo) was treated for 14 years with growth hormone, and I feel that the possibility that this was a factor in his getting Creutzfeldt-Jakob disease should be considered. A careful follow-up of all patients treated with pituitary growth hormone in the past 25 years should be carried out, looking for any other cases of degenerative neurological disease.[1]

Events then moved very fast. The Rodriguez case was just one in about 10,000 children treated since the early 1960s. Hintz's letter was filed at the FDA on March 4, 1985. Four days later Dr Mortimer Lipsett, the director of the National Institutes of Diabetes and Digestive and Kidney Diseases, which distributed hGH, convened a high-calibre meeting of scientists and officials. They decided to notify endocrinologists about the possible connection between Joe's CJD and his lengthy history of hGH injections. In addition they would begin a look back for similar cases among other hGH patients. All non-therapeutic uses of hGH were stopped. The big step — suspending all use of hGH among the 3,000 children then being treated across the United States — was to be considered after Joe's CJD diagnosis was independently verified and further information was sought that might show he was infected via another source. A large meeting, scheduled for April 19, 1985, would decide the fate of hGH use in America.

The heads of other countries with hGH programs were also alerted to the unfolding drama in America. In April, Dr Salvatore Raiti, the Australian head of the American NHPP, telephoned his equivalent in Australia, Leslie Lazarus.[2]

"Although my colleagues at Stanford were fully supportive of my action, many of my other paediatric endocrine colleagues clearly felt that I was an alarmist, and they did not hesitate to tell me so," Hintz wrote a decade later. "The pressure increased when it appeared that the therapeutic use of GH in the United States might be halted because of this apparently unique case."[3]

But there was more than one case of CJD in hGH recipients. Dr Robert Blizzard, an endocrinologist, mulled over the letter he had received from Wayne Tatlock's parents about the death of their son in February. He wrote to the NIH about it on April 11, 1985. One day before the scheduled April 19 meeting, troubled by the recent death of her former patient in Buffalo, Dr Margaret MacGillivray also wrote to the NIH to relate her patient's case history. It was an "incredible coincidence", according to Hintz, that three deaths from CJD in former hGH recipients occurred in such a short space of time.

Dr Paul Brown, the medical director of Gajdusek's re-named Laboratory of Central Nervous System Studies put it this way in his seminal article on the topic published three years later:

> The effect of this new information was like two thunderclaps and forever sealed the fate of native human growth hormone therapy. The next day, on April 19, the hormone was officially executed: among the spectators at graveside, only Genentech was not in mourning.[4]

Genentech, manufacturer of the first synthetic growth hormone drug used in America, stood to gain handsomely.

Some at the April 19 meeting, which had broadened to include paediatric endocrinologists from several overseas countries and members of pharmaceutical companies that marketed commercial versions of hGH, argued that the problem was isolated to NHPP hGH, or to America. They were over-ruled. After an emergency meeting in Stockholm on April 20, KabiVitrum formally followed the American example. On April 22 its Crescormon production was discontinued and, in the days that followed, withdrawals occurred from all pharmacies and client countries and Swedish treating doctors were informed of the decision.[5] On April 22 Canada also suspended its hGH program.

Commercial hGH manufactured by Nordisk, who found the connection between CJD and hGH tenuous,[6] and Ares-Serono were withdrawn in the United States within two weeks. Distribution of both commercial brands continued elsewhere, however.

At the State Vaccine Institute in Cape Town, Emlyn Hitchings, unaware of any hint that CJD could contaminate pituitary glands, had freeze-dried the twenty-fifth batch of hGH made in South Africa on March 21, 1985. However, once the CJD deaths had been reported and the FDA alerted him to the halting of the program in the United States on April 19, 1985, Professor François Bonnici moved immediately. "We shut down that day. Just stopped it," recalls Bonnici.[7] All patients and treating doctors using either locally-manufactured or imported hGH were told to stop immediately due to the deaths from CJD. Remaining hGH from Kabi and Serono was returned.

At the State Vaccine Institute at least 2000 pituitary glands, painstakingly collected or posted in from mortuaries as far flung as Port Elizabeth, Bloemfontein, Durban, Johannesburg and Pretoria, lay in various states of production. Some were still lying in acetone, others were about to be ground up, the hormone not yet extracted. Others had spent up to 20 hours in a filtration column, the next step in the process. More again had been processed right up to the stage where they lay like a tiny little biscuit in the bottom of a 2 ml glass vial — just waiting to be reconstituted with a saline solution and injected into a short child. All of it was incinerated. Mortuaries were told to stop collecting glands.

News of Alison Lay's death, which occurred in February 1985, reached a symposium of European endocrinologists and health authority representatives in Copenhagen on April 27. On May 5, Britain's Dr Derek Bangham telexed Lazarus in Sydney about the death of Alison Lay.[8] Because Alison's treatment originated from glands processed in Great

Britain, a potential worldwide problem had arisen. Based on the American cases and their own, the British closed their program on May 8.

In a report on the topic prepared on May 13, Kabi official, Mr Gunnar Degerman stated:

> If we also [in addition to the three cases in the restricted hGH recipient population worldwide] take into consideration the rare occurrence of patients in age groups below 35 years, there is no possibility whatsoever but to accept a direct causality from the previous hGH treatment.

On May 29, 1985, although the problem was perceived as "overseas" and unrelated to their Chapman purification method, the AHPHP was "temporarily" halted and a letter requesting an urgent drug recall was sent to all treating doctors of both hGH and hPG in Australia. Although 256 children were then under treatment with hGH, an exception was made for about six children with potentially life-threatening hypoglycaemia. With the written consent of their parents, they were allowed to continue receiving cadaver-derived hGH. Infertile couples were told of the expensive alternative of hMG, which replaced hPG in 1986 as a government-sponsored drug. As Lazarus concluded in an article on the temporary — later permanent — shut down of the AHPHP,

> … it is a cautionary tale of considerable importance for transplantation in general, because it would now appear to be important to avoid the transplantation of any tissue or organ from a patient with any type of dementia.[9]

National and private hGH programs in New Zealand, Hong Kong, Belgium, Finland, Greece, Sweden, Hungary, West Germany, Argentina and the Netherlands also shut down. Everyone, however, was bolstered by the knowledge that synthetic hGH would soon be available. This occurred quite promptly. In October 1985, Britain became the "first country in the world" to license a biosynthetic preparation of growth hormone. Called Somatonorm, it was produced by KabiVitrum and cost £4000 to treat one child for a year. Clinical trials about to begin on pituitary-derived prolactin, the hormone that produces breast milk in new mothers, were "quickly abandoned" when the dangers from hGH were revealed.[10]

However, there were exceptions where authorities "inexplicably" continued to use pituitary-derived hGH.[11] In a bold decision that raised eyebrows in the world of paediatric endocrinology, France decided to continue its pituitary-derived hormone production, but with an additional purification chemical, 8 molar urea, which at the time was thought to eradicate CJD infectivity. Japan, Austria, Italy, Denmark and Norway also continued with pituitary-derived hGH for varying periods. Nordisk, the Danish commercial manufacturer, continued manufacturing pituitary-derived hGH until 1987, supplying the drug to both Denmark and France.[12]

Israel also continued with commercial hGH. When Kabi's Crescormon was withdrawn in 1985, Israel continued using Nanormon and Grorm hGH manufactured by Ares-Serono — until 1992 when patients were switched to synthetic hGH.[13] Later, it was found that even 8 molar urea did not totally inactivate CJD. But in France, as would be seen, the damage had already been done.

In Britain, a health ethics committee decided in 1986 not to tell hGH recipients of their CJD risk. The Health Department agreed. Telling patients and their parents would create undue panic when there was no cure or treatment if they contracted the disease. The decision effectively entombed the contamination episode within the medical profession. Dr Bryan Matthews, retired professor of clinical neurology at the University of Oxford and the man who sent the first sliver of human brain that caused CJD in a chimpanzee in 1969, was one of the four ethics committee members. "I have often thought about it subsequently," he told a TV documentary on the CJD tragedy in 1992, "and I think it was the wrong decision."

In Australia, CJD deaths continued to be perceived as an overseas problem. The Federal Department of Health notified treating doctors about the deaths but the decision whether or not to tell patients was left to their discretion. Some endocrinologists told the parents of children undergoing treatment at the time that the AHPHP was shut down. Others thought the same as their counterparts in England and decided against worrying former patients about a disease they would probably not get. Few gynaecologists in Australia told their patients about CJD. It was hoped that the Chapman production method, which differed from the production methods used in both America and Britain, was protection enough against CJD contamination in Australian recipients.

These decisions — not to trace and inform past recipients of their CJD risk when it was revealed in 1985 — have become known by the bitter relatives of the dead, as well as those living in fear of contracting CJD, as "walls of silence". The walls, erected with great success in Britain and Australia particularly, kept families who needed to know all about CJD when it affected them, in chaotic ignorance and without help, either financial or health-wise, at the very time it was needed. Some recipients of human hormone drugs learned of their risk years later via the media, or when they tried to donate blood, or when it reached them on a local grapevine.

In South Africa, children and parents on current treatment were told why the program was stopped and were re-contacted in 1986 when synthetic hGH became available. "It took us about a year or two to decide to warn people who had previously received growth hormone and we were slow in doing that," admits Bonnici. "But then so was everybody. We didn't want to create panic unnecessarily."[14] Most, but not all, of the hGH recipients in this highly migratory country were traced centrally via a national register of patients that had been built up over the life of the program. They were told of their CJD risk via mail, by their GPs or by their original paediatricians. South African neurologists were notified in 1985 and again in 1990 to watch for CJD patients that might have received growth hormone as children. No follow-up study of all hGH recipients was instituted.

In America, where parents had actively campaigned for the collection of more pituitary glands via autopsies and inclusion of donor acceptance on drivers' licences, it was a different story.

A full-scale investigation, including laboratory investigations to test the risk of infection in pituitary glands processed for treatment, began in the second half of 1985. It also included a massive epidemiological tracing study by the NIH, the FDA and the Centers for Disease Control in Atlanta in an effort to find all 7,000-odd hGH recipients on the American NHPP. It was discovered that, although the annual mortality of CJD in the world was about one per million population, in America in 1988 an estimated one in 10,000 deaths each year could be accounted for by CJD. Another estimate, based on an informal survey of several large university pathology departments, took into consideration that not all deaths result in an autopsy and that some cases may have been missed. This study found that one CJD death per 1,000 might be a reasonable assumption. Paul Brown of the NIH suggested that pituitary pools containing 10,000 glands had a good chance, therefore, of containing between one and 10 CJD-infected glands. In America about 500,000 glands were processed between 1966 and 1977. It followed that between 25 and 250 infected glands may have been included in batches processed in that 11-year period alone. "Thus, the question was not whether an infected gland had been processed but whether any infectivity remained after processing."[15]

The results of Alan Dickinson's scrapie elimination experiment on British biochemist Philip Lowry's hGH production process were not published until August 1985. This was in line with the tacit official policy in Britain of not publicising the potential for CJD contamination in hGH — until it became real. Most pituitary programs had been shut down by this time however. So while the experimental results were interesting, they had already been overtaken by events.

Dickinson had, in fact, had preliminary results as early as late 1981, and these had been confirmed in March 1983. British doctors and administrators who shut down the HGHP in May 1985 had known the results for more than two years but had not shared the information. In any case, Lowry's contract to produce hGH had not been renewed beyond 1981. When production switched to CAMR at Porton Down that year, acetone-stored glands (as well as the frozen glands used in Lowry's method) continued to be used.

Dickinson's test had involved adding a massive scrapie contamination at the start of the Lowry processing method. This contamination was progressively removed during the first three steps in the chemical extraction process. Less and less mice died when injected with the contaminated hGH solution at the end of each of those steps. No infectivity at all was found after either of the last two steps of the five-step Lowry method. All mice deliberately infected with hGH from the last two production steps had lived. So Lowry's protocol worked. Dickinson's results suggested it was possible to deliver a safe hormone to the patients, at least when processed by those with a proven ability to work safely with agents that caused scrapie or CJD.

But the infected material had merely been removed from the final drug; it had not disappeared. The infectivity at the start of the experiments had either been concentrated and removed, along with the lumpy material from other pituitary hormones, after each processing step — or worse, it had become trapped and allowed to build up in the machinery used in the processing. That machinery was either the blender or the chromatography column. Between each production step, then, ample opportunity existed for cross-contamination.

"We just used common sense," Dickinson says of the vital, highly aseptic standards that were normal at his Neuropathogenesis Unit laboratory, housed in a building dedicated solely to scrapie investigations. "In our research it was essential to keep strains of scrapie apart, and if you could achieve that, you could trust your methods."[16]

When the final results of Dickinson's test were put before the DHSS/MRC advisory committee in March 1983, it was regarded as reassuring news. However, the committee paid no attention to the possibility of cross-contamination by laboratory staff using the protocol. The whole procedure was just assumed to be safe. Departmental officers "therefore assumed that the acetone method was also safe", one said years later. This assumption was based on no more than Dickinson's own guarded words six years earlier — in his February 1977 warning letter — that the rougher treatment of glands stored in acetone might leave them less open to contamination than the frozen glands used in the Lowry method.[17]

The Hartree method of acetone-stored gland production was never tested in the same way as the Lowry protocol. Firstly, by the time the Lowry method experiment had begun, the Hartree method was longer in use. Secondly, at the time the experiment was commissioned, the concern was directed at the perceived gentleness of the Lowry method. Despite Dickinson's experiment still being in its early stages, from 1981 a modified Hartree–Wilhelmi method was used at the new production facilities at Porton Down. Dickinson's group, long accustomed to working with TSE agents, could purify pituitary extract from very contaminated tissues using Lowry's method current in 1980. But what about all those other laboratories where there was little, if any, knowledge about the highly resistant properties of TSEs?

In 1985 other experiments aimed at finding out whether the virus could be detected in the hormone already distributed in America, and received in particular by the three unfortunate CJD patients, were undertaken at the NIH. Vials of all 76 lots of the hormone still on file with the NHPP were injected into three monkeys and several chimpanzees by a variety of routes — intramuscularly, intracerebrally and intravenously. Despite the chance of finding a vial with an infective amount of CJD being small, the experiment still had to be done. It took years. Eventually one of the three squirrel monkeys developed CJD. Only one of the hGH recipients in America, known to have died of CJD at that time, had been exposed to the particular lot of hGH given to this monkey.[18]

In Australia, an epidemiological study on hGH recipients, begun in late 1985, had "petered out" by 1987 when requested resources from the Department of Health in Canberra did not materialise. The study was begun on hGH recipients because it was thought that delayed treatment was more serious in that group than in hPG recipients. Steps were never taken to extend the study to hPG recipients anyway.[19] A preliminary experiment with mice injected with samples of CSL batches of human hormone drugs was conducted by Professor Colin Masters, who by mid-1985 was back in Australia after his stint in Gajdusek's laboratory and working in his home city of Perth. The tests were inconclusive. If the hormone program was ever reactivated and synthetic hGH was not available, the mouse experiments would have provided valuable data on which to base clearance rates of infectivity.[20] But pituitary-derived human hormone drugs were never again used in Australia.

In June 1985, once the link between hGH therapy and CJD was confirmed in the first two American cases, it was decided that the indelicate task of exhuming the remains of Wayne Tatlock were necessary to confirm whether he had been a third in the apparent cluster of CJD cases. "The fate of treatment of thousands of individuals needing the hormone will be determined by decisions reached in the next few weeks," his neurologist, Ron Tintner, wrote to his parents.[21] Two weeks later the Tatlocks granted permission. Paul Brown remembers the exhumation as "a tricky situation". Although his parents lived in Texas, Wayne had been buried at the Woodlawn Memorial Park on the outskirts of Orlando, Florida.

> You know Florida has a water level that is about two feet below the surface of the earth and there was very little likelihood that anything worthwhile would be found. But we did it. And son of a gun, the brain was perfectly preserved, beautifully preserved. We were really surprised because this [brain] was not just OK. This was impeccable. This was like the brain had been taken out within 30 minutes of death and perfectly saved.[22]

Wayne Tatlock had died of CJD, an autopsy confirmed. In their July 1986 report in the journal *Neurology,* Tintner, Brown and four others described the case as "pivotal to the concept of a potentially serious problem of random contamination by CJD virus of hGH produced in the United States because only one of the lots received by this patient was shared with the San Francisco patient and none with the Buffalo patient."[23] Both Joe Rodriguez and the Buffalo man had shared nine other lots of the hormone.

The conclusion was inescapable. At least two different American lots of hGH had been contaminated and, coupled with Alison Lay's contaminated hGH in England, it meant random contamination may have occurred worldwide. The spongiform change in Wayne Tatlock's brain, as well as in the other three, was mainly in the cerebellum and basal ganglia areas, a different pattern to that usually found in sporadic CJD cases. Tintner and colleagues concluded that his case "together with other cases of iatrogenic disease, suggests that the virus enters the brain from the blood, rather than along neural pathways".

Doctors who had treated patients with hGH, and who had followed reports of the deaths in the September 19 issue of the *New England Journal of Medicine,* or who had listened with growing horror to Paul Brown's presentation on the topic at the World Congress of Neurology in Hamburg in the same month, wondered how many more cases would emerge.[24]

It didn't take long. In December 1985 Deborah McKenzie, a 31-year-old former hGH recipient in New Zealand, began staggering around her home in New Plymouth, watched anxiously by her mother Julia. Deborah, at 12 years of age, had been diagnosed with hypopituitarism and mild intellectual retardation. From October 1970 to October 1973, when she was 19, she had received American-manufactured hGH.

Deborah's job when she first became clumsy was in a centre that made teddy bears. The last toy teddy bear she made, poignant in its imperfection, was held up to a television camera years later. Its eyes were not level. By mid-1986, 12 years since her last treatment, she had been diagnosed with suspected CJD. "What's wrong with me, mum?" she asked her mother, Julia, bewildered as she fought the terrible symptoms. "I don't think I will ever get better. Do you?"

Deborah McKenzie's symptoms were similar to those of the American CJD victims. She developed short-term memory loss, forgetfulness and incontinence. After six months she was sleepy and unable to speak. Her limbs jerked and she experienced brief seizures. Her condition worsened without remission until her death in February 1987. A pair of unusual proteins was later found in her cerebrospinal fluid.[25]

Deborah's hGH treatment preceded the establishment of New Zealand's Human Growth Hormone Program in 1978. Dr Alfred Wilhelmi made her six lots of hGH in his laboratory at Emory University in Georgia.[26] Those batches, sometimes containing up to 15,000 glands, did not necessarily correspond to the lots of hormone assigned to patients. Of this, Paul Brown wrote later:

> Various fractions of the processed glands were often remaindered and later reprocessed with other batches of glands, with the result that material extracted from a given batch of glands often found its way into several different lots of distributed hormone.[27]

Later it was found that none of the lots used by Deborah McKenzie had been given to the three Americans who had died of CJD by that time. Cross-contamination was initially deemed unlikely because production runs for the New Zealand lots were not performed close to runs for any lots received by the American victims. But a later review of his records by Wilhelmi, who produced the majority of hGH in America between 1966 and 1977, showed that one particular batch of glands "had in fact found its way into at least one lot received by every US patient with Creutzfeldt-Jakob disease".[28]

Fractions of pituitary glands used in the production of hormone sent to Deborah McKenzie were also constituents of different lots given to American patients — including the first three that died of CJD. So there could be no distinct cut-off of the source of the contamination between the lots distributed in both countries.

American endocrinologists were keeping a sharp eye out for emerging cases of neurological disease or CJD in their patients. Dr Maria New was one of them. From her office at the Cornell Medical Center of the New York Hospital, nearly 100 growth hormone patients were contacted. Of several patients who had died, one was a 16-year-old girl with learning disabilities. She had had a patchy response to three different periods of hGH therapy between 1969 when she was aged six, to 1979. Two months after her last injection, the girl developed a flu-type illness that progressed over six weeks to a lethal pneumonia. She died on May 22, 1979.[29]

At her original autopsy severe atrophy had been noted around her hypothalamus, the area which dictates some hormone release from the pituitary gland and plays a role in mood and motivation. A re-examination of slides kept of sections of the girl's brain was carried out by the original pathologist in December 1986 — following the news that Wayne Tatlock had died of definite CJD. Amazingly, the pathologist found a single focus of CJD pathology in the corpus striatum that he had not noticed initially. A colleague who reviewed the slide, but had no prior knowledge of the case, verified that pathology.

The girl became the first recorded case of CJD identified in a human before the actual onset of the illness. It might have taken another five to 10 years for her to become symptomatic had she, as it was supposed, been infected quite early in her hGH treatment. In experimental animals, microscopic indications of CJD can be detected long before the onset of symptoms. Dr New and colleagues warned in a paper on the case published later.

> The practical significance of this case is that no patient treated with natural human growth hormone can be assumed to have escaped infection with the virus of CJD, no matter what the cause of death, without a complete neuropathology examination directed specifically at the detection of spongiform encephalopathy.[30]

According to Paul Brown, this discovery did not cause undue panic. The girl had died seven years before the review of her case had produced its astonishing result. And apart from Deborah McKenzie in New Zealand, no new cases had emerged in America in the 18 months since April 1985.

More bad news came soon enough. After the death of a patient in March 1987, Pennsylvania neurologist Dr David Marzewski rang Dr Judith Fradkin, the chief of the division of endocrinology and metabolic diseases program branch at the National Institute of Diabetes and Digestive and Kidney Diseases. Marzewski's 37-year-old patient had been treated with growth hormone in cycles from February 1964 when he was 14 to November 1967.[31]

In November 1986 the patient showed some disturbing signs reminiscent of initial symptoms in other patients. In December he consulted Dr Marzewski, who found he had mild ataxia of his arms, body and eyes. Within two weeks his inability to coordinate his arms and body had worsened and moved to his legs, causing staggering. A magnetic resonance imaging (MRI) scan of his brain showed some atrophy. Five weeks later the patient had trouble speaking clearly and swallowing, developed jerks in his limbs and needed a cane to walk.

The deterioration was relentless. Nine weeks after he first saw his neurologist, the man was bedridden and unable to eat by himself. He died, still mentally alert but having contracted pneumonia, 13 weeks after his first medical consultation. This man was also found to have two abnormal proteins in his cerebrospinal fluid.

So now there were six cases. But their clinical symptoms were different, appearing in a different order than those seen in sporadic CJD. Dementia or mental deterioration is usually a dominant first sign of sporadic CJD in mostly elderly patients, with muscle jerking and definitive periodic EEG activity, or spikes, appearing later as almost set diagnostic markers. In the American victims, at least, visual disturbances, ataxia and coordination problems were the first signs. There was little or no dementia, or muscle jerking or periodic EEG activity.

The symptoms of sporadic CJD and centrally-infected CJD (when CJD-infected tissue is injected straight into the brain) are remarkably similar. When the infection is introduced via another route, such as by injection into a muscle, as was the case for hGH recipients, or by ingestion or through mucous membranes, as was the case with kuru, it is called peripheral infection. Symptoms common in a central infection, such as dementia, are often late or absent altogether in peripheral infection. Cases in which transmission of CJD has occurred accidentally, as in hGH contamination, invariably start with physical symptoms such as ataxia. They are more like kuru than sporadic CJD.

Paul Brown has since proposed that it was the different origins of infection rather than the timing of the infection itself that could explain the major differences between sporadic and iatrogenic (accidental) infection that occurred between elderly patients and hGH recipients. It was the unique case of the 16-year-old girl who had died of pneumonia while in the pre-symptomatic stage of CJD that provided support for his contention.[32]

Dr Mike Harrington, an affable, talented Scotsman, became interested in proteins while studying medicine at the University of Glasgow in the mid-1970s. Fascinated by cerebrospinal fluid, what it contained and how certain proteins in the fluid might be indicators for disease elsewhere in the body, Harrington abandoned his medical studies for a career in biomedical research. He was offered a job at the NIH, in Carl Merril's laboratory, part of the biochemical genetics section of the clinical neurogenetics branch of the National Institute of Mental Health. Soon after his arrival in 1983, Harrington phoned a very interested Gajdusek, whose laboratory was on the same campus, to ask for spinal fluid samples from CJD and kuru patients. As neither scrapie-associated fibrils (SAFs) nor prion proteins could be identified in spinal fluid, Harrington was keen to "to look for any markers that might be useful".[33] Six months later he was collaborating with Dr David Asher at Gajdusek's laboratory after a graduate student in Merril's lab, alarmed at the infectious nature of the material Harrington was working with, told him "you'd better not bring that stuff in here!"

By 1985, working with 100 samples of spinal fluid, Harrington had isolated two separate proteins that appeared to the non-scientist, in test results on paper, like two blurred dots. The two proteins, called 130 and 131, were found in the cerebrospinal fluid of all 21 CJD victims from whom Harrington was able to obtain samples before death. The proteins also showed up in all five cases of herpes encephalitis in samples obtained before death. None of the three kuru patients, nor the more than 71 other mainly neurological disorder cases had these two proteins in their spinal fluid. CJD and herpes encephalitis both affect the brain, but the symptoms of each are quite distinctive. The herpes simplex virus causes herpes encephalitis. It is the same virus responsible for cold sores, shingles and the dreaded genital herpes. Acute illness follows within hours of infection.

In preliminary results published in July 1986, Harrington and colleagues stated:

Despite the unknown origin of proteins 130 and 131, these preliminary findings of their apparent specificity in Creutzfeldt-Jakob disease and herpes simplex encephalitis suggest that their presence in spinal fluid may be of considerable help in differentiating Creutzfeldt-Jakob disease from other common types of human dementia, particularly Alzheimer's disease.[34]

But developing a test from these results required time, effort and money — and too much of each. Not only was it was expensive and inconvenient to get the spinal fluid from patients, it was not predictive. It couldn't be used to tell who would develop the disease and who would not. It was put to its best use in adding to tentative diagnoses of CJD, before sufferers died. Confirmation still depended on telltale microscopic holes, plaques, other degeneration in the brain and transmission to laboratory animals where practicable.

The test in that limited form of 1986 became known as the Harrington spot test. Its distinctive protein duo was used initially to assist in the diagnosis in 1987 of the Pennsylvania patient and Deborah McKenzie. But until it could be simplified, and the time it took to analyse the results was shortened, it would remain merely an aid to diagnosis, and not a test marker. In 1988 Harrington moved to the California Institute of Technology (Caltech). He did not lose hope that his test could one day be improved and marketed as a useful diagnostic tool.

Also by 1988, when seven cases of CJD had appeared in former hGH recipients in America and Britain, it was hoped that the extent of the "micro-epidemic" was over.[35] This perceived "fall" in the number of CJD cases resulting from hGH use was noted by endocrinologists far away in New Zealand. Attempts were made to trace and offer information to all 350-odd New Zealand recipients of human hormone drugs in 1985. But some members of the clinical subcommittee of the National Hormone Committee were reluctant to cause "unnecessary alarm" by tracking everyone and warning them in 1988 not to offer to donate their organs, blood or tissue. Instead it was deemed that the Department of Health should notify blood banks and transplant units of the risk of using donations from pituitary hGH recipients.[36,37]

Joe Rodriguez, with his years and years of hormone treatment and horrible but quick decline and death, became known in the scientific literature as the index case of CJD in a growth hormone recipient. Had his parents not kept in touch with his treating doctor, Raymond Hintz, the tragic string of cases that followed him may have remained hidden for much longer.

CHAPTER 10

Jane Allender:
The price of infertility

A SUDDEN HUSH DESCENDED over the audience. All eyes were fixed on the woman with glossy shoulder-length hair who struggled to haul herself out of her wheelchair. As she leaned heavily on two attendants, one of them adjusted the blue tie of her black graduation gown. The other tried to steady her jerky movements. In contrast to the other graduating students who strode purposefully across the dais of the University of Adelaide's Bonython Hall, this 40-year-old woman staggered, looking as if she might fall as she attempted to cross the floor.

What struck the audience most of all was her radiant smile. For no-one who shook hands with Dame Roma Mitchell, the university's vice-chancellor, during that ceremony looked happier than Jane Allender. On that clear, crisp autumn day in 1988 Jane had fulfilled her life's dream of becoming an architect. And seated under the vaulted arches of this imposing hall, witnessing her halting progress with a combination of pride and pain, were her two children.

Lee, two years older than his 10-year-old sister Kate, found it hard to watch his mother. He saw the way her head lolled, and how easily she could slip from the grip of the two attendants. "This is horrible," he thought.[1] But a moment later, he was cheering inwardly when she shook hands with the regal-looking Dame Roma, the first Australian woman to become a judge and later the Governor of South Australia, who gave his mother the piece of paper he thought he would never see.

She had worked so hard for this. For years all he could remember was seeing her bent over her books, always studying. Lee had often resented the time she had spent, consumed by her goal. But with maturity beyond his years, he realised she had done it so that she could give him and Kate whatever they needed.

So now she was an architect at last. A feeling of unease trickled over him, like it had so often recently. Would she ever be able to work now? For months he'd watched her deteriorating — initially just staggering occasionally, later pushing herself along with a walking frame. Now she was mainly restricted to the wheelchair. He'd noticed her speech becoming slurred, and the way she began to forget things, needing more and more help with everything she did. It upset him to see her stuck in bed, fed mulched-up food. Lee couldn't understand what was going on, but he had a gut feeling that she'd never be her old self again.

For one woman in the audience, Jane's graduation was a bitter-sweet moment. Pam Mayo and Jane went back a long way. They had been good friends and bridesmaids to each other, Jane marrying first in December 1969. As the next graduate was called, Pam catalogued the years in her mind. Before each had married there were the parties, the boyfriends and the interior design course at the South Australian Institute of Technology. When they had finished there had been the short, fun stint when they had set up business together. Jane had gone on to work her way through the ranks of the South Australian Public Buildings Department as an interior designer. Later there had been all that trouble Jane had had falling pregnant, and then the decision to take a course of some miracle drug to help her conceive. The injections had worked, and Pam could still remember Jane's delight at finally becoming a mother. Then in 1980, only two years after Kate was born, Jane and Ted Allender had divorced. In recent years Jane had wondered aloud to Pam about whether the fertility treatment had contributed to her failed marriage.

Pam remembered Jane talking her into doing a refresher course and upgrading her design qualifications to a diploma in 1982. Jane had then decided against doing the same herself, in favour of using exemptions available from the interior design course to study architecture. Pam watched her friend stumble down the stage and lurch heavily into her wheelchair. "What an incredible waste," she thought angrily, as her mind flicked over Jane's six long years of hard work, struggle and determination. All for what? As the rest of the students accepted their degrees, Pam tried to sort out the course of her friend's illness. Her first inkling of something wrong had been six months earlier.

Jane had completed her thesis and had arrived for lunch and a chat. Jane had refused her offer of a second glass of wine. "No, I don't want any more. I feel drunk already," she had said before adding, "in fact I feel drunk all the time."[2] Pam had also noticed that Jane had put on weight around her arms and upper body, a marked change from her usually enviably slender figure. When Jane mentioned a problem with her sense of balance, Pam had rejoined: "Maybe it's all due to the stress of exams and coping with kids. Your holiday in Singapore after Christmas will probably be just what you need." Jane had nodded, brightening.

Another friend present at Jane's graduation had noticed her movements becoming slightly clumsy about the same time — just before Christmas 1987. Michael Cant, who had intermittently dated Jane from the time she began her degree course, had promised her a night out when her studies were over. But as he twirled her around the dance floor at the Grand Hotel at Glenelg — a famous coastal suburb in Adelaide — he was surprised how heavy she was on her feet and how her movements were slightly awkward. "You're dancing like a duck," he'd teased, meaning that she was waddling rather than dancing. Now, watching her lurch across the dais, the memory of that remark made him wince.[3]

Unfortunately, the holiday in Singapore that Pam had prescribed as a cure did not have the desired result. In fact Jane felt so ill with headaches and tiredness that she was forced to cut the trip short. Kate, who at 10 already had her mother's good looks, well remembers those frightening episodes in a strange country when her mother grabbed hold of her crossing the road to steady herself. Instead of shopping and sightseeing with her daughter and mother, Ruth Iliffe, Jane had put herself to bed in the hotel, too tired to stir. Nan had told Kate in her matter-of-fact way that it was probably just stress from her exams and that Jane would feel better if she rested. But Kate thought it odd that her mother couldn't even come shopping.

Kate craned her neck to see her mother, her head nodding slightly, sitting in her wheelchair beside the other graduates. This should have been a great day. It wasn't fair. She'd done all that work, for so long, and now she couldn't even walk. She needed help to do just about everything. Nan was worried that Mum was putting on too much weight. Sometimes Kate used to sneak in extra food when Nan wasn't looking, because her Mum would get really hungry. She felt her father's gaze on her and looked away.

Ted Allender, a tall striking man, his hair lightly sprinkled with grey at 40, was also thinking back to the Singapore holiday. It was just after Jane's return that he had first noticed something badly wrong. While Jane and Kate had been in Singapore, during Australia's bicentenary "celebrations" in January 1988, he had taken Lee on a sailing ship. They'd had a great time standing on deck as the *Failie 3* forged its way through the waves for more than a week from Sydney, south through Bass Strait and west to its home base in Adelaide. But the day he returned Lee to the comfortable home in Bracken Road, Stirling, a suburb in the leafy Adelaide Hills where he had lived with Jane and the children for most of their 11-year marriage, Ted saw that Jane wasn't herself. As she walked towards them, he was immediately struck by how unsteady she was, clinging to the wall for support. "I feel tired and dizzy and my legs ache," she told him.[4]

Despite their divorce seven years before, they had remained on good terms. Watching her, Ted felt a surge of admiration for this gutsy woman who had somehow found the strength to attend her graduation despite her obvious ill-health. For the thousandth time Ted wondered how it was possible that a healthy, vital woman could be grossly afflicted with a condition that had baffled a phalanx of doctors during her hospital stays in both February and April that year.

Initially she had been admitted to the Wakefield Street Memorial Hospital and, shortly before the graduation, there had been a second stint at the Flinders Medical Centre. Now, watching her doped to the eyeballs with Valium to control her wild involuntary muscle contractions, Ted puzzled over the other mystery. The Jane he had married had been a happy-go-lucky, quiet but fun-loving woman. But after the children were born she had changed. Thinking back over their marriage he had to admit that the fertility treatment had not helped.

Jane had kept a diary of her treatment with FSH through the Queen Elizabeth Hospital. Each visit was noted, each consultation. Under the page May 23, 1975, Jane had noted "QEH injection". The same notation was made for the next day, and the next, and the next. May 27 had the simple entry "fertile". On May 28, 1975, Jane had noted "QEH ov. injection — fertile". And the next day she was still fertile.[5] As more students got up to receive their degrees, Ted remembered with a wry grin having to rush home and perform husbandly duties when the hormone levels showed Jane was about to ovulate. This went on month after frustrating month, and was not conducive to a relaxed and spontaneous relationship. It had put enormous pressure on them both.

But, Ted remembered, September 29, 1975, had been the day that made it all worthwhile. "Pregnancy test through," Jane had written in her diary. "Pregnant for four weeks." Jane's dream of being a mother was realised with the birth of Lee Michael Allender on May 14, 1976. Jane was equally keen for another child. Treatment at the Queen Elizabeth Hospital fertility clinic this time resulted in a pregnancy with the oral ovulation-stimulating drug, Clomid. Kate Louise Allender was born on New Year's Day, 1978.

Jane was depressed after Kate was born. But even when she improved she was uncharacteristically insecure. She seemed unable to make her mind up about anything, even which shoes to buy. Sometimes she bought shoes only to change her mind later and have to return them. She consulted her mother about the smallest things, a habit that irritated Ted intensely. He put it down to continuing hormonal changes, not really knowing what else to think of her increasingly restless and irrational behaviour. "You need a break, why don't you have a holiday?" Ted suggested.

So Jane went to Paris for a month to stay with friends in late 1979 while Ted remained in Adelaide with the children. But when she returned, Jane, giving in to tears, told Ted she wanted to return overseas. Communicating became a strain and the relationship deteriorated to the point where Ted and Jane separated in July 1980.

In the months that followed, a male photographer called Jan, whom Jane had met while in Europe, came to stay. They got on well and the relationship took a serious turn when Jan suggested Jane and the children go to live with him in England and see how things developed. And things went well for a time. They travelled, spent some time in Greece and took pictures of the children among the ruins in Athens. Jane and Ted were divorced while she was away. The decree nisi was confirmed by telephone to Jane in England on December 21, 1981.

But living arrangements in Jan's bachelor flat in London with Jane, the children and, for a period, Jane's mother, Ruth, were not ideal. An English winter dampened everything, including the relationship and Jane returned with the children to Stirling.

Ted, who by that time had formed a new relationship, saw them often. As time passed, he noticed a gradual evolution away from the quiet, considerate, selfless person he had married. Jane, he felt, had become an obsessive, compulsive worrier — aspects of her new character that had played a significant part in his leaving the marriage. It was as if Jane's whole personality had been altered. The shoe-buying problem, enough to drive anyone mad, was later extended to haircuts. How much to cut off, what style, when to make the appointment. Jane still seemed incapable of making the smallest decisions without consulting her mother.

But it was not only that. Ted noticed that her worrying had extended to not allowing the children out in the sun, even for a few minutes, without being slathered in sun cream. Lee had wanted a bike, like all his other friends, but Jane worried that he might fall and hurt himself. When Ted had finally bought one after weeks of Jane considering it, she insisted that he wear a helmet — merely to ride around in the back yard. Even the children were irritated.

Home security became a big matter, which alternately staggered and amused Ted when the children told him of it during visits in late 1986 and early 1987. Kate remembers that Jane would check and recheck each door and window in the house every night, ticking off each one on a plain waxed card. Given that the house was set back slightly from the road, and was almost invisible to neighbours because of native bush and trees, Kate thought that perhaps this was natural.[6] Jane even asked a neighbour to park his car next to hers in the carport, to give the impression that more than one adult lived there. Even Jane knew this was a bit extreme. On one of their semi-regular lunches with the children, Jane told Pam Mayo she knew she had an obsession, one that was causing her to lose sleep. "It's crazy. I can't bear it," Jane said. "I get into bed and I can't remember if I've bolted the door, locked the door, locked the windows and done this and that so I have to get up and check it. Then I get back into bed and I'm still worried."[7]

As Pam Mayo made her way with the Allender family group from Bonython Hall to the celebratory gathering at the university canteen following the graduation ceremony, she recalled that Jane's Singapore trip had highlighted, rather than improved, Jane's deteriorating health. She remembered clearly that scorching day in February 1988 — was it only three months ago — when Jane had telephoned her. "I'm in the Wakefield Street Memorial Hospital, having all sorts of tests to see why I'm lurching instead of walking," Jane said in a matter-of-fact tone. "They're trying to find out what's wrong with me. Can you pop over for a visit?"

Although doctors had taken blood samples, performed a lumbar puncture and subjected her to a series of EEG scans to measure the electrical activity in her brain, they had not been able to diagnose her problem. Various conditions including MS and a brain tumour were suggested. Pam, who hadn't seen her friend since their December lunch, had been shocked when she'd seen Jane. Only two months had passed, yet Jane had had to lean against a railing just to walk down the hospital corridor.

Michael Cant also had visited Jane in hospital, and had once taken a bottle of champagne to cheer her up, but she'd hardly touched it. She was too upset at the prospect of having to cancel a job interview for a position she had hoped to fill with a firm of architects. All those dreams, all that work, and now it was within her grasp, she was too ill to work.

Jane had attempted a letter to her friend Angie, an architecture student from Singapore, in March, describing what had happened to her the previous December 1987. But by then her handwriting was barely legible and it was never posted.

"This illness finally reared its ugly head during the last weeks of my B. Arch Degree," she wrote. "I was at the time working on my final project … marking the finish of the Degree. I was suffering from a virus at the time. I had a migraine, vomiting and severe aching legs and joints. I was," she began in a jerky scrawl, crossing out the word "bed" until the next occurred to her "refined [sic] to bed".

"I rang the uni, told them that I'm not going to get the final project in — requested an extension. I was knocked back! Worked hard to get it finished, another mistake but I ended up getting the project in, however not coloured." Jane underlined the last two words and went on to explain how she had later completed the colouring. "The results I received 70% for the project — the year's work 68 — I had done it … I went to see Dr Brummitt, my local doctor. I complained of dizziness and he took my blood pressure. It was normal. Asked me to walk in a straight line — I could not …"

In April there were more tests when Jane was admitted to the Flinders

Medical Centre, where she came under the care of Professor Richard Burns, the senior director of neurology. She also talked several times with the neurology registrar, Dr Jeffrey Cochius, who was only a few months into his neurology training.

"My dear Angie," Jane wrote from the hospital. "I have been here since Monday. I am now starting to get fed up with hospital routine and would like to be home — but the tests are still going on! I am at this hospital purly [sic] for seeing Professor Burns, Professory [sic] of neurolo" she trailed off without finishing the word.

"Tests! I am fed up with tests. I have had everything from brain scans, lumba [sic] punctures, electric shocks, brain current measurement etc etc — I OK. No tumours — a relief. My problem is one of walking and stability. When I try to walk it's very wobbly and easily fall — it's so crazy when 2 months ago I was normal."

"I had an interview offered to me at Woods Bagot [an established large architecture firm in Adelaide]. Unfortunately I had to ring them and explain the situation — but they were very good saying they will hold it open for me. I have to ring them on Friday — I don't want to turn it down but may be I will have to ..."

The tests again failed to result in a definitive diagnosis. Jane's family became increasingly worried. There were new and disturbing developments. Her speech was becoming slurred and she often lost concentration. Every time she returned home after a new bout of tests, she grew physically more frail.

In April, when Pam Mayo made her first visit to Jane at the Flinders Medical Centre, her friend was agitated and slightly confused. "They've told me I've got this weird disease," Jane confided, "but it's not true. I know I've got a brain tumour and they're just not telling me." Pam was nonplussed. She had spoken with Jane's mother on the phone that morning and Mrs Iliffe, a former nursing sister, had told her there was definitely no sign of a brain tumour. But Jane would not be put off by Pam's denials and kept insisting in a panic-stricken voice that she had a brain tumour. "Look, it is," she kept insisting. "They are just not telling me. They're trying to fob me off."

Upset at her friend's state of mind, Pam decided to investigate the situation herself. She left Jane in her shared room and strode over to the nurses' station. She spoke to a nurse there. "Look, Jane's really in a state because she's convinced she's got a brain tumour, and I've been told it's not, so could you come and explain to her while I'm here what it actually is?"

The nurse came to the point quickly. "Your friend has a deteriorating disease of the brain." She paused. "And it's fatal."

Pam's head swam. It was too much to take in so suddenly. "How long will it take?" she whispered.

"It could be six to nine months," was the reply.

Pam was stunned and disbelieving at the same time. This was Jane the popular, the one with all the boyfriends, the girl whose long, slim legs Pam had envied when they went shopping for hotpants while studying for their interior design course. The one with the big brown eyes and smooth honey-brown hair that had given her the Jean Shrimpton look just when it was all the rage in the late 1960s. How could Jane be dying? And from what?

The nurse mentioned a strange foreign-sounding name, which she abbreviated to CJ disease. When Pam and the nurse returned to the ward, Jane looked up. The nurse had told Pam that Jane's condition had been explained to her by several doctors the previous day. This time she was determined Jane should understand and accept the news. "You don't have a brain tumour," the nurse began slowly but clearly. "As the doctors explained to you, they think you have a brain disease called Creutzfeldt-Jakob disease, which means that your brain will deteriorate further and further until it stops functioning altogether and you die," she said flatly.

Jane's face was stony. When the nurse finished speaking, Jane said in an expressionless voice, "So I'll just become a vegetable?"

The nurse was direct. "Yes, that's what's going to happen."

Jane looked up at her friend, who was still mute not only from the news of Jane's condition but from what she considered the brutal frankness of the nurse. "Pam, just pick something up and hit me over the head will you?" Pam understood what she meant. After leaving school, Jane had worked for a time at the Spastic Centre, nursing children with severe brain damage. "I don't want to end up like that," Jane whispered, almost to herself, "and as far as I know, that's going to happen. So just hit me over the head. I can't bear the thought of that happening."

"Let's get a coffee," Pam suggested, helping Jane into a wheelchair.

In the coffee shop downstairs, above the clatter of cups and saucers, the murmur of muted conversations, and in spite of her impaired speech and broken concentration, Jane succeeded in communicating her shattered feelings. She cried because she realised that what lay ahead was not the hope of recovery, but certain death.

The memory of that conversation brought a lump to Pam's throat a month later as she gazed at the cool and lofty arches of Bonython Hall as Jane was wheeled outside. She could still hear the agony in Jane's voice as she accepted that her condition meant there was no brain tumour but something infinitely worse. "Oh God, this is terrible," Jane had said. "I can't believe it. All I want to do is see my children grow up. It's not fair. That's all I want out of life — just to see them grow up."

Watching her daughter's graduation ceremony, Ruth Iliffe's heart was breaking. Jane was her only child, and they were very close, especially since the divorce. Jane needed their help, and she and her husband Michael, gave it unstintingly — whether it involved financial assistance, minding the children, or Michael, a retired university lecturer in maths and physics, helping Jane with the harder mathematical component of her course. In the past months, they had devoted themselves to caring for her because she could no longer look after herself. In the natural scheme of things, children bury their parents, not the other way around. Watching Jane deteriorate before their eyes had been unbearably painful.

As Ruth's anxious eyes rested on her daughter, by now bloated from over-eating and unable to walk properly, she clung to the hope that Jane would pull through this. Deep down, however, she knew the moment of triumph had come and gone, and the worst was yet to come. At the postgraduation gathering, Jane smiled widely but was clearly only partially aware of her surroundings. When Lee, referring to Dame Roma, asked what "the Queen lady" had said to her while she was on the dais, Jane frowned momentarily. "I can't remember," she replied.[8]

Watching her and noting Jane's worsening short-term memory, Ted was thinking back to the first time he had heard doctors put a name to the condition. The personality changes he had noted since their divorce had become profound by the time Jane's physical symptoms appeared. But was it really only a few short weeks ago that they had learned, by persevering with their questions, the tentative but probable and shattering diagnosis?

On a visit to Jane's house he had come across a note lying on the dining table that Ruth explained had been left for her by one of the doctors who came so often to see Jane. "The cause for the unsteadiness and the memory problems is most probably a slow virus. Unfortunately there is no specific treatment for this infection of the brain," the note had stated.

On behalf of her daughter, Ruth had then written some questions on the back of the piece of paper.

1. Name of virus?
2. How common is it?
3. What part of the brain is it in?
4. Do you know definitely what course it will take — or is it an unknown quantity?
5. How did I catch it?
6. Are there any ways to help — antibiotics?

On the next medical visit and beside the first two questions, a doctor had written in bold capitals "Possibly JAKOB CREUTZFELDT".

Ted had been in Sydney on a business trip when the answer was filled in. While showering in his hotel room, the phone had rung. It was Ruth, and her usually controlled voice had sounded shaken. "They've found out what caused Jane's illness," she'd said. Before he could say anything, she'd continued: "They say she got it as a result of that fertility treatment she had. It's some sort of virus, apparently, a foreign-sounding name I've never heard of. They said she'll be dead in two to six months".[9]

With that knowledge, the request for him to come into the Flinders Medical Centre the previous month made more sense. Although confined to a wheelchair with her head wobbling in a disconcerting way, Jane had still been mentally alert. The social worker sat Ted and the children down with her and explained that Jane was suffering from a non-specific disease of the cerebellum — the part of the brain that controlled all motor function and movements like walking — which was incurable, untreatable and irreversible. He would have to look after the children from then on.

By that time the father of another daughter, Morgan, who had been born in 1983, Ted had realised his own life would change dramatically. He told a friend who was a GP. "Are you sure it's Creutzfeldt-Jakob?" asked the GP. At Ted's nod he was clearly shocked. "She's too young for that. That's very bad news. There's no treatment and it's always fatal. She won't live, you know." He explained to Ted in as much detail as his limited knowledge would allow that the disease usually attacked people in their late fifties and sixties. It could not be treated or cured because it had a long latency period — decades sometimes — during which time the brain was damaged to the point where the physical symptoms, including staggering and jerking, arose.

It was Professor Rick Burns at the Flinders Medical School, who made the vital connection between Jane's illness and her past history. After discussions with the QEH fertility clinic and an examination of her medical records, he found she had been treated with hPG in 1975, the drug that Ted and Jane had known as FSH. Burns remembered several medical journal articles back in 1985 and 1986 that had reported cases of CJD in young people treated in the United States with hGH. If his suspicions were correct, Jane would be the first person to have contracted CJD as a result of taking pituitary hormones to induce fertility. Certainly her symptoms were consistent with CJD, but Burns knew he had to be circumspect as there was no diagnostic test for CJD.

Ted had talked about the case with Cochius, the neurology registrar who had first assessed Jane on admission to Flinders Medical Centre. Cochius knew about her obsessive-compulsive behaviour with the windows and doors at her home, and had initially thought her staggering walk might have been hysterical, in other words part of some underlying psychological problem. Cochius was just 30 years old and in his first year of neurology training, fascinated by all types of diseases of the brain and central nervous system. He particularly remembered Jane telling him that when she was holidaying in Singapore in January she had realised she was swimming crookedly, veering off to one side. "That's weird," he'd thought, "I've never heard of that problem before".[10]

Cochius had never seen a case of CJD, although he'd heard about it. He was interested when Burns took Jane's history again, conducted all the same tests and proposed CJD — a possibility that had not occurred to him. And the diagnosis seemed to fit. This was despite Jane's relative youth at age 40, and not having obvious signs of dementia, a common early symptom in elderly sporadic victims of the disease. To diagnose CJD definitely, they both knew Jane Allender's brain would have to be examined after her death. It was agreed that such an unusual case should be reported in the medical literature.

Almost as if the anticipation of her graduation had buoyed her up and kept her going, once it was over, Jane went downhill rapidly. The family hired two nurses to provide 24-hour care. Jane lost her sense of time, and her sleeping cycles varied constantly. One by one her bodily functions stopped. She lost her speech, her sight, became partially paralysed and incontinent. Her jaws seized and periodic convulsions and fits of uncontrollable tremors left her exhausted. Her facial expressions were deranged and shocking to family and friends who visited. Worried in case she caught the severe flu that was rampant in Adelaide at the end of May 1988, her parents bundled her off to their holiday cottage on Kangaroo Island, off the coast of South Australia. It overlooked the unique tidal Pelican Lagoon and conservation park where she had spent many happy days as a child.

They made a sad entourage on the ferry from Cape Jervis to Penneshaw, the worried elderly couple, the two children and the woman so incapacitated that she could not manage to get out of the car, but spent the entire crossing sitting inside it. Ted, who didn't accompany them to Kangaroo Island, loaded Jane's stainless steel hospital bed and wheelchair on to the ferry. He waved at the two children Jane had so desperately wanted to have, and felt a pang to see her so helpless inside the car, her head rolling around, her eyes not focused, and her hands curling up like claws. She looked like an elderly person with Alzheimer's disease, not a woman in the prime of her life.

The beauty and tranquillity of Pelican Lagoon were usually uplifting. But by now, Jane was unaware of anything going on around her. Two months later, on August 10, 1988, Jane developed pneumonia and was taken by air ambulance to the Flinders Medical Centre.

Ted rushed to the hospital from Mildura, hundreds of kilometres to the east on the Victorian border where he was working. All the weight she had gained had gone. Jane had become skeletal and lay curled in a foetal position. Cochius, too, was shocked to see her so wasted physically on her admission to the emergency department. She was not eating, talking or understanding anything. Large abscesses had broken out on her neck and she could hardly breathe. Burns sought permission from Ruth Iliffe to perform an autopsy to enable confirmation of CJD. She gave it on the understanding that the results would be forwarded to her when available.

Two days later, Ted received a telephone call from the hospital. "If you're planning to bring the children in to see Jane this afternoon, it's probably better if you don't," he was advised. "Jane is in the throes of passing away and it's not a pretty sight. It will be very disturbing for them to see her like this." At 11 p.m. that night Ted had the distressing task of telling his children that their mother had died.

Just before they left for Kangaroo Island where he and Kate temporarily attended a local school, Lee had had a sudden premonition that his mother would never come home again and had run for his camera to take a photograph of the hospital bed in their lounge room. But his conscious mind continued to deny what his instincts already knew. "The doctors can make her better," was his constant thought as he watched his mother slide into a coma. But on August 14, 1988, when Ted broke the news, the blow was sudden and terrible for Lee and Kate. They heard the words that their mother was dead, but it didn't make sense.

On a wintry August day, Jane Louise Allender, just 41, was cremated. It was a sad, simple and restrained funeral. While the minister spoke movingly about a young life snatched away, Ted kept a watchful eye to make sure everybody was all right, especially the children. He'd taken them to counsellors when it was clear Jane was going to die, to help prepare them. They had resisted. They didn't want to talk about their mother with outsiders, and on this day too their distress was too deep to find a release in tears.

Jane's ashes were taken to the American River Cemetery on Kangaroo Island. As if the enormous stress of Jane's illness had sapped their strength, her parents' own health declined rapidly after her death. Michael Iliffe, then 78, told Ted after the funeral that he had nothing more to live for. He was soon diagnosed with Alzheimer's disease, went blind and died in May 1994. Ruth, then still a spritely 74, later suffered a stroke that left her speech impaired. She died in April 1995.

It took several years for Lee to start letting out some of the pain he'd bottled up about his mother's death. By that time he was so severely depressed he needed psychiatric treatment, which finally allowed him to acknowledge that he blamed himself for his mother's death. If not for him, he reasoned, she never would have received those hormone injections that had infected her with the deadly disease.

Ted's anger was immediate and closer to the surface. From the moment that Jane died, he had the conviction that something was seriously wrong with the whole story. Various officers of the Federal Department of Health denied knowledge of Jane's case, which Ted found more than strange given that the hPG she had received had been Federal-Government sponsored. But his attempts to establish a definitive link between Jane's fertility treatment and her death were met with a deafening silence — a silence that would not be explained for another four years.

Like a frustrated detective who discovers that most of the clues are missing, Ted immediately embarked on his own investigation into how Jane contracted CJD. His first problem was to find a way to penetrate the arcane world of medical jargon and legal procedure, where the answers to his questions lay hidden. A first step was acquiring the post-mortem report, since the family had not been told officially the cause of Jane's death. Apart from that scrap of paper mentioning the possibility of CJD, which one of the medicos had left on the kitchen table, there would be and could be no confirmation without the pending autopsy report.

Ruth Iliffe was never contacted again by any doctor. Ted wrote to Burns requesting Jane's pathology reports in September 1988. The following month he was given a letter by Jane's GP, Dr Peter Brummitt. In the letter Burns stated that the cerebellum had yet to be studied in detail.

This is just a short note to let you know that the diagnosis of Jakob-Creutzfeldt Disease has just been confirmed at post-mortem examination. I have reviewed the slides today with the pathologists. We are undertaking the process of writing her case up because of the very important social implications amongst other things.[11]

Certainly the health authorities were aware of a link between Jane's hPG treatment and her death. It was clear from the bottom of Burns' letter that a copy had been forwarded to Professor Leslie Lazarus, the former head of HPAC, which oversaw the AHPHP under which Jane had been treated.

Six months after his initial request, Ted received the full post-mortem report from Professor Burns. It had just become available to him from the pathologist, Dr P. Blumbergs. It detailed the widespread spongiform destruction of the brain, which confirmed again "the features are those of Jakob-Creutzfeldt Disease".[12] Ted also wrote to the Centers for

Disease Control in Atlanta. The reply was unequivocal. Never had they seen a report of a single case of CJD following hPG injections.

On March 30, 1989, the day he received Jane's full post-mortem report, Ted again rang the Federal Department of Health and was referred to the Australian Drug Evaluation Committee (ADEC). Ted wanted to know if a report had been made to its Adverse Drug Reactions Advisory Committee (ADRAC) because Jane's death would surely come under that category. He also mentioned that he was about to seek legal advice. Promptly the next day, a letter was sent from ADEC to Ted Allender. It stated that ADRAC "cannot involve itself in matters of legal redress", that a formal written report providing all details would have to be provided for assessment, and that he should approach Jane's treating doctor to provide a report to ADRAC.[13]

If Jane did contract CJD as a result of treatment she had received in a public hospital, it occurred to Ted that there could be a case for compensation. A healthy woman had undergone treatment to have a baby and had died as a result. Two young children had lost their mother. In early April he contacted a prominent Queen's Counsel in Adelaide. The opinion, however, was not encouraging. One isolated case of disease and death was insufficient to prove any link with the fertility treatment, Ted was told. Even if compensation was possible, because Jane was not working when she died nor was she the sole provider for the children, the payout was likely to be small.

In April 1989 Ted also paid for a Medline database search in America of all medical journal reports on CJD. As the computer spewed out reams of paper filled with every reference to a scientific or medical publication on the condition, he discovered what had happened in 1985, when the deaths of three young men from CJD first alerted American specialists to the lethal link between the disease and hGH.

In the meantime Jeffrey Cochius, Jane's neurology registrar, had written a draft letter to the *Lancet*. He thought the world should be alerted to this unusual probable cause of CJD. His submission, among the thousands of letters received annually, "just failed to win a place" despite its subject matter being of interest to readers, a reply from the *Lancet* stated.[14] Undeterred, Cochius sent a reworked article to the *Australian and New Zealand Journal of Medicine*. But it would be late in 1990 before it was published.

In the long, cold winter of 1989, Ted felt discouraged and isolated. He had moved back into Jane's home at Stirling with the children. He found it distressing to see Lee and Kate so disturbed and frequently reduced to angry tears. He organised more psychological counselling, but they baulked at attending. It was too painful. And as a family they felt isolated. Many friends and acquaintances shunned them in the months after Jane's death. They felt uncomfortable, not knowing what to say following such a tragedy. So former friends said nothing at all.

Ted's requests for Jane's fertility-related medical records from the Queen Elizabeth Hospital in April 1989, after the advice from ADEC on reporting adverse drug reactions, met with shrugs and denials. No-one, it seemed, knew anything about a woman called Jane Allender who had spent much of 1975 being treated with a hormone called hPG. "By now it was obvious something was really wrong," Ted recalled.

On May 22, 1989, a letter did arrive, not from the hospital but from the Crown solicitor. Ted was informed that on the information provided to the Queen Elizabeth Hospital, it appeared that Jane had been a private patient of Professor Lloyd Woodrow Cox. After a consultation, Cox had referred her as an outpatient to the Queen Elizabeth Hospital where she received FSH. The letter stated that it was believed that Cox was still in possession of her case notes. It included an explanation about the source of the FSH. It was of human pituitary origin, produced, tested and packaged at CSL. The drug had been distributed with the permission of HPAC by the Commonwealth Department of Health. A register of all ampoules and their batch numbers had been kept by HPAC's head, Dr Leslie Lazarus, by then director of clinical research at the Garvan Institute in Sydney.

That was the only official information sent to Ted Allender, despite all his inquiries in the aftermath of his former wife's death. And so, preoccupied with other personal problems, Ted ran out of steam and reluctantly gave up his investigations. He had a gut feeling the silence was conspiratorial, designed to hide any mistake that may have been made, and that his efforts to break it would never reveal exactly how Jane had been exposed to CJD.

Unknown to Ted Allender, Jane's death was of major concern, both to neurologists and gynaecologists who had treated several thousand women and men with hPG throughout Australia, New Zealand and

Britain in the 1960s, 1970s and 1980s. Nor did Ted know that quite a lot of people — including the very peripherally involved chief health officer of the Department of Health, Dr Tony Adams, who had been informed of the CJD diagnostic confirmation in November 1988 by Lazarus — were aware of the link between Jane's hPG treatment and her death. Her own former gynaecologist, Cox — who had been another of the hundreds present at the University of Adelaide graduation ceremony where Jane had to be helped to and from the dais — told a later inquiry that he did not know the reason for her obvious ill-health.[15]

In August 1990 Jane Allender's case history was published in an article in the *Australian and New Zealand Journal of Medicine*. Cochius, Burns and colleagues from the Flinders Medical Centre described her case as "unique in that it is the first report of CJD occurring in a recipient of human pituitary-derived gonadotrophin" and added that "approximately 90 women received injections from this particular batch".[16]

The reference to only one of the three batches from which Jane Allender was treated related to an inquiry in 1988 by Dr C. Alderman, the clinical pharmacist at Flinders Medical Centre. He had rung HPAC advising of a patient who had apparent CJD, and was told she had received hPG only from batch 44 when she in fact received hPG from batches 34 and 36 as well.

From the moment in August 1990 that news of Jane's case spread throughout the medical fraternity world-wide, doctors and scientists held their breath and hoped that hers would remain an isolated medical anomaly. None of them could foresee the tragedy already unfolding in a quaint little village in the English countryside.

CHAPTER 11

BSE and brains:
Transmission spreads

T HE TOLL from the mystery disease in cows climbed steadily after Kent vet Colin Whitaker saw Daisy the cow stumbling around in April 1985. But it was not until 18 months later, in 1986, that the Ministry of Agriculture, Fisheries and Food (MAFF) acknowledged the disease with an article in the *Veterinary Record*. In the time leading up to this report, there was no official warning that cows in largely dairy herds in southern England were dying of an exotic new disease. The disease was not included among those reported in the annual government report *Animal Health 1986*. And government vets employed by MAFF were firmly told not to speak publicly about the disease or associate it in any way with that dreaded scourge of sheep which it resembled — scrapie. At least not at first.

It was not until November 1987 that statistics on the diseased cattle were officially kept and that MAFF gave the condition a name: bovine spongiform encephalopathy, or BSE for short. It was another TSE, or so-called "prion" disease, and a relative of scrapie. Before long the British press had its own title — "mad cow" disease. The name stuck and soon became the euphemism for the best known of these mysterious diseases.

Charting the progress of the epidemic was difficult. Separate areas of government continually cited different figures. When BSE was named, 20 cattle were reported as infected. In June 1988 the *British Medical Journal* cited a government spokesman as saying there were 246 cases of BSE.[1] Yet only a month before, an editorial in the *Veterinary Record*[2] reported nearly double that number — 455 cases among the 12 million cattle in Britain. By summer, 731 BSE-affected cattle had been reported on 560 farms in Britain and the Channel Islands. Less than a year later, in February 1989, 2160 were reportedly confirmed on 1667 farms. Up to 400 new cases were being reported each week. Affected cattle at that stage ranged from three to 11 years old, and had been born between 1979 and 1984. They all had one thing in common — they had been fed commercial protein concentrates. These concentrates came in pellets of calf feed, a protein cake or protein supplements in mixed feed rations.

In the lean post-war years British cattle had been fed a protein supplement to increase milk yield. Beef herds were less likely to have eaten the protein supplement. The supplement came from meat and bone-meal extracted from sterilised animal waste that had been discarded from abattoirs, boning-out plants, butchers, knackeries and restaurants.

By 1988, 41 rendering plants were operating in Britain, producing 350,000 tonnes of meat and bonemeal and 230,000 tonnes of tallow for soap and candle manufacture from cattle, sheep, pigs and other animals, including poultry.[3]

During the first year of the outbreak — from the time Colin Whitaker saw the first cases in April 1985 — until November 1986 when it was first officially recognised by MAFF's Central Veterinary Laboratory,[4] BSE-infected cows were themselves sent to knackeries, rendered down and added to protein supplements being fed back to dairy herds. Naturally herbivorous cows were turned into carnivores. But eating the rendered down remnants of their own species turned them into cannibals and isolated BSE outbreaks became an epidemic.

Scientists continue to speculate on various theories for the cause of the BSE epidemic. The semi-official view is that some of the sheep carcasses rendered down and mashed up into a protein feed for cows and other animals had scrapie. As a result, a rare break occurred in the species barrier between sheep and cows. Changes in rendering practices introduced in the 1970s and particularly the early 1980s, when the rendering industry was deregulated, may have helped foster this break. One change was the elimination of fat-removing solvents when animal fat was no longer in demand for industry. The other and more important difference was the introduction of a "continuous flow" method of cooking carcasses. This method used lower temperature cooking over less time than for the previously used "batch" method of cooking animal remnants. One or both of these changes may have allowed the highly-resistant scrapie agent to survive the "cooking" with ease.

Another, similar, theory was that a single mutant strain among the more than 20 already known in scrapie had overcome the species barrier in cattle and had spread. From 1987, scrapie expert Alan Dickinson shared the view with colleagues that transfer of scrapie from sheep to cattle on many occasions was not the most likely possibility and that earlier cases than MAFF had identified had been recycled for longer than was appreciated. The species barrier to commonly occurring scrapie strains had been effective for centuries, with cattle and other animals co-grazing with sheep without problem. Dickinson claimed that equally likely was that BSE, rather than having occurred as a single transfer of a scrapie strain or spontaneous eruption in British cattle, came instead from an imported cow from another country: "Mechanically recovered meat [flayed from the spines of cattle and used as filling in meat pies, sausages, hamburgers] from these cattle was going to be hooching with infectivity. Absolutely socked, packed full of it, stuffed to the gills, yes".[5]

A fourth scenario according to Brian Ford, the sector chairman of the British Institute of Biology and science editor of the *Guinness Book of Records*, is that BSE had long been a disease of small incidence in cattle in Britain, quite distinct from, although similar to, scrapie. Feeding of the diseased cattle back to themselves, under changed and lower-temperature rendering practices, had caused the epidemic, he argued.[6] The use of dangerous organophosphorus compounds to control the warble fly pest, the over-use of fertilisers, and the lack of a particular dietary acid are other theories.

Critics of the British Government's performance in relation to the BSE epidemic point to little being done to stamp out the epidemic at the beginning. They say that BSE could have easily been controlled by slaughtering the herds it appeared in and stopping protein supplements being fed to cattle. They say the lack of any bold initiatives hangs on the fact that any such slaughter would have alienated farmers, traditionally Conservative voters, in the lead-up to the June 1987 general election. The Tory Party, led by Margaret Thatcher, was re-elected for a third straight term. A month later, government vets having already been gagged on the BSE resemblance to scrapie, Colin Whitaker — a non-government, independent vet — was asked not to mention the phrase "scrapie-like syndrome" during his presentation on BSE.

It was not until after the election that the Neuropathogenesis Unit in Edinburgh, one of the most knowledgeable bodies in the world on scrapie and similar TSEs in animals, was asked for help by MAFF's

Central Veterinary Laboratory. In April 1988 the British Government set up the Working Party on Bovine Spongiform Encephalopathy (WPBSE) with a group of appointed members. Chaired by the professor of zoology at the University of Oxford, Sir Richard Southwood, it had three other distinguished members and an adviser. Not one of them was an expert in TSEs, despite the presence of a body of such experts working in Britain in the scrapie field.

Around the same time, the first warning about possible transmission of BSE to humans appeared in the medical literature. Under the heading "For debate...", Tim Holt, then an intern at St James's Hospital in Balham, and the hospital's senior dietitian, J. Phillips sparked outcry with their letter to the *British Medical Journal* of June 4, 1988.

In strong language they warned that the new cattle disease currently affecting dairy herds could pose a serious risk to humans. They introduced the concept of kuru, which was diet-linked, and revealed that although animal brains were classified as prohibited offal in uncooked meat products, no such restraint applied to cooked cattle brains. In fact cooked products like meat pies, consommés, patés, tinned stews and stock cubes had brains and other mechanically recovered meats added to them almost routinely. It couldn't be listed as added meat, but it could be used for extra bulk. "... this is little comfort to those of us aware that the Creutzfeldt-Jakob disease agent can survive high temperatures."[7]

Holt and Phillips pointed out that farmers were not obliged at that time to report cases of BSE. Dairy farmers, those most affected, could either continue milking the cow until symptoms became unmanageable and they had to be culled, or send them straight to the abattoir as soon as the first signs of disease appeared. With the numbers of BSE cases probably under-reported, and brains available from butchers and frequently added to low cost canteen food, it was likely that the most infective parts of BSE-affected cattle — including those which were pre-symptomatic and killed while incubating the disease — were abundant in various parts of the British food supply. Another highly infective part of the animal, the spinal cord, was not routinely removed from chops, according to Holt and Phillips, who were most concerned that brains should be abolished from British food. At the very least, they should be more clearly defined on labelling.

That same month, June 1988, BSE became a notifiable disease. On June 21 that year, the day after the new WPBSE first met, it urgently recommended the slaughter of BSE-affected cattle and the banning of scrapie-contaminated meat and bone-meal feed supplements. At first temporary, it came into effect on July 18. Then, on August 8, 1988, a compulsory "slaughter with compensation" policy came into effect — the government ignoring the WPBSE recommendation of the working party for full compensation. Farmers received only 50 per cent of the value of a cow if it had BSE. Those who slaughtered healthy cows, later found not to have the disease when their brains were examined at autopsy, were paid the full value.

This economic solution by politicians bent on saving money encouraged non-reporting of BSE cases and the quick off-load of affected cows at market, so BSE still entered the food supply. And after the ban on meat and bonemeal in Britain, the feed was still exported to European countries, notably France.

Politicians were initially dismissive of both the Holt letter to the *British Medical Journal* and the campaign by a concerned retired London neuropathologist Dr Helen Grant, who wanted cattle brains banned from human consumption. Sheep's brains were not routinely added to our food, she argued, "so why should we be made to eat their [cows'] beastly brains?"[8] British beef products were perfectly safe to eat, the politicians argued. Scrapie-infected sheep had been eaten for centuries and there was no increase in Creutzfeldt-Jakob disease, so the same would apply to BSE-infected cattle. It became a standard refrain.

But in November 1988, after its second meeting, the WPBSE recommended the permanent discontinuation of the use of protein feed for ruminants — cows and all cloven-footed animals — due to fears that current rendering practices would not eliminate the BSE agent. It also recommended the precautionary destruction of milk from suspect cows as well as continued surveillance of the offspring of affected animals. If the species barrier could ostensibly be broken between sheep and cows, some asked, why it couldn't it be broken between cows and the humans who ate the cows.

The report of the working party noted the death of two African antelopes in a British wildlife park from a spongiform encephalopathy — a nyala, in June 1986 and a gemsbok in July 1987 — after being fed a meat and bone-meal concentrate. The committee was told this concentrate had not been incorporated into the feed of animals at the park until March 1986. If BSE had killed them, this meant an incredibly short incubation period.

The committee speculated that domestic animals exposed to sheep and cattle offal might not be susceptible to contracting BSE because high temperatures were used in pet food manufacture. Nevertheless, it recommended transmission experiments in cats and dogs and surveillance on the health of domestic pets.

In humans, the report said, the risk of transmission appeared "remote". A caveat was added that has been repeated many times since. If BSE was transmitted to humans it would probably resemble CJD, with an incubation period theoretically spanning decades as in kuru. "It cannot automatically be assumed that animals and man will react to BSE agent exposure as they have done to scrapie, which in the human case has not led to any clear association with disease," Sir Richard Southwood and committee members concluded.

Almost immediately beef consumers were reassured that British beef was perfectly safe to eat. To politicians "remote" risk, apparently translated as no risk at all. But in June 1989, Dr Hugh Fraser, a scrapie researcher of note at the Neuropathogenesis Unit in Edinburgh, admitted publicly that neither he nor several colleagues would be eating sausages, pies or other foods that contained the nervous tissue of cattle from then on. The media seized on this. The government was obliged to take note of human consumption — rather than concentrate on cattle consumption of infected animals. Fraser was told to keep his opinions to himself.

In November that year, the government finally introduced a ban on specified bovine offal — the much touted SBO — designed to eliminate cow brains, thalamus, spleen and tonsils from the human food supply. It excluded offal from calves under six months old, because they had never been seen with BSE.

The political platitudes worked. BSE was something that affected cows, not people, most thought. Like lung cancer, it was something that other smokers contracted. BSE was invisible. To the average consumer, their beloved hamburgers, sausages and meat pies were OK. But the SBO ban was not policed and the consumer was not protected.

While MAFF dragged its heels in the summer of 1987 in the lead-up to and following the general election, another outbreak of CJD from a sinister new source was revealed. Dura mater is the tough membrane that encases the brain and separates it from the hard outer helmet of the skull. Almost pure collagen, it looks and feels like stiff parchment. The marbling of blood and lymph vessels, the faint network of veins and capillaries through the dura mater, gives the effect of a delicate shadow motif on sailcloth. But this vital membrane is not elastic, and has no give at all. Once it is cut or torn, accidentally or in surgery, its edges cannot be drawn together. It must be patched.

Neurosurgeons found decades ago that the best substance with which to patch human dura mater is more of the same. Synthetic materials do the job, but healing is far quicker with human dura mater. Like pituitary gland extracts before the advent of synthetic growth hormone, there is only one source — cadavers. In 1958, the same year that Maurice Raben and Carl Axel Gemzell first published their successes with trials of their extracts of hGH and hPG, neurosurgeons in America reported early use of freeze-dried dura mater from the US Navy tissue bank.

A decade later, several types of dura mater were available commercially, either freeze-dried or dehydrated with organic solvents. They were sterilised by various methods including gamma irradiation and liquid ethylene. Two of the major brands were Lyodura made by B Braun Melsungen AG and Tutoplast by Lyofil-Pfrimmer GmbH of Erlangen, both German companies. Between them they sold hundreds of thousands of packages of dura mater around the world. Use of this product was not limited to neurosurgery.[9] Dura mater was useful in hernia repairs as well as orthopaedic, ear and larynx, urologic and gynaecological operations, plastic surgery and heart and spinal procedures. Dentists sometimes used it. With the commercial availability of dura mater, neurosurgical operations to remove tumours, repair injuries or correct congenital malformations in the brain became commonplace.

In Australia, where both Lyodura and Tutoplast were imported from 1972, a 56-year-old meat worker from the state of Queensland underwent the removal of a tumour on his acoustic nerve in 1982 after two years of increasing deafness. The opening in his dura mater was patched with a graft of Lyodura. Then, in early 1983 36-year-old Mrs Pauline Nuttall, a stock controller from South London, weary of four years of headaches and visual disturbances, went to the National Hospital for Neurology in Queen's Square, London. She was diagnosed with a brain tumour, which was growing inwards from her inner skull lining and causing her symptoms. On removal it was benign. The cut in her dura mater was patched with a graft of Lyodura.[10,11]

In April 1983 a 10-year-old Spanish boy was given a Lyodura graft to close the wound created by the removal of a benign brain tumour. In November that same year, a 17-year-old Spanish youth had the same operation and his dura mater was also patched with a Lyodura graft.

Again in Spain, in quick succession, a 34-year-old man and a 53-year-old woman both underwent operations in December 1983 and January 1984, respectively, to widen the big hole at the base of the skull where the spinal cord joins the brain stem to allow more room for a Chiari malformation. This is a rare congenital condition in which the cerebellum, the part of the brain that controls motor function, pokes down into the spinal canal. Uncorrected, it can cause slowly progressive incoordination of limbs and difficulty walking. Each of these two patients also had a fluid-filled cavity in the spinal cord drained. Lyodura was used to close the dural holes created in each operation.[12]

In March 1984 a Japanese woman underwent the removal of a brain tumour and was given a Lyodura graft to seal the incision into her brain lining. And in America in April 1985 a 28-year-old woman was admitted to St Francis Hospital in Hartford, Connecticut, for the removal of a potentially destructive lump in her right inner ear. Her dural opening was closed with a Lyodura graft.

In May 1985, a 27-year-old Italian man underwent an operation to remove an abnormal growth of bone on his head again with a Lyodura graft. And in September a 22-year-old American woman with a Chiari malformation had adhesions around her cerebellar tonsils cut. Again a Lyodura graft was used to patch her dura mater.

Then in October 1985, on opposite sides of the world, two young men underwent neurosurgery. Brian Bowler, a 26-year-old builder from Luton, in Bedfordshire, underwent an operation to widen an existing hole in the skull for the insertion of a drain in a fluid-filled cavity in the spinal cord and to release a trapped nerve. A sizable piece of Lyodura was grafted from the base of the skull down to the third vertebra in his neck.[13] And as spring warmed the land of the long white cloud, a 22-year-old man from Dunedin, in the south of New Zealand's stunningly picturesque South Island, suffered extensive tears to the dura mater on both sides of his head during a bad fall. These were repaired with Lyodura. Almost a year later, in September 1986, the Dunedin man's compatriot, 21-year-old Neville Trainor had a brain tumour removed.

Every single one of those people — the Spanish boys, the Spanish man and woman, Mrs Pauline Nuttal of London, the Japanese woman, the Italian man, the two young American women, the meat worker from Queensland, the two New Zealanders and Brian Bowler — had been given a death sentence. Whether it took 18 months or more than a decade, those dura mater grafts would kill them.

Tutoplast and non-commercial dura mater were also used in neuro-surgical operations. An estimate of Lyodura sales in the decade after its release in 1969 placed usage of the product at "over half a million packages".[14] By 1991 almost one million packages had been sold around the world. In Germany, the biggest market, up to 10,000 preparations were sold annually.[15]

The first official sign of trouble with dura mater grafts was an item in the *Morbidity and Mortality Weekly Report (MMWR)* published by the Centers for Disease Control (CDC) in Atlanta in April 1987.[16] It alerted the world to the fact that the 28-year-old Connecticut woman had died during the previous month from CJD and that her dura mater graft, in the absence of any other risk factor, was strongly implicated in her death at such a young age.

An extended report in the *Journal of Neurosurgery* in November 1988 detailed her decline, which coincided tragically with an early-stage pregnancy. The symptoms of both appeared around the same time in November 1986. By December, after a month of nausea, vomiting and abdominal cramps, she developed slurred speech and a staggering walk. Before Christmas she had declined mentally, her speech had worsened, she had visual hallucinations and all four limbs jerked involuntarily. After admission to the Yale–New Haven Hospital in January 1987, an EEG showed periodic waves characteristic of CJD. At the family's request, her pregnancy was terminated at 16 weeks. A later biopsy showed spongiform change.[17]

A CDC check at the hospital where the original operation was performed showed surgical instrument sterilisation was acceptable and no neurosurgery had been performed on any person with unexplained dementia in the three months preceding the woman's operation. A joint CDC/FDA investigation concluded that Lyodura might carry a higher risk of transmitting CJD than other dura mater products used in America.

In April 1987 the United States FDA issued a safety alert, which recommended the destruction of all Lyodura packages that began with the numeral "2", indicating packaging in 1982, as well as all unmarked packages. Soon a general warning was issued to health authorities, colleges and specialist societies in Australia. The Neurosurgical Society of Australasia alerted neurosurgeons in Australia and New Zealand, and import permits for both Lyodura and Tutoplast were withdrawn by the Federal Government. But stocks of Lyodura were not recalled because lot 2105, used in the American woman's operation, had not been imported. Nor was dura mater from that particular lot imported into New Zealand, where the next reported death occurred.[18]

Another patient on whom a graft from that lot number had been used was Richard M. Nesom, who underwent ear surgery on April 8, 1987 at the Meadowcrest Hospital in Gretna, Louisiana. A series of ear operations over the years had left scar tissue, which was removed. At the same time a cyst was removed. Nesom's dura mater was cut and required a patch of Lyodura.

A lot number indicated processing of dura mater on the one day, but not necessarily from the one cadaver. It was later revealed that 75 boxes of dura mater from lot 2105 were sent to B Braun Melsungen's Canadian distributor, Tri Hawk International. Tri Hawk sold the Lyodura to St Francis Hospital in Connecticut in April 1984 and to Meadowcrest Hospital in October 1984. Other boxes from lot 2105 were sent to six other countries.[19,20]

After the FDA alert of April 28, 1987, Nesom was told of his CJD risk by his neurosurgeon, who estimated his chances of contracting the disease from his dura mater graft were one in 1000. The estimate was based on calculations by FDA doctors, using the number of cadavers and boxes that comprised lot 2105.[21]

Nesom, a Catholic priest in his fifties, filed a law suit against Tri Hawk in the United States District Court for the Eastern District of Louisiana on March 16, 1988, claiming damages for mental anguish and emotional distress as a result of his possibly contracting CJD in the future from his Lyodura graft. He later added B Braun Melsungen. That particular additional claim was dismissed on the grounds that the company had no link with the state of Louisiana.

Although the man from Dunedin in New Zealand died on July 31, 1988, only two months after a rapid decline into dementia, his death was not reported in the *MMWR* until early in 1989. His became the world's second reported case of CJD following a dura mater implant. The *MMWR* report was reprinted in various publications afterwards, including the *Journal of the American Medical Association (JAMA)*[22] and the *Communicable Diseases Intelligence (CDI)* bulletin issued by the Federal Department of Health in Australia.[23]

The New Zealander, then 27, developed symptoms 31 months after the graft. He died two weeks before Jane Allender. The report of his death was used in Richard Nesom's court case as evidence of a second CJD death following Lyodura use. But it added little, as lot 2105 had never been used in New Zealand. Dr Carl Culicchia, Nesom's neurosurgeon, told the court in Louisiana that it was highly unlikely that Nesom would contract CJD because the longest recorded incubation period for the disease was 31 months. Nesom's case was dismissed in 1991 through lack of proof that his own Lyodura graft was contaminated with CJD.

Yet a letter in December 1989 — more than a year earlier — published in the *Journal of Neurosurgery* told of the first CJD death linked to dura mater in Italy. The man, who had the abnormal bone growth removed from his head in May 1985 and was now aged 30, had developed symptoms in January 1989, 44 months after his operation. CJD was confirmed from a biopsy in a Rome hospital in April 1989. The authors of the letter warned of the current potential risk of more cases in grafts of Lyodura manufactured before May 1, 1987. "… after that date, according to representatives of B Braun Melsungen AG, their procedures for collection and processing of dura mater were revised to reduce the risk of CJD transmission, including in the manufacturing process a one-hour exposure of 1N sodium hydroxide, a treatment known to inactivate the CJD virus in brain tissue".[24]

In a response published in the same issue of the *Journal of Neurosurgery,* Dr James W. Pritchard of Yale University, one of the authors of the paper on the Connecticut woman, stated that "transmission of CJD by that route should now be considered established". Pritchard didn't even know at that stage that the Spanish youth who had had his benign brain tumour removed in November 1983 had lived only another three years. He had died of CJD at 20, in December 1986, at a time when no other cases had emerged and doctors were not sure of the link with his dura mater. This case remained unreported in mainstream literature until 1993, when details were first published in a paediatric journal.[25]

Nor was it likely that Dr Pritchard was aware, and clearly Dr Culic-chia was not, of the death of the Queensland meat worker. The report of his death was limited to the *Communicable Diseases Intelligence* bul-letin, circulated from Canberra, and was not included in mainstream lit-erature until nearly a decade later. It had preceded the deaths of the two young men from New Zealand and Italy, and far outstripped them in terms of incubation period. The Australian's symptoms appeared 58 months after the removal of the tumour on his acoustic nerve. He died seven weeks after dizziness, blurred vision, disorientation and memory loss first appeared — in August 1987.[26]

And it was not until 1991 that the death of the Japanese woman was reported.[27] She had developed progressive ataxia in December 1986 and died in August 1988 — the same month as Jane Allender, and shortly after the first New Zealand victim.

In 1989 neurosurgeons were concerned enough with the three cases on record. Then the illness struck again, this time in Luton, outside London. Brian Bowler was only 30 when he became unusually with-drawn in August 1989. Strangely, the affable builder suddenly had dif-ficulty recognising people. Speaking normally was an effort, and he had trouble maintaining his balance. A month later, when he was admitted to the Royal Free Hospital in London, he could not walk unaided, feed himself, swallow properly or speak without slurring. Soon he could not speak at all. He became permanently drowsy and developed frequent jerks in his limbs.[28] In the weeks before his death from CJD in Decem-ber 1989, aged 31, intense pain caused him to bite away his lower lip. An inquest in 1990 linked his death to the use of Lyodura during his operation in October 1985.[29]

In Britain, once Brian Bowler's death was reported in the less main-stream *Journal of Neurology, Neurosurgery and Psychiatry* in 1991, the weight of this and other similar cases led the Department of Health to allow the 20-year import licence for Lyodura to lapse. This was four years after its first warning about potential CJD contamination of that brand of dura mater following the first death in America. Britain's Department of Health had issued a second warning after the 1989 report of the Lyodura-linked death in New Zealand.[30]

The warnings and the end of Lyodura imports were far too late for Pauline Nuttall. A report in the *Journal of Neurology, Neurosurgery and Psychiatry* alerted the world in early 1993 to her death, eight years after her tumour removal. She had developed the symptoms of CJD and was admitted to the National Hospital for Neurology in Queen's Square, London. Five months after her initial visual disturbances, difficulty standing, dyslexia, slurred speech and trouble finding the right word in conversation, she died on May 18, 1991. An inquest into her death in August that year confirmed that she had died as a result of the transplant of a CJD-infected piece of dura mater.[31] About 600 Britons a year had been treated since 1971 with National Health Service-issued imported Lyodura, so potentially 12,000 of them were at risk of CJD from this source.[32]

Only in 1994 did neurosurgeons learn officially of the nine-year incubation period in the man from Spain, who was 25 when he underwent brain surgery.[33]

And it was five years after her operation in September 1985 that a second American woman from North Carolina showed horribly familiar symptoms. In 1990 she complained about blurred vision and depression. She became pregnant, gained a lot of weight and was confined to bed with high blood pressure. Towards the end of her pregnancy she became unstable on her feet. A healthy baby boy was delivered at 39 weeks gestation in February 1991. She deteriorated over the following year and died at home in May 1992. An autopsy confirmed CJD changes.[34]

When this case was reported in the journal *Neurosurgery* in April 1994 a Washington doctor, Norman H. Horwitz, warned in a short item following the case report that "these misfortunes should energise the neurosurgical community to reassess the sterilisation precautions used for all cadaveric tissues in current use, such as bone implants for interbody vertebral column fusions, to preclude the transmission of other pathogens".

The longer incubation periods did not stop. It was seven years after his brain tumour removal that Neville Trainor's parents, Margaret and Ron from Dunedin, suffered the anguish of watching their son, by now 28 and an aluminium joiner, deteriorate rapidly. His symptoms began with speech and walking difficulties in December 1993.

"He suffered terrible hallucinations, epileptic fits and motor control loss," his mother told a local newspaper soon after his death from CJD. "It was horrific to see him on his bad days. His fingers and legs were all bent up and he would jump and twitch and his whole body would double over."[35]

Neville Trainor was disconnected from a life support system at Dunedin Hospital at the request of his family in late June 1994.

One interesting case did not involve a graft, but a German orthopaedic surgeon who had worked with sheep and human dura mater between 1968 and 1972. During that time he had handled up to 150 ovine brain linings and 12 human dura mater for research. He had opened the skulls with a band saw, removed the dura mater and tested them for mechanical qualities. The dura mater handled was mostly fresh, but sometimes it had been preserved or freeze-dried.[36]

This orthopaedic surgeon's own symptoms of disorientation, staggering walk, vision problems, jerking and threatening visual hallucinations began in May 1992 — the same month that the new mother in North Carolina died at home. By September he was dead. Neither the surgeon nor his wife could remember any lacerations of his skin during his dura mater handling period that might explain transmission of CJD via either the sheep or human dura. He was 55 and his age suggested he may have developed sporadic CJD. However, the clinical course of his disease mimicked the course of peripherally infected TSE transmission (like that of kuru and hGH-related cases of CJD particularly) with initial staggering. Sporadic CJD was often dementia-oriented, as had been previous dura mater-related cases.

All these cases of dura mater-linked CJD were thought to have occurred between about 1982, when the Queensland man had his operation, and around 1987, when sterilisation methods were improved by B Braun Melsungen. That was until the revelation in 1993 of what is thought to be the earliest probable case of dura mater-linked CJD. Old medical records, traced in a retrospective study of CJD in England and Wales between 1970 and 1979, revealed the death from probable CJD in 1978 of a 51-year-old woman. Her death occurred nine years after a piece of bone was removed from the base of her skull to relieve pressure on the upper end of her spinal cord. The opening in her dura mater was patched with a cadaveric dural graft of unknown origin. Although no autopsy had been performed, she had died after a six-month deterioration, which began with loss of balance and speech slurring, and descended into mutism.[37]

An Italian woman, who had an incubation period of 111 months, was another case that fell outside that 1982–87 period. She died in mid-1992, eight months after the onset of CJD symptoms. In November 1981 she had undergone neurosurgery at Rome University's La Sapienza for the removal of a protrusion of brain lining into the air-filled space between the eyes. The dura mater used to close the opening in the right frontal area of her brain lining was made non-commercially at the university.[38]

And a third case of CJD outside this time frame was identified in a Canadian who had been given a Lyodura graft in a Toronto hospital in 1988 and who died in September 1992.[39] A fourth case, reported in 1996, was mistakenly thought by its authors to be the fourteenth reported case of dura mater-linked CJD. In fact, although some cases had not been reported at that stage, the 41-year-old Spanish woman who received a Lyodura graft in May 1991 and died of CJD in February 1993 would at that time have been about the twentieth known victim and the fifth reported Spanish citizen to die of CJD in this way.[40]

The doctors who reported the case from the General de Cataluña Hospital, in Barcelona, pointed out that the incidence of CJD in neuro-surgical patients may be far greater "if we think of the potential trans-mission of the disease to patients with severe head injuries and malig-nant brain tumours, who, due to the short period of survival after surgery, do not surpass the theoretical incubation period of CJD".[41]

The incubation period for dura mater-related CJD stretched and stretched. By 1995 it had reached nearly 13 years with the death of the Adelaide boy who received a dura mater graft when his benign tumour was removed in 1982.

About the time Jane Allender was buried at Kangaroo Island off the middle of the massive southern Australian coastline, Jan Blight began stumbling and falling over about 2000 kilometres west. Doctors thought she might have MS. But as Christmas 1988 approached, her retired parents, Frank and Doris Wright of suburban Perth, did not like the way their daughter's limbs shook or that she had become irrational and bad-tempered — and incontinent. Her stumbling walk deteriorated to the point where her right leg dragged, she continually caught her foot on the mat, and she needed a stick to support herself.

Soon, to her parents' disbelief, Jan was confined to a wheelchair. Examined by a Perth neurologist in February 1989, she complained of light-headedness in addition to her other obvious neurological problems. Admitted to Royal Perth Hospital in March 1989, doctors saw a lady with a mask-like face who spoke in a monotone. Shortly before she lost her power of speech and eating because of her difficulty swallowing, her mother remembered her hitting the hospital bed with her fist. "I do not like having to go through this," she screamed.[42]

In early April, during a mini mental-state examination, Jan could not subtract seven from 100, or seven from the result. Nor could she, when asked, touch the tip of her nose and then her ear with her index finger without the commands being broken into separate stages. Finally, asked to close her eyes and write a sentence on a dotted line on the page presented to her by the examining doctor, she wrote in a wobbly hand "I am going home today". Tragically, she never went home to the small country town where she lived with her husband.

In May 1989, just before her 50th birthday, Janice Elizabeth Blight died in a South Perth nursing home. Her death certificate stated she died as a result of two days of pneumonia with months of underlying "idiopathic multiple system atrophy" or non-specific neurological disease.[43] In other words, no-one really knew what was wrong with her.

August 1989 marked the beginning of the horror story that continues in France today. Three months after Jan Blight died from an unknown cause, half a world away in cosmopolitan Paris a small boy called Nicolas Guillemet complained to his father, Alain, of double vision and trouble walking straight. Diagnosed with total growth hormone deficiency at only 18 months of age, he had been treated with hGH from December 1979 to 1988, when he began taking synthetic hGH. In September 1989, a neurological examination of Nicolas, then 11 but still small compared to his elder brother, revealed that his staggering walk had worsened. An electroencephalogram was abnormal, and by January 1990 his EEG readings were characteristic of the periodic sharp waves that often help to diagnose a CJD patient. Two months later he could barely talk, was almost blind and was bedridden. He died in November 1991, unable to live in his new home in Normandy. CJD was confirmed at autopsy and hamsters injected with his blood developed a neurological disease.[44,45] He was thought to be the youngest person ever to contract CJD.

But Isabelle Norroy, another French youngster of only 10, from a small town near Orleans, changed that notion when she began losing her balance for no apparent reason in May 1990. She had been treated from the age of two with several drugs, including hGH, to overcome her panhypopituitarism, which meant she had little or no secretion of vital anterior hormones from the pituitary gland. In 1988, like Nicolas and any other French child under treatment, she switched to synthetic hGH.

In April 1990, as Nicolas lay bedridden and mute, Isabelle complained of double vision and headaches and later developed a staggering walk. By August 1990 her writing was almost unreadable and her speech was barely comprehensible. Bedridden by January 1991, she died several months later.

These two cases were reported, before their deaths, in a short letter to the *Lancet*, April 6, 1991. Some of the parents of the 1700-odd children treated with pituitary-derived hGH in France up to mid 1985 heard about those first two deaths. But many remained ignorant. Then in the July 20, 1991 issue of the *Lancet,* two doctors at the laboratory of paediatric neurophysiology in the Trousseau hospital in Paris urged colleagues to consider conducting early EEG readings. EEG readings on Nicolas, Isabelle and a 20-year-old former hGH recipient with apparent CJD had been abnormal. Double vision might also indicate CJD, they warned, because experiments with scrapie-infected rodents had revealed that the retina was affected early in the course of the disease.[46]

In August 1991 the parents of 15-year-old Ilyassil Benziane, a fifth hGH recipient suffering from probable CJD who was by now bedridden, consulted a lawyer. Maitre Giselle Mor, who had her law office outside Paris in Franconville, listened with horror to the story of Ilyassil's deterioration. His parents had been told little by doctors, but enough to know that he was dying of the rare and fatal CJD. They wanted to know if it was linked to his hGH therapy. Maitre Mor lodged a complaint of unintentional injury, which under French law meant that an examining magistrate could investigate the matter. This preliminary investigation phase, often lengthy, establishes facts, responsibilities of various people and aims to identify any breaches of law that may have occurred. By the end of 1991, Ilyassil was dead. The complaint was amended to unintentional homicide.

He was not the last. In December 1990 Jean-Philippe Mathieu, a vivacious 17-year-old in his last year of school, was suddenly persistently tired. A popular young man, he hoped to study mathematics at university in Grenoble when he left his local school in the tourist town of Thonon, on the shore of Lake Geneva near the Swiss border. Soon his jokes dried up, his personality changed and he suffered several strong fevers.

Jean-Philippe had been treated with hGH, both pituitary-derived and synthetic, for 10 years until 1989. His treatment, his father Jean-Bernard says, was "cosmetic" because he was not as tall as his sister, cousins and parents. Throughout 1991 Jean-Philippe had trouble walking straight. A neurologist thought he had MS. In May 1991 it was the family doctor who correctly suspected CJD, a diagnosis backed by doctors at the Trousseau hospital.[47]

By July 1991 Jean-Philippe's parents had transformed their home into a hospital. Their beloved son, unable to walk or feed himself, was tended by his mother, who had left her job. In 24-hour rotating shifts, family members, girlfriends, his sister and other family friends sat with him, talked to him, unable to believe Jean-Philippe was turning into a vegetable before their eyes. With medical costs soaring, and feeling isolated in his grief and anger at his son's impending death, Jean-Bernard Mathieu contacted reporter Jean-Yves Nau at *Le Monde*. On February 2, 1992 the newspaper published its investigation into the scandal and revealed publicly for the first time that 10 French child recipients of cadaver-derived hGH had contracted a fatal brain disease. The media and government reaction was swift. A government investigation was ordered immediately but it was too late for Jean-Philippe, who died in the early hours of February 4, 1993 as his father dozed beside him. He was 175 centimetres tall.

Endocrinologists around the world were puzzled at the extremely young ages at which the disease had manifested itself in France. They hoped — in vain — that there would be no more cases. But among the 1700-odd French families that would be most affected in the aftermath of the hGH program — many still ignorant of the deaths, articles in medical literature, further television coverage of Jean-Philippe's tragedy and Ilyassil's family's legal action — an attractive, raven-haired university student called Benedicte Delbrel was enduring her own hell.

CHAPTER 12

Jenny Halford:
A pattern emerges

JENNY HALFORD STUMBLED even though she had hold of her husband's arm. "What's the problem?" asked Noel, concerned as he watched Jenny grimace and stare down at her legs.

"Oh, I can't walk. I can't coordinate."

It was June 1990 and they were on their treasured evening walk. Their pleasure at living in the tiny Berkshire village, quaintly named Inkpen — a derivative of the original Hinge Pene listed in the 1086 Domesday Book — had not diminished in their 16 months of living in England. Every night when Noel Halford returned from work in nearby Swindon they would leave their house with the duck pond in the garden and walk up Bell Lane for about half a mile. From the top they would look out over the valley towards Shalbourne as the summer sun set, turning the wheat fields in the west into a shimmering, swaying mass of gold. The sky would darken to reveal a mass of stars so foreign without the familiar Southern Cross constellation visible at home.

Noel's posting to England as human resources manager with the Courtaulds packaging company was a new direction for the Halford family. He didn't really have to ask Jenny when the job offer came. They had always wanted to travel overseas and this was their opportunity. So, with daughters Penelope, then 10, and Lucinda, then seven, they had left Melbourne's Tullamarine Airport that scorching first day of February 1989 and arrived, as most Australians do, to a bitterly cold dawn at Heathrow 26 hours later.

They were determined to enjoy the experience of living in another country for the first time. With Noel away for several days at a time running personnel, industrial relations, training and welfare for the company, Jenny wrote often to her mother, Margaret Knight. Jenny was lonely at first, reading and re-reading the welcome letters from home and worrying about the girls settling into school life at St Gabriel's at nearby Newbury. She drove them there and back each day. The traffic, rain, wind and weather were all so different, even though Melbourne could be quite cold in winter. Among the first of 131 letters to Margaret from then on, Jenny wrote in February 1989: "Missed seeing you on your birthday. Must be 23 years since I missed seeing you mum — you seem so far away."[1]

In early March Jenny wrote of gradually making more friends, in particular Chris and Kay, two mothers with two girls each at St Gabriel's, women she described as "a lot of fun". "We get on so well and the six girls do too, so I am beginning to feel a bit more settled." A month later the Halfords prepared to move their 49 cartons of belongings into a comfortable red brick house in Inkpen, aptly named "Cobwebs".

Although they married in the Presbyterian church in 1967, the Halfords did not worship regularly. One Sunday in spring, as the church bells pealed across the valley, Penny said suddenly, "let's go to church". "What a good idea," said Noel. They walked the half mile to the Anglican Church of St Michael and All Angels, wheat fields in the distance striking a blaze of yellow along the valley cut by a prehistoric road known as the Wayfarers' Walk.

The moment they walked into church with its thirteenth century high-pitched roof was a turning point in their lives. "Something just happened," Noel recalled later.[2] Although it was an ordinary service, the welcoming smiles of the congregation and the atmosphere inside the flint and stone building with its church registers dating back to 1633 brought a special feeling of warmth and belonging that the Halfords had never experienced. Afterwards they met and became close friends with some of the parishioners, like Anthea and Roger Hunt — friends who would soon be indispensable. Their first year in Inkpen was the happiest of their lives.

It was from the beginning of February 1990, after the week-long storm that killed 45 people in south-eastern England, and another 35 in Western European countries, that Jenny began to feel unusually tired. But she kept up her busy life, which revolved around taking the girls to and from school and activities, a voluntary job helping with the local Meals on Wheels service and working part-time as a library technician.

Just before the much anticipated arrival of Margaret and Jenny's step-father John Knight on May 26, the Halfords made their final move, to a big old farmhouse called Beacon House. It had a curved courtyard wall and beech trees on each side. With extras like donkeys, cows and chickens, it had a huge garden and plenty of room inside for visitors. The girls loved it.

Jenny invited 20 villagers for coffee to meet Marg and John the morning after their arrival. It was a cheerful introduction but one which noticeably tired Jenny, already exhausted by the recent move. Marg noticed that her daughter found it hard to summon up her normal quiet efficiency and enthusiasm. But Jenny said she had been to the doctor about her occasional "poor week" and blamed menopause for her stomach pains and headaches.[3] But most noticeable to Marg, and a fact remarked on later when Jenny's older sister Barbara watched a video of Marg's holiday, was that Jenny's brown eyes seemed somehow bigger. And her voice was slightly louder, more strident, unlike her usual gentle tone.

Margaret and John left England on June 1 for a bus tour of the continent, not knowing that Jenny was becoming increasingly ill. In bed at night, Jenny's arms and legs jerked occasionally, waking Noel. He had noticed her sometimes stagger, although Jenny never said much more than, "it's ridiculous, I'm losing my balance". On several nights Noel had to pacify her after nightmares. After one particularly bad one Jenny had cried out that spiders were crawling all over her.

But it wasn't until the night in June 1990 when they were confirmed as Anglicans in the lovely old church in nearby Lambourne that Noel noticed for the first time that Jenny could not walk in a straight line. Confirmation was a significant step for the couple, who were not church-goers until their arrival in Inkpen. It was a commitment, a seal on their new faith and community belonging, and had followed the christening of Noel and the girls a week earlier at St Michael's. During the confirmation ceremony Jenny's balance was so bad that she had to hold on to Noel as they knelt before the altar. Her symptoms, whatever they meant, were becoming very worrying indeed.

During the three weeks Margaret and John were in Europe Jenny saw Dr Jeremy Bray, the local GP. He could find nothing physically wrong with her, although whatever the problem, it was apparently neurological. Signals from her brain were not working properly, giving rise to her difficulty with coordination. Puzzled, Noel and Jenny refused to worry until they knew exactly what was wrong. Dr Bray, concerned by her obvious and deteriorating balance problem, suggested further tests, including one for MS. He referred Jenny to a neurologist and an appointment was made for July 9.

The walk along Bell Lane that summer night in June was the last evening stroll for the Halfords. As Jenny struggled to walk straight, Noel sensed her symptoms were bad news indeed. "Let's try it again," he said gently, helping her forward. MS was not so bad, he mused, as Jenny leaned on his arm. People lived with it. That night Noel practically carried Jenny home.

Jenny never complained about any illnesses, but she did tell Marg, when she returned on June 21, 1990 from her European trip, about her increasing difficulty with balancing, especially descending stairs. She also felt lethargic and had intermittent bouts of double vision. Sometimes she had the sensation of her eyes swinging from one side to the other. In addition, Jenny's handwriting had deteriorated slightly from its usual very neat script.[4]

By late June Jenny was finding her job at the library difficult. She was becoming oddly clumsy, dropping things. Villagers like Anthea Hunt were aware she had problems with her eyes because she told them. "The ground keeps coming up at me," she complained several times. Noel hoped the problem was simply a persistent inner ear infection. "I feel everything's closing in on me. The ground, the walls," Jenny burst out uncharacteristically during her mother's visit after falling over yet again. "It's pretty frightening."

On a day trip to Donnington Castle on June 24 Jenny was so tired and her legs so sore that both Noel and John had to help her walk up to the castle. In early July Jenny appeared to cope, still driving the girls to school and to music lessons in Hungerford as well as mounting shopping and tourist expeditions with Marg and John. One night the four adults went to a local pub. Noel and Marg were the only ones game enough to order the beef and Yorkshire pudding in the wake of media stories at the time that "mad cow" disease might cross the species barrier to humans.

But Marg noticed that although she prepared a beautiful dinner party for eight on Friday night, July 6, Jenny had accomplished it "with a certain amount of holding on to chairs and benches". Jenny told her mother: "I've got to keep moving, Mum. It's just a nuisance." Noel was worried she might have an accident during one of her dizzy spells, and convinced a reluctant and continually tired Jenny to give up driving.

While Noel was at work, Marg and John took Jenny to the outpatient clinic at Newbury Hospital for her July 9 appointment with Dr Nigel Hyman, a Yorkshire-born, Oxford-based neurologist whose daughter Emma, coincidentally, was in Penny's class at St Gabriel's. Marg and John watched Jenny walk crookedly towards the door when her name was called. Inside, Hyman, a tall thin man of 42, looked up from his desk and gestured that she be seated. He took her recent medical history, scribbling down the poor balance she complained of for the past seven weeks and a "vague" feeling Jenny felt she could not shake off. In the past month she had been tired and her legs had been a bit "twitchy".[5] During the physical examination he noted that she was slightly off balance.

"Now, can you please walk in a straight line over here putting your heel to your toe each time?" The simple exercise proved fruitless.

"Can you just touch your finger to your nose," said Hyman, indicating that she follow his lead. Jenny couldn't do it well. Her hand jerked its way toward her face. She tried again and again. Her finger eventually hit the end of her nose but it took a lot of effort. Nor could she carry out the requested heel-shin coordinate, a test in which the patient, while lying down, attempts to move the heel of one foot up and down the shin on the opposite leg. Hyman, who had been fiddling with the paper clips on his desk as he watched, was very worried. Among his notes he wrote down "mild incoordination".

Hyman's busy scribbling made Jenny anxious. Finally, he stopped writing and gave her news she had been dreading. "There is something definitely wrong," he told her gently, fiddling with his paper clips once again. "I think it's an infection of some sort. It could be one of a number of things. It could be an infection in the cerebellum, which is part of the brain. Or it could be multiple sclerosis or even a brain tumour." [6]

Hyman wrote to Dr Bray, Jenny's GP, saying he thought she was developing cerebellar ataxia, balance trouble caused by a problem with the cerebellum, the part of the brain that controls motor function. The recent onset of symptoms possibly indicated MS, a cerebellar tumour, even an underactive thyroid gland, although Bray had already discounted a thyroid problem with a specific test. Hyman ended his letter with the suggestion that Jenny undergo a brain MRI scan, which is the best way of looking at the cerebellum.[7] Because he was also attached to the Radcliffe Infirmary in Oxford, Hyman suggested Jenny travel to the famous university town for the MRI scan. He suggested a longer stay as soon as she could be booked in so some additional tests could be conducted, a prospect that Jenny found inconvenient as well as slightly frightening. The Halfords had planned a family holiday to the south of France the following weekend. "I wouldn't let my wife go if she were in your condition," Hyman told her baldly. "You may not be able to walk without help in another week."[8]

Once outside, Jenny's shocked expression, said it all. John and Marg had to take her arms to steady her as they walked across a road. Penny and Lucie were disappointed at the cancelled holiday, especially since Jenny still looked well. They wanted to know why the doctor couldn't give their mother some tablets for her legs.

A few days later Marg was startled when Jenny dropped a glass that she was replacing on the kitchen bench. She got another and it, too, smashed to the floor before both of them realised that she had completely misjudged the distance. The bench was a good 10 centimetres further away than she thought.

Double vision was also becoming a big problem and, true to Hyman's prediction, Jenny soon needed a stick to walk outside. Crossing roads was dangerous without Marg or John to help her. At night, the pain and jerking in her legs nearly drove her mad, as well as lost her valuable sleep. She complained to Hyman, when she returned to see him at Newbury Hospital on July 30, that she was sleeping more during the day and that her balance was worse. The MRI scan, conducted on Jenny as an outpatient at the Radcliffe Infirmary on July 18, 1990, was normal, revealing no tumour and effectively eliminating MS as a possible cause of Jenny's problems. The Halfords were relieved that the "worst case scenario" was ruled out.

On July 19, Jenny walked by herself for the last time. With Noel, Marg and John, she spent a lovely day at Stourhead, a beautiful old building with picturesque lakes and gardens on the Stour River in Wiltshire — something she had always wanted to do.

While appearing to cope day by day, Jenny was deteriorating rapidly and was constantly tired. But she continued the hectic round of visiting friends and taking the girls for outings with friends, sometimes accompanied by Marg and John. Jenny worried that her mother and step-father were not seeing enough of Britain. At night she was so tired she would nod off in her chair. Reading her library books became too much. "The back of my neck is getting sore, mum," Jenny said one night. "I feel like a hypochondriac, what with my legs and the back of my neck. I don't know what's wrong with me. I'm sick of complaining, mum," she told Marg, who didn't think she complained at all.

By the end of July, as Marg and John's return to Australia loomed, Jenny was barely able read or write but still enjoyed outings in the car. There were plenty of invitations from friends to swim in the unusually hot 30 degree Celsius heat, but Jenny swam only a few times. Naps after breakfast and lunch became routine. Marg bought her daughter two much-needed walking sticks because Jenny was very slow getting around and still needed someone's arm to help her walk. Jenny appeared fed up with her symptoms rather than frightened.

Seated at the table during a farewell tea for Marg and John, Marg marvelled at her daughter, so attractive, looking younger than her 44 years. It was hard to think there was something so wrong with her. She thought Jenny would merely be in a wheelchair until doctors found the problem. Whatever it was, Marg resolved to return to England as soon as she could.

Marg and John left for Melbourne on August 3, 1990. At the airport, Jenny and Marg were in tears as Jenny told her mother how much she loved her. "You're the best mum in the world." Marg, who promised to return soon after sorting out the building of her new house on the coast outside Melbourne, thinks now that Jenny must have known she was very ill.

Noel drove Jenny back to the Radcliffe Infirmary several days later. There she was put through a host of routine motor function tests before an auditorium full of doctors. The jerks in her arms and legs were very apparent. Ever the prolific correspondent, Jenny wrote from her hospital bed about being examined by a succession of doctors and medical students, answering innumerable questions, and having to lie on her back for 12 hours after a lumbar puncture. "Dear Mum," she wrote.

"This is my first big attempt at writing a letter. I really can't see what I've written so it's very hard. It's really very difficult to concentrate and I have to stop every now and again ..." Marg was shocked at how Jenny's handwriting had become so alien.

On her second day at the Radcliffe Infirmary, as Jenny lay in bed mulling over what horrors the lumbar puncture, blood, cerebrospinal fluid, EEG and chest radiograph tests might eventually reveal, a dark-haired, bearded doctor she hadn't seen before strode into the ward with Hyman.

"This is Dr Cochius," Hyman said preceding him into Jenny's spartan room. "He's from Australia too but working with us at the moment as a registrar and will be helping to look after you."[9] Hyman left them and Cochius sat down beside Jenny. They talked about their common nationality, how she loved living in Inkpen with her husband and two daughters since her husband's transfer but that she had been having trouble walking properly, had double vision and had developed soreness and jerks in her legs.

Jenny was bewildered by what was happening to her. It was in her eyes. She was becoming increasingly unwell and no-one seemed to know why. She explained to Cochius how, when she was reading, she would scan the line and then have trouble getting back to the next line. Sometimes she would leave one line and think she was reading from the next line down when it was in fact three lines down and she had lost the thread of the story. This, Cochius knew, was a sign that her eyes were not moving in a coordinated way. While she talked he noticed subtle muscle spasms in her fingers. He could see that she would look at him and suddenly her eyes would move away from him, darting from side to side. This was not good. It was also horribly, uncannily familiar.

Jeffrey Cochius was struck by the similarity between Jenny Halford and Jane Allender, the first patient he had ever seen with the rare Creutzfeldt-Jakob disease. Here was a woman a little older than Jane, with two children, presenting at a hospital with remarkably similar symptoms — vision disturbance, jerks, staggering walk over several months and a recent history of falling over. It was almost like they were the same patient except that Jane Allender had had the added obsessive/compulsive disorder on top of her symptoms.

Cochius thought Jenny Halford had CJD too, even though it was only the second case of the disease he had seen. If he was correct in his diagnosis, Jenny had only months to live. He had to ask the question.

"Have you ever had trouble getting pregnant?"

"Yes," she answered, puzzled that a neurologist would ask her a gynaecological question, "as a matter of fact I did have."

"Were you treated for it?"

"Yes, I had some injections before I had Penny."[10] Jenny asked why he was so interested in her fertility history.

"I've seen a case like yours before," he told her.[11]

Later, Noel remembered Jenny's haunted eyes as she recounted her conversation with Cochius. Jenny said, "I think that other lady must have died."[12]

Hyman, when he related his bad news to Noel a few days later, explained that Cochius had been working at a hospital in Adelaide where a woman had died two years beforehand. The circumstantial evidence for their probable diagnosis, was strong. "It doesn't look very promising," Hyman said. "We suspect it might be Creutzfeldt-Jakob disease. The woman in Adelaide had the same gonadotrophin fertility treatment as Jenny and Jenny is showing all the right symptoms. It's incurable."[13] Noel had feared that whatever was wrong with Jenny was very serious. Here was the confirmation.

Talk of the fertility program so many years ago that had produced their Penny raised the same old mixed feelings in Noel. The excitement of the pregnancy, the pain and worry when Jenny became ill, that frightening call from the doctor when Jenny went into premature labour and the eventual delight when they took their new daughter home.

Jenny, 156 centimetres tall and normally weighing about 50 kilograms, suffered from anorexia nervosa, which was the cause of her fertility problem. One particular dramatic weight loss had caused her to stop ovulating because her oestrogen levels were so low. But after seven years of marriage, Jenny wanted to become a mother. Tablets to correct her problem had not worked so Jenny was referred to Dr Noel de Garis. "Now if you can get your weight up ..." the doctor left the obvious unsaid. She knew well enough that she needed to be healthy enough to conceive and carry a pregnancy.

Dr de Garis referred her to Dr James Evans at the Royal Women's Hospital in Melbourne who reviewed her history, carried out tests and eventually explained that a drug containing FSH might work by

replacing the lack of Jenny's own hormone and triggering egg production. "It's a very expensive program sponsored by the Federal Government and you've got to be sure you want children," he told both Jenny
and Noel. They were sure. "Well then, I think this will work," he said
with a reassuring smile.[14]

Between September 1976 and May 1978 — three times longer than
many couples — Jenny received 14 courses of injections from CSL
batches 38, 43, 45, 60 and 67.[15] The Halfords knew of no problem with
the treatment. No health risk was mentioned. Nor was the source of the
drug revealed to them. And there was certainly no talk about trials or
experiments. About the only problem they understood — short of it failing — was the chance of a multiple pregnancy. "Look, it's not going to
be multiple, multiple," Evans had assured them. "There may be two.
You have to expect that there is a chance of that."[16]

The Halfords' lives changed in May 1978. Noel was part-managing a
printing plant in Cobram, a town north of Melbourne. The phone rang
with a very excited Evans on the other end. "I know you've been
coming a long time but I've finally got good news," he told Noel almost
breathlessly. "Your wife's pregnant."

Noel drove the 220 kilometres home in world record time, chuckling
all the way, but knowing they would have to be extremely watchful of
Jenny's weight to ensure the baby received enough nourishment. When
he arrived home Jenny gave him the news, not knowing Jim Evans
could not contain his own. "You knew didn't you!" she said mock
accusingly when Noel's feigned surprise failed to fool her. When a twin
pregnancy was confirmed at two months it was double the joy.

While only six months pregnant, Jenny fell gravely ill and was hospitalised. She wasn't eating properly and her weight had fallen danger-
ously low. She went into premature labour. Noel was in a meeting on
November 3, 1978, when a very worried de Garis rang. "It's a disaster.
I can't guarantee that Jenny will survive." Then he added: "You might
lose them all." By the time Noel arrived at the Royal Women's Hospital even Jenny thought she would die. "I've got to live," she told him
determinedly. "I've just got to do this."

The next morning at 9.36 a.m. Penelope Halford was born, followed
shortly afterwards by Jacqueline. The girls were given oxygen to help
their immature lungs but Jacqueline, not strong enough, died two weeks
later. Penelope struggled on, each new day a dreaded waiting game to

see if she gained or lost precious grams necessary to build on her two pound birth weight.

After three months Noel and Jenny took their treasured daughter home and, after a bout of post-natal depression, partly because of Jacqueline, Jenny took on her long-awaited role. She put on weight and took to motherhood with gusto. Two years later Jenny was fully occupied with Penny and — incredibly — slightly overweight. Unaided by medicine, she fell pregnant again, and when Lucinda was born on June 13, 1981, the Halford family was complete.

Noel was distressed by Hyman's tentative but horrifying prognosis of CJD. He had trouble remembering how to pronounce it. As he tried to grasp the implications of Jenny having possibly contracted such a lethal infection, he decided not to upset her straight away with the news until the doctors were more certain.

Hyman, as usual tremendously supportive, told Noel all he knew about the disease and the symptoms that led inevitably to death. But how could it be linked to that tedious but ultimately successful course of injections? The birth of Penny had been proof that it worked. It was not until Hyman took the trouble to explain that the drug was made from an extract of hormone taken from the pituitary glands of dead bodies that Noel began to understand. One or more of those dead bodies must have been harbouring CJD. The infected pituitary glands severed from those bodies had contaminated the drug Jenny eventually received. Hyman explained to Noel that the disease was very rare, that it could be latent for years before it showed up. The only possible reprieve would be if Jenny had taken hCG or hMG, both of which were extracted from urine.

"Mum could you ring Dr Evans at the Royal Melbourne and ask what type of gonadotrophin I was on?" Jenny asked her mother during a phone call, hoping that her drug had not been manufactured from the third source, pituitary glands.

"Oh, Jen," Marg replied. "I don't think Dr Evans would remember me."

"Mum," Jenny insisted. "It's a matter of ... I could end up a vegetable if I don't know which one I was on."[17]

Marg decided to ring her nephew, Robert Moulds, first. Coincidentally, he was associate professor of clinical pharmacology at the University of Melbourne and the Royal Melbourne Hospital. "I knew Jenny wasn't well," he told Marg when she explained Jenny needed to know what type of hormone she had been given during her fertility treatment. Straight away he asked how old Penny was, thinking she might be about six. If she was, Jenny might not have been treated with hPG, which was withdrawn from Australia in 1985 after deaths from CJD in America and England.

"Well, she'll be 12 in November," Marg replied.

"Oh my God." Aware of the case of CJD following fertility treatment in Adelaide, Moulds explained that there was probably nothing the doctors could do.

"Should I go straight back?" Marg asked, knowing her husband had booked them a return flight at Christmas, three months away.

"Time will tell but it won't be long," he said heavily. "I don't think she'll be there at Christmas."[18]

On August 30, 1990 Jenny Halford wrote her last letter to her mother. As usual she included snippets of family life in Inkpen and was pleased to relate how the junior school head had suggested she attend school in her wheelchair to help junior students with their reading.

> It was lovely to go and see the children and feel that I was a bit useful again. Mum I can't read what I am writing so hope you can. Will try and write more slowly. Delighted to receive your letters. Noel and the girls race in with them for me ... I can't write letters any more to anyone. I'll just try and write to you, mum, and to the whole family.[19]

But she could not. A few weeks later, in the September school holidays as the evening air turned crisp, Noel took Jenny and the girls to stay with friends who lived at Budleigh Salterton, the former home of Sir Walter Raleigh on the Dorset coast. By then Jenny was almost totally confined to a wheelchair. As Noel ran, pushing her along the beach and watching her hair fly in the wind, he realised that it was possibly the family's last holiday together.

Jenny deteriorated rapidly after the holiday. She had been through the stage of sitting on a stand to shower. And to get up in the mornings she had to swing her legs over the bed. But she fell and cut her hand. The stairs became too much for her. Rather than continuing to bump her way downstairs on her rear end, she and Noel began sleeping in single beds downstairs in the library. It was the only spare room they had, but also the nicest. Friends and village neighbours rallied around, cooking nightly meals on a roster basis, visiting each day with Jenny, who tired very easily. Sometimes they would take her on outings in the wheelchair, charging the doors in the supermarket, yelling "Do you think this is an automatically opening door, Jenny?" Noel went to work and each day Anthea Hunt drove the girls to school. Jenny, popular and admired by all, received as much help as everyone could give.

In addition to almost daily telephone calls during each week, Noel took over Jenny's weekly letter writing to the family in Melbourne, stressing the importance of remaining positive despite Jenny's periods of feeling low. He included all the news, like the joking at the September Inkpen Common monthly working bee. It had been suggested that cutting blades be put on Jenny's wheelchair to save time. Then a friend chipped in with the thought that it might look "too much like the return of Boadicea and frighten the community. It is difficult to adjust to your limitations when you have been as active as Jenny," Noel wrote, "and I know she would not mind me saying that attempting to cook the evening meal is beyond her point of endurance at this time."

By late September Jenny's balance had deteriorated so badly that she was advised to stay in bed. Her bodily functions began to fail and nursing help became necessary. Mentally, however, she remained sharp, if a little forgetful, and she slept a lot. Short outings to the hairdresser and a heroic appearance at the annual general meeting of the school parents' association meant a lot to her, even though her deathly pallor shocked those who hadn't seen her for a while.

Jenny thought of her childhood in northern Tasmania as she and Noel watched the rain through the library window one typical English autumn afternoon. She told Noel how her father cooked waffles and about the fabulous taste of her mother's golden syrup dumplings with ice cream.

"You know," she told Noel another day as they sat and looked out over the pond in the back garden, flanked by the post and rail fences behind and the paddocks beyond, "I could have lived this life out in a wheelchair. But there is no way known I could be bedridden for the rest of my life. I just couldn't do it."

On October 15, 1990, the day before Noel turned 48, he and Jenny travelled to London by ambulance for a consultation with Dr Anita Harding, a neurologist at the National Hospital for Nervous Diseases,

Queen's Square. Hyman had suggested a second opinion. They knew it was their last hope. After another EEG examination and more tests, Harding sat them before her in her office. In her straightforward way she explained both frankly and courteously that she was almost certain it was CJD. It was terminal and there was nothing that could be done.

On the way back to Inkpen they both cried for the first and last time. Noel sat next to Jenny's stretcher in the ambulance and held her hand. "Well, if that's got to be it, we've got to walk towards it and not be afraid," he told her. Jenny nodded as the tears coursed down her face. "Well at least I've had 12 years of motherhood and nothing can take that away."

Noel rang their families in Australia and urged Margaret to return to England as soon as she could. It almost broke her heart when Jenny came on to the phone. "I'm so glad you are coming back, mum. I don't know how long I've got."

Still able to reason, Jenny worried about what to tell the girls, who could see their mother falling apart in front of them. Penny was almost 12 and Lucy was nine. "How can I tell the children I'm going to die when I'm not giving up?" she asked Noel.

He replied, "Well that's a fair question. What we'll tell them is that the doctors believe that Mummy is going to die but we have faith and we're going to tough it right out."

After a roast dinner the next night, cooked by a neighbour in honour of his birthday, Noel wrote to Marg.

"What can one say in a situation we are now in other than we will still maintain a positive attitude and take one day at a time. Even in her present state Jenny is an inspiration to all who see her and I'm pleased to say she has retained her humour. Please be assured that I will take the best care of Jenny and make sure she is comfortable and secure at all times. Believe me, I know the anguish you are going through — it's a very, very tough time."

Soon after, Jenny's speech, until then fairly normal, began to slur slightly. Her neck had to be supported by a brace. She lost the use of her right hand and made poor use of her left hand as a substitute.

"I felt I was never a good enough wife to you," Jenny told Noel before she lost her ability to talk entirely.

"Oh God," he replied taking her hand, "Don't be so silly."

And then, when it was the last thing on his mind she told him: "I hope you meet someone else. You deserve something in life."

"What will be, will be. We've got the children to think of and I never want them to forget you."

Marg returned to Inkpen from Australia on October 26 with Jenny's siblings: sister, Barbara and brother David. David could only stay a week before flying to America on business. Jenny was determined to enjoy an outing with her brother so the family went for lunch to a local pub. David and Noel helped her in and out of the car because Noel couldn't manage her on his own. But the trip was hopeless for Jenny. She could barely swallow and had to be fed by her mother. Her extreme tiredness meant her head flopped from side to side. Marg had to help hold it up.

David left on November 4, 1990, Penny's twelfth birthday. Jenny appeared to be distancing herself from them — letting go, Noel thought, by not taking great interest in the opening of the presents, which was usually a big celebration. It was as if she was avoiding becoming too emotionally involved.

Saying goodbye, when he knew he would never see her again was distressing for David. Jenny did not cry. She couldn't. She had no moisture in her eyes and was not even able to blink. Noel hired a nurse experienced in caring for terminally ill patients, to give her constant care while he continued to work and the girls went to school. Visits from friends continued. A week later Barbara had to leave.

"I'm sorry I can't get up to say goodbye to you," Jenny said, slurring, as family members struggled to keep their composure. "I won't see you again but I am so pleased you came. It's the best thing that happened to me."[20]

Noel knew she did not have long to live. He frequently marvelled at his wife's bravery and secretly hoped she could hang on for another 12 months. But Hyman, who visited in October, and the GP, Bray, a frequent visitor, shocked him with the news that Jenny, by now drinking through a straw and unable to speak, would definitely not see Christmas.

It was a terrible blow, heightened soon after by a letter from his old boss in Melbourne who had enclosed a clipping from the *Age*, a local morning newspaper. Dated October 31, 1990, the article had warned that hundreds of Melbourne women may have been exposed to the slow-acting virus CJD after the death of a South Australian woman in 1988 and the initial diagnosis of a Melbourne woman currently living in England.[21]

Noel wondered if the other woman's family had gone through the hell his family was experiencing. The newspaper article had followed the publication in the *Australian and New Zealand Journal of Medicine* of the report written by Cochius and colleagues in Adelaide about Jane Allender, the first case of CJD in a recipient of hPG. Noel knew Jenny was soon to become the second.[22]

Jenny, meanwhile, still mentally alert in her wakeful periods, continued to be the centre of village gossip sessions. Eight or nine local women would surround her bed each morning drinking coffee and including her in the general natter. By this time Jenny was addicted to chocolate and large blocks of it were greeted with smiles of delight by the patient and frowns from the nurse.

When they had gone and she was left with Marg during the afternoon until Anthea Hunt returned with the girls from school, Jenny would worry about her children. "I feel as though I've got the weight of the world on my shoulders, mum," she slurring told Marg at the beginning of November. "I don't know what's going to happen to the girls." As Marg recalled, Jenny then shut her eyes. "She wanted to talk to me but she just couldn't keep going. She didn't have the strength."

Soon her tongue became paralysed, she could no longer speak and by mid-November Jenny was slipping in and out of consciousness. She lay there unblinking and seemingly aware, as the morning coffee sessions went on regardless. An impromptu service was held around her bed one night with villagers and her children praying and singing hymns around the piano led by their next-door neighbour, Gabriel Cave, then in training for the Anglican priesthood.

Jenny Halford died on November 29, 1990, surrounded by her family. Noel remembered then that telling moment before she suddenly lost her speech. He had walked into the library to find her gazing out the window. She had turned to him and said: "This is where I really wanted to be in my life."

And so his adored wife stayed in England. He left her where they had shared the happiest time of their long union. After the autopsy, which confirmed CJD, Jenny was cremated in Oxford. Her memorial service at St Michael's in Inkpen on December 4, 1990 was packed beyond its seating capacity of 120. Former neighbours travelled from France and a couple holidaying from Australia who had heard about Jenny through

Rotary squeezed in alongside mourners from all over England as the four bells in the St Michael's bell tower pealed out over the valley.

In the church cemetery, shaded by a rosebush, stands a simple memorial stone dedicated to Jenny Halford, 1945–1990. Penny helped word the inscription. "The flowers may fade, the sun may set, but we who loved you will never forget."

Noel, a gentle, soft-spoken man not given to sudden outbursts, subsided into anger. Anger that his wife was gone, that his children were motherless and that they were never told there was a risk of CJD involved in hPG treatment. On occasions in the months following Jenny's death, when he collected his girls after work from the Hunts' home at the other end of Inkpen, he would talk about his frustration. That his wife had died under a program that was supposed to be so good and so safe, that it was supplied free by the Federal Government was almost unbelievable. "I'm going to do some digging and try and make sure that there is compensation available to all those mothers who were infected," he told Anthea's husband, Roger Hunt, in early 1991.[23]

None of them knew it then but soon Jenny Halford's name and what happened to her would become headline news in a scandal worse than the thalidomide tragedy of the 1960s.

CHAPTER 13

"Forget the cows, what about the kids?"

By THE BEGINNING of the 1990s, the BSE epidemic became a political as well as economic nightmare. By December 1989, 25 countries had declared bans on the importation of British cattle, cattle semen and embryos. Then in January, American military bases banned British beef. By February 1990 the number of infected cows reported had risen to hundreds each week. This was possibly a direct result of the British Government finally agreeing to pay full compensation for each BSE-infected animal culled. Veterinary checks, supposed to include a thorough inspection of each animal, were inadequate, and the specified offal ban (SBO) on cattle over six months old was "too little too late" — and was never properly policed.

Then in April 1990, after developing a staggering walk and incoordination, a Siamese cat called Max died of BSE. The death, one in an estimated seven million cats in the British Isles, sparked another round of consumer anxiety. Within a week of the cat's reported demise, farmers, doctors and the Labour Party had accused the British Government of failing to take effective measures against the spread of mad cow disease. Doctors claimed that pathologists were refusing to carry out postmortem examinations on CJD victims for fear of contracting the disease, and schools in Humberside, Staffordshire, Oxford, Liverpool, Surrey and Westminster had struck beef from their menus.[1] Meanwhile, columnists scathingly dismissed the latest round of BSE scare stories as another big food scare along the lines of the 1988 salmonella and listeria scares from eggs and paté. Only this time it was beef, the traditional British fare.

After Tim Holt's prophetic letter in the *British Medical Journal* in June 1988, retired neuropathologist Helen Grant began her successful campaign via letters to newspapers in 1989 to have cattle brains, which were not allowed to be included in animal food, removed from the human food supply as well. She and her family stopped eating beef products — sausages, pies, pasties, patés. So did Professor Richard Lacey, who exploded into the media in 1990. In a series of dire warnings, the professor of microbiology at Leeds University suggested that, to minimise the chances of contracting CJD from BSE, no-one under 50 should eat British beef, that all of Britain should be quarantined, all exports should be halted and six million cattle should be slaughtered to stem the epidemic. He forecast that the first cases of CJD resulting from eating BSE-infected beef products would start in 1996.

Lacey was a headache for the government, which put him down as an ignorant man who liked his face on television. Meanwhile the government promoted the idea, propped up by the Southwood Committee's finding, that BSE presented "minimal risk" to humans and that there was no evidence that the disease could cross the species barrier. The then Agriculture Minister, John Gummer, in particular will never be forgotten for the political stunt he pulled in May 1990. In front of a large media scrum at an Ipswich boat show Gummer fed a beefburger to his four-year-old daughter, Cordelia, to show consumers how safe he thought beef was.

In August 1990, when Jenny Halford had her fateful meeting with Jeffrey Cochius and when the CJD Surveillance Unit in Edinburgh was just a few months old, Alan Watkins, a reporter with Rupert Murdoch's tabloid newspaper, *Today*, rang an eminent British neurologist. BSE was a story on the boil, the kind of consumer horror story that *Today* loved. Hoping to drum up a news story on the BSE crisis, Watkins asked his contact if there was anything new to report. "Forget the cows," was the neurologist's terse reply. "Why don't you start looking at the kids who have died? It's the same thing." Watkins' only clue was that the dead children had received human growth hormone.

Working nights on the *Today* news desk with little time for reporting, Watkins plugged away at the story in his spare time. It became, he now acknowledges, not the biggest, but the "most important story in my career". He became known in the office as "the mad scientist" and because of all his stories on the BSE crisis, colleagues took to greeting him with "moo" calls on his arrival each day. Six months later he had the story. In a series published over two days in May 1991, *Today* exposed the "Scandal of the timebomb children — cover-up over youngsters injected with killer disease".

In what is easily one of the worst, most harrowing interviews he has ever conducted, Watkins heard in detail the horrendous implications of CJD on a young man and the rest of his immediate family. In his series he charted the story of Terrence Newman, a former Air Training Corps cadet who had died at 21 from CJD. His symptoms began nine months before his death on December 3, 1990. By August 1990, seven years after he was last treated with the hormone that helped him reach 166 centimetres, Terry's balance was awry and he walked as though drunk. In September, by which time he couldn't walk without help and after tests at the Middlesex Hospital had ruled out MS and other neurological conditions, he was tentatively diagnosed with CJD. His parents were told he would die but that it could take 12 months.

Eric Newman recalled in the newspaper series how he had sat in the kitchen of their home with his first-born son. "My life's been one big disaster hasn't it Dad? Does this mean I'm going to die?" As Eric put it: "No-one could have told such a thing to a lovely boy who'd never hurt anything or anybody in his life. So I lied. I told him he would be all right but that he might have to be in a wheelchair. After that we all lied to him. We lied every single day for the rest of his life".[2]

Terrence Newman was one of six former hGH recipients who had died a horrible death, their families ripped apart and ignorant of the cause. In the months leading to his death in 1990, even the family GP had no idea what was wrong — as he had no idea that Terrence was at risk of CJD. The *Today* series revealed publicly for the first time that the Department of Health and Social Services (DHSS) in London had decided not to notify anyone. It did not notify the parents who gave their permission or the children who received hGH of the very real risk of CJD to recipients. There was little point in worrying people unnecessarily. "The doctors who gave that advice were adopting, in my view, an old fashioned paternalistic view of medicine: I suppose it is a sort of we-know-best approach," said Professor Michael Preece, head of the London-based Institute for Child Health, and member of the clinicians' committee which oversaw part of the program.[3] He and other doctors maintain that all relatives and doctors should have been advised immediately.

The DHSS, in response to Watkins' series, responded only that it was "not current policy to contact patients or their relatives directly" and anyone worried about being at risk of CJD from hGH injections should contact their GP or specialist.

Meanwhile, Maureen and Eric Newman had contacted Sheffield solicitor David Body. After listening to one of the saddest stories he had ever heard, he thought they had a very good case with which to sue the British Government for negligence.[4] He applied for legal aid on behalf of Terrence in November 1990, but the certificate lapsed with Terrence's death in December 1990. Body then advertised in the *Law Society Gazette* for lawyers with similar cases.

As Body painstakingly assembled his complicated case against the might of the British Government — and learned a lot more about science than the average lawyer — he would not have been surprised to find that, in the years it took to get the trial to court, that initial death toll from hGH would triple.

Stephen Cummings noticed the personality changes in his wife gradually. By 1988, 16 years after their wedding, the former army cook had gone through a series of jobs — on the railways, in a canning factory, dealing with concrete water tanks and in an intensive piggery. Vonda had, after the birth of their daughter Lauren and an apparent subsequent bout of post-natal depression, settled in well in her husband's home town, Albany. She made friends, wallpapered whole rooms herself, tended a large garden, played the organ, and tinkered with the car. Then a series of medical mishaps and two operations in 1986 and 1987, one to correct carpal tunnel syndrome in one arm, the other to fix a crack in a knee bone, seemed to precipitate a change in Vonda.

Stephen noticed the perpetually worried look that had settled on his wife's face. "God Vonda, what's wrong?" Stephen said to her more than once.

"I don't know," she replied. "I don't feel right." She told Stephen's sister at the time that it was like "the walls were closing in" on her.[5]

Vonda's belief in God, strong enough to sustain weekly outings to church, vanished. When her husband asked why she no longer went to church, she remarked that "there's no such thing [as God] anyway". Her twice weekly voluntary sessions at the local Yakamia Primary School testing pupils ended abruptly. "Maybe that's the thing that I noticed most," Stephen recalled years later of the dreadful slide in his wife's health in 1988. "She lost her interest in life. It just went." Vonda rarely went out, much to her husband's frustration. Stephen often visited, alone, the home of a friend where he would have few quiet drinks and listen to music. The friend sometimes would ask Stephen: "What's wrong with Vonda?" It was a question he couldn't answer.

Sometimes Stephen would come home from a week away working to find Vonda sitting in a lounge chair, the house a mess around her, and no food prepared for the family. Cosy marital chats in bed became a thing of the past and arguments took their place. "When you finally find out what it finally is that's caused the problem you go through all these guilts — oh why did I say that to her," Stephen said in anguish much later.

Vonda, always a good reader, became voracious in the habit. But often Stephen would find her reading or watching television with a hand over one eye, to correct the double vision that began to plague her.

"Things that really mattered to Vonda, her principles, and her normal way of thinking suddenly changed," Stephen recalled. She became paranoid at one stage that year about Gareth's poor eating and tried to force feed him. She began walking sideways. Her double vision was constant. "Stephen the back of my head is hurting," she would complain of repeated bad headaches throughout 1988. Her weight began to see-saw. Concerned that she was too heavy for her 165 centimetre height and medium build, Vonda lost so much weight her husband began to worry about her.

Vonda kept a diary in which she chronicled important dates and events of the family. In neat handwriting she had recorded her cartilage removal operation on October 13, 1988, her husband's resignation from the piggery on September 19, 1988. Vonda had her first appointment with a doctor "to find out what's wrong" on February 1, 1989. Her GP referred her to a specialist who took X-rays that revealed nothing wrong. She was tentatively diagnosed in March 1989 with chronic fatigue syndrome after a CAT scan showed nothing.

Later Vonda complained of lower back pain. She also stumbled when she walked, fell over frequently, ran into furniture and looked ill from her constant headaches, worsening double vision and general feeling that something was radically wrong. "Look," Stephen exploded, "you've had your wrist done, you've had your knee done. Try a chiropractor. Maybe he can find something."

"Well he (the chiropractor) took one look and said 'You don't need me. You need a neurologist'."[6]

By late 1989 Vonda's weight had soared by more than 17 kilograms over her pre-diet weight of about 57 kilograms. Always hungry, she snacked constantly. When she literally squeezed herself into some good clothes to attend a family wedding, everyone noticed. In South Australia, her mother-in-law, Muriel Cummings, who was in regular contact by telephone, received a stream of phone calls from West Australian relatives about Vonda's decline. Some thought she had been drinking. Vonda herself seemed to be giving up and told Stephen he would have to take over looking after the children.

"How are you Vonda? Are you feeling any better?" Muriel Cummings asked each time she rang. "No, if anything, I'm feeling worse, Mum," was Vonda's usual reply. In her diary on Tuesday November 21, 1989 Vonda wrote, in handwriting that had deteriorated noticeably: "This illness I have has been with me 18 months. It is really tiring me out so that everything is a real effort."

Previously a prolific correspondent to family and friends and a person who never forgot birthdays, Vonda sent her last Christmas card in 1989. In an accompanying letter she wrote: "Please tell all the other rellies that I can't. Whatever is the matter with me, I can't think, I can't write and it's all been too hard."

"That was when I really knew," Muriel recalled, "that whatever she had was really dreadful."

On December 23, 1989 Stephen took Vonda to see a Perth neurologist, the same specialist who had examined Jan Blight 10 months earlier. As with Jan, he admitted her to Royal Perth Hospital that day. Vonda had walked, with help, into the hospital. She did not emerge for nine weeks and by that time she was in a wheelchair, no longer able to read, feed herself or watch television. Her body shook from the violent jerking muscle spasms in her limbs and trunk.

In hospital she had undergone a battery of tests including more CAT and MRI brain scans and a lumbar puncture procedure, wondering the whole time if her condition was due to a brain tumour. The MRI scan showed some atrophy of the outer layer of the brain, which underscored the eventual diagnosis of cerebellar degeneration caused by some sort of virus. The condition could stabilise or even improve, an outcome that Stephen in his ignorance, believed would occur.

Vonda returned to Albany and stayed in the local hospital until Stephen could organise some home care. In March 1990 Vonda made her last diary entry. Her handwriting was barely legible. "Gareth's first school social."

"If people could understand," Stephen Cummings said in 1993, reliving in detail for the first time the demise of his wife, "when your wife, mother of your children is deteriorating before your eyes, it's horrific … Our lives, our normal lives, were taken from us." In May 1990, with the children greatly affected by their mother's illness, he sold their house and returned at Vonda's request to her father's farm near Ardrossan, a town in rural South Australia where she grew up.

Stephen, who had become the target of abnormal outbursts of anger by a now-demented Vonda, as well as pointed questions from family and friends, returned to Western Australia for two weeks. While there on personal business he revisited the Perth neurologist and was told that Vonda's condition might not be treatable and that more tests in the hope of a miracle cure or new drug might not help. By the time he returned to South Australia Vonda had been transferred to the neurology department of Queen Elizabeth Hospital in Adelaide. This was the same hospital where she received her fertility treatment 15 years before.

After more than a month in hospital and another round of inconclusive tests Vonda asked Stephen to take her home. The request coincided with the suggestion that Vonda undergo a brain biopsy in order to rule out anything at all that could be treated. Stephen refused. Vonda had told him she didn't want any more tests and wanted to go home.

On July 16, 1990, the Queen Elizabeth Hospital successfully applied for Vonda to be placed under the custody of the South Australian Guardianship Board. This was carried out under an archaic law in which a person suffering from a mental handicap and incapable of looking after their own health and safety can have their custody taken over by the board, regardless of the wishes of the next of kin or immediate family members. With Vonda's further deterioration, the hospital decided not to proceed with further diagnostic tests that had been approved by the Guardianship Board. Stephen Cummings appealed to the Mental Health Review Tribunal, which revoked the previous guardianship order.[7]

Totally incapacitated, Vonda returned home to rotating carers, including Stephen, a district nurse and relatives. In the dry heat of early December 1990, a month after Jenny Halford's death in the wintry countryside of Berkshire, Vonda stopped eating. She was readmitted to Maitland Hospital, and spent her second Christmas in two years away from her family, almost skeletal compared with her previous obesity.

On the day of her death, January 17, 1991, Vonda Cummings was surrounded by her grieving family. Her death certificate stated she had died of cerebellar degeneration. But after two post-mortem examinations in February and March 1991, the second pathology report listed cause of death as "general debility (CJD)".[8]

On March 21, 1991 at Sydney's Westmead Hospital, 27-year-old "Stephen" died. He became what is regarded as Australia's first and — at the time of writing — only CJD victim following hGH therapy. Adopted soon after his birth in January 1964, Stephen suffered from the blood disorder hypogammaglobulinaemia, deafness and later the debilitating Crohn's disease. He was also growth deficient, resulting in a decade of hGH therapy starting in 1973.

In 1989, as Jan Blight deteriorated in Perth and young Nicolas, the first French hGH recipient, developed the symptoms of CJD, Stephen began suffering severe headaches. He walked around in a daze, ate his food in a demented manner and uttered strange things. At the time of his death, he was an invalid pensioner living with his elderly adoptive mother. None of his hospital notes referred to CJD. No autopsy was performed. And like Vonda Cummings, despite admission to Westmead Hospital, one of Sydney's largest public teaching hospitals, no-one considered CJD from his previous hGH history. Not even when most of his hGH treatment and his death were at the same hospital.

Meanwhile, CJD had claimed another hGH recipient — this time in Brazil. In May 1991 doctors in Rio de Janeiro reported the death in the *British Medical Journal*. The young man had received hGH extracted and purified by the hGH pioneer Maurice Raben and was treated for 11 years, between 1968 and 1977, before the extra purification of column chromatography was introduced in American-manufactured hGH. He died of CJD after a 33-month illness. The diagnosis was made on clinical symptoms and the presence of the two proteins in his spinal fluid identified under a Harrington spot test.[9]

It was late autumn 1991 in England when Paul Andrews, a handsome 26-year-old company executive began to vomit every morning. He also felt lethargic and unenthusiastic about his highly paid marketing and promotions job. From the age of 11 to 17 he had received three injections weekly of hGH and had grown to a height of 165 centimetres — too short for his original ambition to be a police officer, but fine for his next aim — politics.

While washing his car on May 10, 1985, he had learnt of the CJD deaths of American hGH recipients on a BBC Radio 4 item reporting the shut down of the British hGH program. His mother, Ann, who rang the Great Ormond Street Hospital for Sick Children where her son's treatment had begun was told by a secretary that there had been deaths only in America. This was totally incorrect. The first British CJD victim, Alison Lay, had died in February 1985 and it was her death that had shut down the British program.

Reassured, however, Paul Andrews went on to university, completing a degree in international politics and history. He travelled the world and settled into his job in 1989. But two years later, when a series of tests did not reveal a cause for his lethargy and vomiting, he wondered if it was at all rooted in his hGH therapy. Referred to an adult endocrinologist, in December 1991 the specialist told him that the deaths from CJD that Andrews had briefly referred to in the consultation were not limited to America. They had occurred in Britain as well. The toll was then six and rising. Andrews was shocked and wondered if these strange symptoms were the beginning of his end.

He found subsequently that the endocrinologist was one of those on the ethics committee who had decided, over several objections, not to inform or trace previous hGH recipients to tell them of their CJD risk. Since Alan Watkins' dramatic series in *Today* six months earlier and the fact that the death toll had risen so alarmingly for such a rare disease, the department had reconsidered its decision. The task of tracing and warning all 1908 hGH recipients had fallen to Professor Michael Preece at London's Institute for Child Health based at Great Ormond Street Hospital for Sick Children. It had begun only two months before

Andrews was told verbally by the endocrinologist that he, too, was at risk of CJD.

Andrews found it hard to concentrate on work, more so when he read a newspaper article headed "Programmed to die — by an NHS blunder" in May 1992.[10] He later found that the CJD hormone contamination story had broken a full year beforehand but that tracing had still to reach many hGH recipients who remained unaware they were walking time-bombs.

Andrews became angry at the actions of the DHSS. With each new media story on the scandal of the "timebomb children" it responded coldly that no compensation would be paid to the families of those who had died on a government-sponsored treatment and that all hGH therapy had been good medical practice based on the best knowledge of the time. It was not lost on many that farmers were by now being compensated fully by hundreds of pounds for the loss of each beast that fell victim to BSE. Farmers were a far more powerful political lobby than the shrinking hGH recipient population.

Eventually, as the death toll rose to eight, Andrews became so concerned that he might contract CJD that he gave up his job. If his life was to be cut short, he would spend the rest of it as he wanted, travelling and being with family. "It was quite a matter-of-fact judgment," Andrews recalls of the end of his marketing career, and the added perks, mobile phone and car. "If I was going to die then I might as well prepare myself for it and try to find out more as to why I was at risk."[11]

CHAPTER 14

Australia confronts its CJD risk

L ATE ON THE NIGHT of November 27, 1991, a politically conservative Liberal Party parliamentarian rose in the House of Representatives, in Australia's capital, Canberra. He suggested that the
Federal Government compensate the families of two women who had
died after fertility treatment on the Australian Human Pituitary Hormone Program (AHPHP). The parliamentarian was Peter Costello, then
the opposition spokesman on consumer affairs. Destined for far greater
heights in federal politics, he had been a neighbour of Noel and Jenny
Halford in Melbourne before they moved to England.

Stunned by Jenny's death, Costello had offered to help Noel in any
way he could. With Halford's permission, in the latter half of 1991
Costello wrote to Jenny's treating doctor Dr James Evans and CSL,
which had manufactured the hPG. When he raised the death of Jenny
Halford in federal parliament it was the first public announcement —
anywhere — naming her as the second tragic victim of CJD attributable
to hPG injections. Costello suggested that the Federal Department of
Health directly notify all women who had received hPG of their CJD
risk status. Many doctors had ignored several departmental letters sent
out in 1985 and again in 1990 when Jane Allender's death had been
reported in the medical literature.

Costello proposed that the department provide counselling to those at
risk as well as to the families of those who had died, and that the families of both women who had died be compensated by both the department and CSL.[1]

Costello's speech was reported briefly in Melbourne newspapers,[2]
with a major follow-up by ABC television reporter Craig McMurtrie,
who recognised the potential for a longer news piece for the Summer
Edition of the ABC's nightly current affairs program, the "7.30
Report". He interviewed Costello on camera in a Melbourne park, and

Halford was filmed in England for the segment. Jenny Halford's original treating gynaecologist, Evans, told McMurtrie that CJD was like a "timebomb". At the time he prescribed the hPG, however, he said all doctors on the program were acting on the best information available to them. They were not aware of the risks of CJD.

The government-owned CSL, which was preparing for privatisation, refused to communicate except by fax. Several doctors warned McMurtrie to "be careful". He knew Jenny Halford was the second case but could not get information on the first death. As he questioned why women were not warned of the CJD risk, McMurtrie was given a standard response from doctors and bureaucrats along the lines of "there are secrecy provisions preventing us from contacting people. We are caring for the patient by not raising needless concern, not causing alarm".[3]

The "7.30 Report" documentary on the AHPHP and Jenny Halford's death was aired on January 16, 1992. The response was immediate and overwhelming. Hundreds of letters streamed into the ABC's Gore Hill studio in Sydney from people who had been treated on the program and had no idea of the risk of CJD. All were worried and desperate for more information.

News of the ABC item and the strange-sounding disease it featured reached Ted Allender the following day via his parents. Ted called the ABC in Sydney. "We've been looking for you," said an excited McMurtrie when referred the call. "The Health Department wouldn't tell us who you were."

With a television crew McMurtrie flew from Sydney to Adelaide and met Ted in the room of an Adelaide hotel. Ted was cautious and unwilling to have his surname used. McMurtrie slipped the video of his ABC "Summer Edition" feature report into the VCR machine in the hotel room. As Ted watched grief-stricken widower Noel Halford being interviewed in England and relating the eerily familiar story of the gradual disintegration of Jenny Halford, his mouth went dry.

Throughout the interview, McMurtrie referred to Jenny Halford as "the second case", and as Noel Halford described the way that his wife's illness was diagnosed, Allender could hardly believe what he was hearing. The reason why Jenny Halford's condition was diagnosed so promptly and linked with her fertility treatment was nothing but the bizarre coincidence that neurology registrar, Jeffrey Cochius, had seen both Jane Allender and Jenny Halford.

Only one question needed answering for an immediate initial

diagnosis. As soon as Jenny Halford admitted she had received an injectable hormone to become pregnant, Cochius had his answer. That remarkable coincidence was one of the key developments that ensured the accidental transmission of CJD through pituitary extracts for infertility would now be confirmed as a definite risk factor for the disease and not a one-off that could be dismissed easily.

It was easy to conclude that if Cochius had not been in Oxford at that time, Jenny Halford's death could have been misdiagnosed. Certainly her fertility treatment would not have been probed. Without it, there would have been nothing to link her case with Jane's. Watching the video, Ted felt the familiar anger, suppressed for more than two years, grow. Scientists and medicos were mucking around with bio-technology and then walking away from the disasters they created without being accountable, he thought. He showed his anger in McMurtrie's second program on the CJD scandal describing the bureaucratic and medical "wall of silence" that continued to shield those he blamed for Jane's death.

The second program, screened the following week on January 23, 1992, featured Ted Allender and radical feminist and University of Melbourne research scientist Dr Lynette Dumble. McMurtrie wanted a comment from someone about the second case. He had tried several feminists and finally found Dumble who, always interested in kuru, was happy to comment on CJD and its relationship to reproductive medicine, a serious issue for radical feminists. Dumble told McMurtrie that the Federal Department of Health was being either "compliant with the medical profession on what might be the cover-up of a frightful disaster or the department has failed to comprehend the implications of what is a terrible debacle".

Two Melbourne women treated with hPG, Sue Byrne and "Heather", also spoke on camera of their anger at being left ignorant of their CJD risk because of the Department's policy of telling former patients through sometimes-reluctant treating doctors or GPs. "It was taking away my right to know," Sue Byrne said. The chief health officer, Dr Tony Adams, said that the department had to work within the system that had built into it strict privacy laws to protect the identity of individuals. Many patients on hPG and hGH had moved or changed their names since their treatment and it had been difficult to track them.

Another stream of letters to the ABC followed the second program,

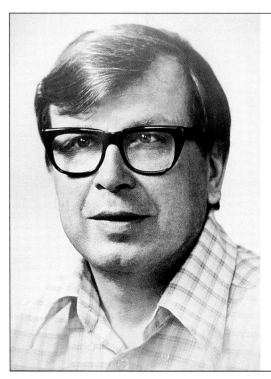

Dr Daniel Carleton Gajdusek, a pioneer in the research of kuru and other transmissible spongiform encephalopathies, was awarded the Nobel Prize in Medicine in 1976. (*Copyright © The Nobel Foundation.*)

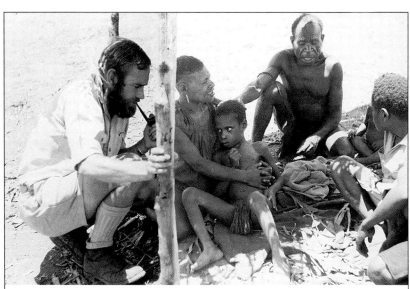

Dr Michael Alpers with a kuru patient in a village near Waisa in 1962. (*Courtesy, Dr Werner Stöcklin.*)

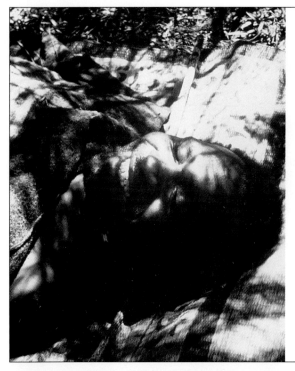

A kuru victim, shaded by a canopy of branches outside his house in the South Fore village of Waisa, finds even filtered sunlight painful, a common kuru symptom. (*Courtesy, Dr Michael Alpers.*)

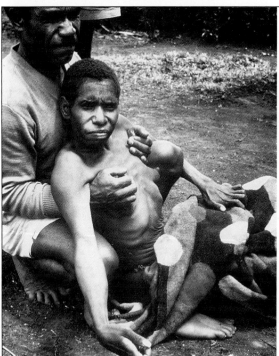

A husband supports his wife, who has an unusual hand posture, in the third or terminal stage of kuru in Ketabi village in the Purosa Valley, Papua New Guinea in 1969. (*Courtesy, Dr Michael Alpers.*)

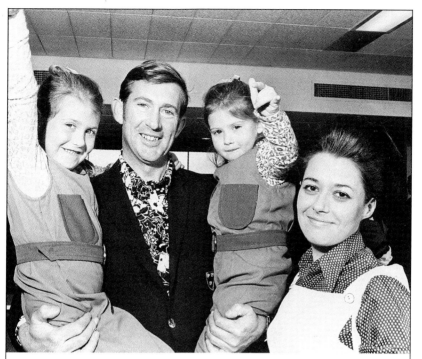

Geraldine Brodrick departs Sydney for a holiday in Honolulu with her husband Len, and daughters Belinda (left) and Jacqueline in July 1971. Geraldine became the most famous recipient of cadaver-derived fertility hormones when she gave birth to nontuplets on June 13, 1971, none of whom survived. *(Courtesy, Fairfax Photo Library.)*

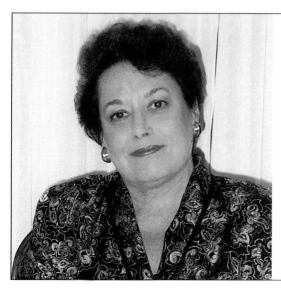

Geraldine Brodrick in 1997.

Spongy holes dotting the brain of a Sydney woman who died of sporadic Creutzfeldt-Jacob disease in 1997. (*Courtesy, Professor Clive Harper, Neuropathology Department, University of Sydney.*)

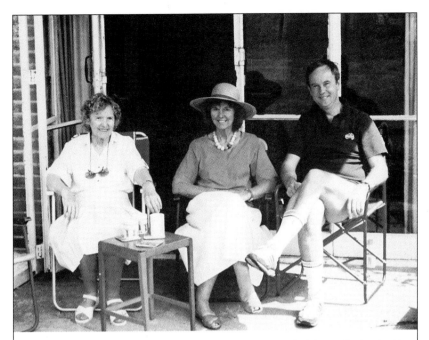

Jenny Halford having morning coffee at Beacon House in Inkpen, England with her husband, Noel, and mother, Margaret Knight, in May 1990. Jenny, who contracted Creutzfeldt-Jacob disease after participating in a fertility program, died six months later. *(Courtesy, Noel Halford.)*

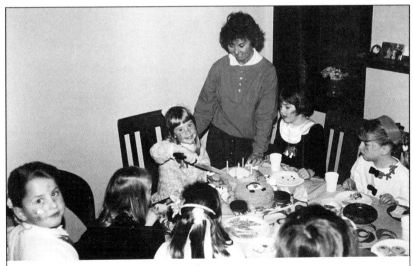

Jenny Halford at her daughter Lucie's birthday party in Melbourne, 1986. *(Courtesy, Noel Halford.)*

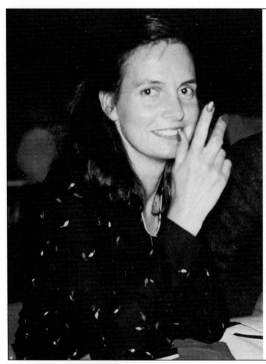

Jane Allender, who contracted Creutzfeldt-Jacob disease after participating in a fertility program in 1974. *(Courtesy, Ted Allender.)*

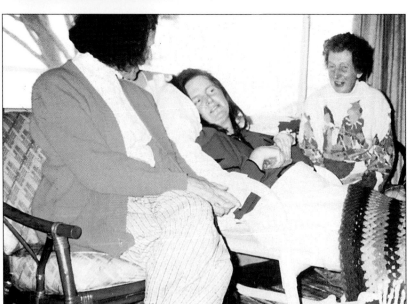

Jane Allender's 41st birthday party at her parent's Kangaroo Island holiday home, June 11, 1988, two months before her death. Jane's mother, Ruth, is seated to Jane's left. *(Courtesy, Ted Allender.)*

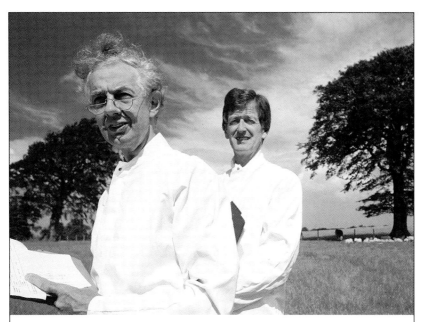

British scrapie expert and founding director of Edinburgh's Neuropathogenesis Unit, Dr Alan Dickinson (left), with collegue Dr Richard Kimberlin in 1986.

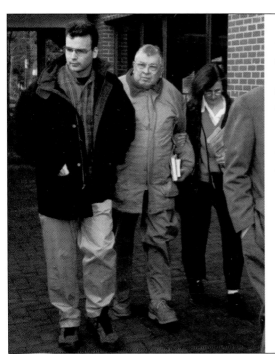

Dr Carleton Gajdusek leaving a Maryland courtroom in April 1997, after being sentenced to a one-and-a-half years in prison for abusing a 15-year-old Micronesian boy he brought to America to educate in 1987. *(AP/AAP Image.)*

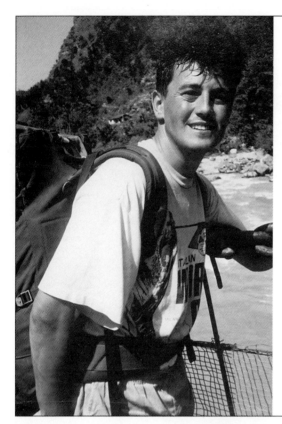

'Just in case' he contracted Creutzfeldt-Jacob disease, Paul Andrews, British LGH recipient travelled to Nepal in 1994 for a walking tour that he had always dreamed of doing.

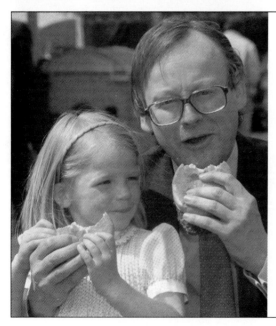

Then British Agriculture Minister John Gummer and his daughter Cordelia, aged four, at a boat show in England in May 1990 demonstrating the 'safety' of British beef burgers. *(AP/AAP Image.)*

with more trickling in for months as further news stories were aired. In one address to a national television audience, Dumble, whose research expertise lay in organ transplantation and women's health, warned that "Frankenstein medicine has Frankenstein results" and that the worst expectations of medical experiments on women had been realised with the administration of the potentially lethal hPG shots.

Many treating doctors were angered by Dumble's remarks, arguing that they were doing their best for their patients at the time and had no idea of the risk of CJD. The knowledge lay in another area of science. Until the small risk of transmission to others from potentially contaminated tissue, organs or blood was raised many doctors did not want to cause unnecessary alarm in people who had only a tiny chance of contracting such a rare disease.

It wasn't until the first request to trace and counsel patients had been sent to treating doctors by the Department of Health in November 1990 that initially reluctant doctors saw the benefit in warning former patients not to donate blood, organs or tissue as a precaution. Some doctors gave up when thwarted by out-of-date addresses, and in some cases changed details, since treatment. Others plugged on, with no additional resources. Some doctors had retired, while others traced the patients of former and dead colleagues. Each had to devise a tracing method and it took time to compile mailing lists. These methods only reached a few hundred of the more than 2000 Australians who had been treated officially. Once the publicity began in early 1992, it led to redoubled efforts to trace those at risk. Primed by media stories, former patients contacted their doctors wanting an explanation and information about CJD.

Many, recipients of hPG particularly, were angered that they had not been contacted by their doctors when the risk became known in 1985. Some wrote to Sue Byrne after the ABC programs in January 1992. Sue, who had conceived her second child on the AHPHP and had then had four more children without medical help, was incensed and had suggested the establishment of a hPG task force. Eventually state-based CJD support groups were established and she took on the demanding role of national coordinator of the CJD Support Group Network Inc.

Ted Allender got Noel Halford's number in England from Craig McMurtrie. In mid-1992, on a blustery winter's evening, the two tall, serious-faced men met with firm handshakes in a Greek restaurant in Melbourne's trendy Chapel Street. Noel, who had returned briefly to

Melbourne to look at job opportunities, was still visibly affected by his recent bereavement and could barely talk about his wife without tears. As far as he knew, Ted was the only man in the world who could empathise with him. Ted, with his energy, drive and growing cynicism towards the medical profession, and Noel, more reserved but resolute, and articulate and determined to stop at nothing short of an inquiry into the whole sorry mess, hit it off instantly.

"We've got to run with this, Ted," said Noel. Ted, just as angry, agreed.

By the time of Ted and Noel's dinner, Peter Costello had asked for and received answers to seven questions from the Minister for Health, Brian Howe. This became the first official release of information about the AHPHP in relation to a link with CJD. The answers revealed that about 1500 women — later revised down to 1400 women — were treated with hPG between 1964 and 1985. Up to 1992, after the decision by health authorities that only treating doctors should contact and counsel those treated under the AHPHP, only 352 women had been contacted. After its 1985 letter to treating doctors and the second letter in November 1990 asking them to trace and counsel former patients and warn them not to donate organs, blood or tissue, a third letter was sent to doctors from the Department of Health in January 1992. A fourth letter was sent in February 1992. Three more letters followed.

Costello's political clout had got the matter moving and it was a bonus for Allender and Halford to have a concerned and interested politician backing a matter they considered of the utmost importance. That night, in the Greek bistro, Ted and Noel made a pact to join forces: to get to the bottom of how CJD had contaminated the hormone drugs, and find out why no-one wanted to know about the consequences.

The meeting between the two was a turning point in what would become known as the CJD scandal in Australia. They were determined to break the wall of silence put up by doctors and bureaucrats — no matter how long it took. Now there were two of them. And soon, when Stephen Cummings contacted Ted Allender, there would be three.

Tracing of the 2100-odd recipients of hPG and hGH in Australia began in earnest in January 1992 after McMurtrie's "7.30 Report" stories on the ABC. A CJD unit was established within the Department of Health, with an initial complement of four. The unit traced death certificates of human hormone recipients and answered inquiries to establish whether callers had received pituitary-derived injectable drugs or some other type, including imported commercial hGH or gonadotrophins extracted from urine or tablets of any sort. Information was sent to the doctors of the former patients, not released on the telephone. If records did not include the name of the caller, it did not necessarily mean they had not been treated. Stimulation tests, IVF and other research uses of both hPG and hGH were not included on the departmental database.

A large problem surfaced — the database itself. Described in medical papers with such pride in the 1970s, not only was it incomplete, but it was written in such archaic computer language that a completely new database had to be created in January 1992. The lengthy exercise took staff from other sections of the department, which contributed to the mess that followed — incorrect entries, the omission of treatment dates, incorrect listings of doctors, incomplete batch numbers and the incorrect inclusion of synthetic rather than solely pituitary-derived growth hormone recipients.[4]

The Australians were well behind the American researchers who by 1989 had traced more than 95% of their 7,000-odd government-sponsored hGH recipients in a massive follow-up ordered in May 1985. The aim was to assess the risk of CJD and other complications of hGH therapy. A contract was given to a company called Westat Inc, which used a telematch service to match addresses and telephone numbers. Forwarding addresses were obtained from postmasters; letters were sent to last known addresses asking recipients to call a toll-free number; employers, landlords and neighbours were asked for help without the reason being given; and motor vehicle administration, voter registration records, tax and school records were also scanned.[5]

The underlying causes of growth hormone deficiency had already led to 254 deaths in the 6,284 patients known to have been treated under the NHPP in the US. Death certificates or medical records were obtained in 248 of those cases and strange neurological symptoms were screened by a committee of neurologists. About half those who had died had not been subjected to an autopsy.

Some of those tracing options used in America were not open to the Australian CJD unit and its small staff. Later in 1992 it was deluged with calls in the wake of more publicity. Department of Health personnel later admitted they were afraid of breaching one section of the National Health Act that provided for a jail sentence if information requested by one individual was released that disclosed information about other parties — including institutions — without their consent.

Depending on which hospital or treating doctor was initially consulted by anxious hPG or hGH recipients or their parents, experiences varied on whether they got requested information on CJD, their own medical records, batch numbers of injections used or all three. Some got what they wanted, some did not. Many of those who rang the CJD unit, the majority of them from among the 1,400-odd female hPG recipients, wanted to be told one thing: that they would not contract CJD. Such reassurance was impossible. All CSL batches were implicated. Jane Allender and Jenny Halford had received no common batch injections. However, the last known batch number from which Jane Allender was treated was 44. Jenny Halford had received hPG from five batches including batch 43 for a stimulation test and batch 45. Vonda Cummings was treated solely from batch 44. Jan Blight was treated solely from batch 25.

Melbourne endocrinologist Dr Garry Warne, chairman of the growth hormone advisory committee of the Australian Paediatric Endocrine Group (APEG), had written a full year earlier, in July 1991, to the Minister for Health, Brian Howe. In the letter he said the group was concerned about the government leaving the counselling of former patients with a risk of CJD to treating doctors who did not have the resources to trace former patients. APEG had no problem with recipients having a right to be informed and receiving counselling, but the group considered it urgent that funds be made available from the government to pay nurse counsellors to trace and counsel the patients.

"In the past two months, the British press has carried some ugly publicity against health authorities there, because of alleged failure to adequately inform former GH recipients of the risk of CJD. The situation here could be worse, because we have done less," Warne wrote. "We urge you to give this matter your urgent consideration."[6]

Although the minister replied in August 1991, throwing the onus back on endocrinologists, nothing more was done until a meeting on June 30, 1992 in Canberra, following both "7.30 Report" features and other media reports. This was attended by the head of HPAC, Professor Leslie Lazarus, five Department of Health officers, one paediatric endocrinologist and an obstetrician. The meeting decided to liaise with the Health Insurance Commission to find addresses of recipients who had not been traced to date and to forward the addresses to their doctors. A single counselling service to handle both hPG and hGH recipients was to be set up in Sydney and Melbourne for three months, it was agreed, "with the aim of completing the exercise if possible before Christmas".[7]

CJD was an alien term to the Cummings family before Vonda's death. In his grief, nothing made sense to Stephen Cummings until he saw a current affairs program on commercial television in early 1992 that linked CJD to the fertility drug hPG. At Stephen's request his local GP made inquiries with the neurology department of the Queen Elizabeth Hospital, but was told that Vonda Cummings had not undergone hPG therapy at the hospital. The Cummings family did not believe this answer. Stephen was positive that Vonda had undergone fertility treatment via injection at the hospital. None of the details of patients treated privately were linked by computer to central medical records until 1980. Vonda's treatment had been in 1975. It was not picked up.

In mid-1992 Dr Lynette Dumble, alerted by the McMurtrie stories, began researching the warnings that had been given to human hormone drug recipients, particularly in view of the theoretical risk to others from accidental transmission of CJD via tissue, organ or blood donations. She found that far too few had been contacted and, with Dr Renate Klein, a lecturer in women's studies at Deakin University in Geelong, wrote to the *Lancet* about it. Dumble wanted doctors from around the world to be aware that CJD was transmitted through hPG and not merely through hGH, the risks of which had been cited in various scientific and medical journals since 1985. Up to mid-1992, despite several articles in the medical literature on CJD and hGH, Jane Allender's case had not been cited anywhere apart from its original report. This meant hPG-linked CJD was not being appreciated worldwide.

Dumble had also found in her reading that HPAC, which ran the Australian program, had broken its own guidelines in allowing the use of hPG on ovulating women undergoing in-vitro fertilisation treatment. Dumble and Klein's *Lancet* letter was published in the October 3, 1992 issue.[8] In it they accused the Federal Government of keeping Australian human hormone recipients "in the dark" about their CJD risk. The letter generated wide publicity in both Australia and Britain.

In line with the decision made at the meeting involving the

endocrinologists in June 1992, the chief health officer, Adams, announced in October that the Federal Government would pay for special services to trace and counsel human hormone recipients. Two-thirds remained officially untraced by their doctors. These services, were to be available only in Sydney and Melbourne.

In a London newspaper article that followed the *Lancet* letter, retired. Birmingham-based Professor Wilfred Butt, one of the pioneers of hPG treatment in Britain, said he had treated up to 200 women nearing the end of their reproductive years. They had been making last attempts to become mothers in the 1960s and 1970s. "They would now be running into the age group where there's a greater incidence of illnesses inducing dementia anyway. It would be hard to diagnose whether they had Alzheimer's disease or CJD," he said.[9]

In late November 1992 Drs Dumble and Klein delivered a paper to the Australian Bio-ethics Association conference in Sydney that received front-page newspaper treatment. In it they warned that Australia faced an "epidemic" of medically induced CJD from human hormone drugs because of official silence; recipients should have been warned long ago not to donate organs or blood.[10]

Meanwhile, Sydney freelance journalist Diane Armstrong had met a woman at a dinner party in mid-1992 who was extremely anxious about her risk of CJD after being notified by her doctor. Armstrong contacted doctors on the AHPHP, as well as women who had been treated for infertility. The subsequent article was published in the *Sydney Morning Herald*.[11] The accompanying front-page news headline highlighted a quote from the company secretary of CSL, who had told Armstrong that hPG was "experimental" and "not established therapy".[12]

This author, who had written about Dumble and Klein's predictions and a run of follow-up stories that continued over a week, was deluged with calls from frightened, anxious, angry, resentful women in particular, who were desperate for more information and critical of the defensive attitude of departmental staff in Canberra who refused to give them information about their own treatment. Some parents of hGH recipients also contacted this author. As did Noel Halford, keen to find another media outlet interested in the story, to broadcast his and Allender's calls for an inquiry.

The CJD unit in Canberra was so overwhelmed with telephone calls it established a hotline on December 3, which in the next four weeks alone took 1800 calls, and had to more than double its staff to 10. In late December the *Hinch* current affairs television program broadcast the hotline number that contributed to the number of calls.

The temporary counselling, announced in October 1992 in only Sydney and Melbourne, and obviously inadequate for the numbers and geographical spread of recipients, was later expanded to professional "anxiety counselling" under the Marriage Guidance Council (later renamed Relationships Australia). CJD support groups were set up in each state to channel information and hold regular meetings for those interested.

Some treating gynaecologists and endocrinologists did not believe the claims that either hPG or hGH use was experimental or being used in a trial. It had been in use for so long it was considered standard treatment. CSL later retracted use of the word "experimental" in relation to human hormone drug treatment in Diane Armstrong's feature article in a later letter to the *Sydney Morning Herald*.[13]

Echoing comments from his colleagues in Britain, the Federal Health Minister, Brian Howe expressed sympathy to the families of the CJD victims, but said there was no basis on which the government or CSL could admit to legal liability for any compensation. These comments followed unsuccessful attempts to settle a law suit against Emory University in Atlanta, where Professor Alfred Wilhelmi had produced the hGH for New Zealand that had resulted in the death of Deborah McKenzie. New Zealand barrister Michael Okkerse was confident that "substantial litigation" would follow his case from other relatives of hGH victims. They may be eligible, he claimed, for damages from a variety of sources including manufacturers, suppliers and government regulatory agencies that approved the use of human hormone drugs.[14]

In the last month of 1992, in a joint letter sent by registered post to Howe, Noel Halford and Ted Allender launched the first salvo in what they expected to be a protracted war in their battle for compensation for their motherless children.[15] They wanted a meeting to discuss government responsibility for the deaths of their wives under a Commonwealth program and from a drug manufactured by the government-owned CSL, the producer of Australian blood products, all vaccines and the anti-venoms for a number of poisonous snakes and spiders. Allender and Halford also wanted to discuss repeated calls for women on the fertility program to be warned of their risk of CJD and to ensure that, as a precaution, they did not donate organs, tissue or blood and inadvertently spread the disease.

But Howe did not reply. A federal election loomed in March 1993 and it was well known that he was unlikely to remain in the health portfolio. Frustrated and disappointed that their attempt to establish high-level dialogue with the government had not even brought an acknowledgment, Allender and Halford realised that calling for an inquiry into the whole saga might be a necessary next step.

His family had always called Patrick Baldwin "smiler", a name he reacted to more than Patrick. He was a happy child, the eldest of Noel and Janet Baldwin's three boys and two girls. He was close to his siblings, loved western movies, barracked for Leeds United soccer team and loved fishing with his maternal grandfather, a sporting angler. But he was shorter than his brothers, and at 14 was diagnosed with growth hormone deficiency.

From October 1977 until September 1980 Patrick received injections of hGH several times a week at Sheffield Children's Hospital, about 60 kilometres from his home in Gainsborough, Lincolnshire. He grew to 163 centimetres (5 feet, 4 inches) by the time he was 18, and was taller than his beloved grandfather, who was only 157 centimetres (5 feet, 2 inches).

After qualifying as a mechanic Patrick joined the British Navy, as his brothers did, in 1983. At 20, training to become a leading marine engineer, he married a Portsmouth girl, Mandy, and together they had two daughters, Nicola and Zara. But the marriage foundered and they divorced in August 1990.

Twelve months later, Patrick began losing his balance as his ship, the HMS *Cottesmore*, returned from a voyage. His brother Mark, rang his parents in October, concerned about Patrick's deterioration in the three months since he had seen him. They drove the 500 kilometres to Portsmouth the next day. To see their son with a patch over one eye due to double vision, and a strange barking cough, holding on to doors and walls to let them into his flat, was a huge shock. Patrick crawled upstairs to the bathroom and returned downstairs by shuffling on his rear end, just as Jenny Halford had done in Berkshire. He told his parents that the Navy was conducting multiple tests on him for a variety of disorders including MS.

But Patrick knew at once why he was constantly dizzy. He told his parents that while on shore leave in America once, he had read an article about deaths from CJD in American hGH recipients. He had also seen the father of 20-year-old Saul Hefferon-Waldon, the second British hGH victim to die, on a television documentary. He had already rung the Sheffield Children's Hospital and, although he didn't tell his parents, he had told the navy doctors that he probably had the beginnings of CJD following his hGH treatment.[16]

Patrick continued to deteriorate as his tests with the Navy continued — CT and MRI scans, lumbar punctures, and tests for brain tumours, congenital malformations, syphilis, and other infections that can affect the brain and balance. In January 1992 he was referred to the National Hospital for Nervous Diseases at Queen's Square in London. There, doctors agreed he was more likely to have CJD than MS because his condition was worsening daily. Soon he could not walk at all.

Patrick was fully aware he did not have long to live. Confined to a wheelchair by February 1992, and unable to work or care for himself, he couldn't stay in Portsmouth, close to his loves, the navy and his daughters. Determined to beat the illness, he told his father when he arrived to take Patrick back to Gainsborough on February 21, three days after his thirtieth birthday: "Dad, I will be out of this chair and back at sea!"

Noel and Janet did not realise their son's illness was linked with his childhood hGH injections until he came home. Each day he gradually lost the fight against the terrible damage to his brain. "You've got a son there and technically he was fit for active duty but he was in a wheelchair. You see him getting worse every week and your mind starts to work and you think there is a reason for this. This did not come from drinking a cup of tea," Noel recalls angrily.[17]

Noel saw a story in the *Sheffield Evening Post* about hGH and CJD and from it contacted David Body, who had already lodged writs on behalf of the families of CJD victims, the first of which was Terrence Newman. In May 1992 he received "a lot of information that was very helpful" from the *Today* reporter, Alan Watkins.[18] "We had a lad dying in the house and those responsible — who knew something about it — never came near us. It's a man-created disease — no two ways about it. There was no follow-up," Noel recalls bitterly.

In the last six weeks of his life, the weather turned cold and Patrick no longer responded. He lay for hours staring mutely at the ceiling. His parents spoke to him and asked questions each time they entered the room. In this terminal vegetative state, he was filmed several times for news items and documentaries on the hGH medical disaster and his parents' calls for an inquiry and compensation for their granddaughters. They remained angry that no official attached to the program — with so many already dead — had offered information, advice on whether barrier nursing was necessary or financial help.

Patrick was nursed 24 hours a day by his mother, fed through a tube in his stomach. His mouth was swabbed every few hours. He sometimes mashed his lower lip, having clamped shut on it as he inhaled during his sleep. His father would slap his face with a flannel to unclamp his lip in the morning as the television blared in the background in the vain hope of keeping his mind active. He had drugs to control the spasms and pain and salve for his cracked lips. Patrick Baldwin lost his fight against CJD in December 1992.

By the end of 1992 the British Government, like the Australians, had ruled out any compensation for growth hormone CJD victims. As the death toll rose beyond seven and publicity was generated around England by the Newmans, the Baldwins and others who were suing the government for compensation, support from opposition MPs bolstered repeated calls for an inquiry into the medical disaster. Each call was greeted with the same governmental reply: doctors treated patients in good faith acting on the best information available at the time.

Another hGH recipient, Stuart Smith, who was also in a wheelchair for his thirtieth birthday, grew to 168 centimetres and received hGH over almost the same period as Patrick Baldwin — from April 1977 to 1981. Bright, handsome, and sporty, he was ecstatic about the lease on life his height gave him. But it would also be a death sentence.

Just like Patrick he knew about CJD contamination of hGH from news stories and knew that when the dizziness and staggering started it meant the end. Watched helplessly by his family, he became blind, totally incapacitated and died in October 1993, the twelfth British hGH recipient to die of CJD. A thirteenth, James Bettinson, was already dying when Stuart Smith's inquest at Northampton in October 1994 found, as with Patrick Baldwin, that he had died of CJD linked to his hGH treatment.

In France, meanwhile, the death toll from CJD, growing at a frightening rate, had topped 30 among the 1700-odd former child recipients treated up to mid-1985. An official investigation into the French hormone program began in 1992 following media claims and legal action taken by parents of the dead, including the 15-year-old youngster, Ilyassil Benziane. The investigation would reveal one of the most shocking scandals in France's medical history.

CHAPTER 15

The genetic lottery

A MILESTONE WAS REACHED in 1989 on both sides of the Atlantic that revolutionised the diagnosis of familial TSEs. Researchers at Northwick Park Hospital in London found a particular mutation in one gene[1] of several members of an English family who died of CJD.[2] Subsequently, in collaboration with the Northwick Park group, Stanley Prusiner's laboratory in California showed beyond doubt that there was a genetic link to TSE diseases. Karen Hsaio and colleagues from Prusiner's laboratory published their discovery of a particular mutation in one gene — what Prusiner and others now popularly describe as the prion protein (PRNP) gene (Gajdusek's group calls it the scrapie amyloid protein gene) — in several sufferers of the inheritable variant of CJD, GSS.[3] That single change, a minute difference when compared to another human without that mutation, was not found in members of the same family who were not affected by the disease.

This was final proof of the genetic role in human TSEs. Although suspected since the 1970s when about 10 per cent of cases of CJD were found to be familial, new molecular genetic techniques had made it official that TSEs were both infectious and inheritable. At this time, the late 1980s and early 1990s, the idea that an infectious TSE disease could be diagnosed solely by genetic testing was highly controversial. The suggestion that it was possible, made by Dr John Collinge, a London neurologist then working with the Northwick Park group, was shouted down, even after mutations were found in cases that did not have typical symptoms of TSE diseases.[4]

One case reported in 1990 was very atypical. A man, brought up by his maternal step-grandmother because both his mother and maternal grandmother had developed presenile dementia, was thought to have familial Alzheimer's disease or Huntington's disease. At age 27 he had declined intellectually, lost his memory, spoken in a jerky, abrupt way and relied totally on others. Symptoms, however, had apparently begun in his boyhood when an anti-social personality disorder, characterised by stealing, fighting and verbal abuse, was noted. By his early twenties he had become aggressive and was particularly violent towards his wife. He was dead at 36, having entirely lost his memory and his ability to speak or to walk without severe staggering and jerking of his limbs.

But when the man's brain was examined after death, no spongiform change was detected. Nor were any amyloid plaques — associated with both TSE diseases and Alzheimer's disease — found. However, a mutation — in this case an insertion or extra chunk — was found on his PRNP gene. This insertion was also found in another member of the man's family. It was identical to that reported by workers at the Northwick Park group. Within three years, another 46 relatives of the man's family covering seven generations would be investigated and reclassified. Some of these relatives had previously been diagnosed by doctors as having Alzheimer's disease, Huntington's disease, Parkinson's disease, Picks disease, CJD, GSS, atypical dementia and myoclonic epilepsy.

In 1990, Collinge and colleagues suggested that "prion dementia" might be "a more appropriate diagnostic term" for cases, such as the 36-year-old man, which were remarkably lacking most of the normally recognised post-mortem criteria of TSE diseases, including spongiform change but who had unmistakable genetic markers for familial TSE disease. Screening by PRNP gene analysis would also help to identify the full range of symptoms in inherited TSE diseases and "may be relevant to the assessment of possible transmission of bovine spongiform encephalopathy to man".[5]

A mystery disease emerged in 1986 that would later be added to the family of human TSE diseases. Fatal familial insomnia (FFI) is just what it sounds like. It's an inherited and terminal disease in which inability to sleep is often, but apparently not always, a key symptom. In its first appearance in the scientific literature the case of a 53-year-old Italian man was recounted.[6] He went to his doctor complaining that his previous ability to sleep soundly had vanished. He could sleep for only two to three hours a night. On top of that, he had lost his libido and had become impotent.

Two months later the patient was down to one hour of sleep a night, which was dominated by vivid dreams. He developed slurred speech, limb tremors and a staggering gait. Although he would slump into a stupor if left alone, he would perform what were described as complex gestures accompanied by noisy breathing while in that state. Bright light could arouse him to wakefulness. Later he developed jerks in his limbs and would breathe irregularly. He died nine months after his symptoms began. Two of his sisters and two other members of his extended family had died after similar symptoms.

In 1992, a specific FFI gene mutation was identified and reported.[7] This discovery meant that FFI could be distinguished from other TSEs by simple DNA analysis of a blood sample. In 1995, FFI was confirmed as a TSE after it was successfully transmitted to experimental mice.[8,9]

By 1997, 10 years after its discovery, doctors and scientists around the world had pinpointed eight families with the inherited killer in their midst. The seventh family was discovered in Australia after the death, in November 1994, of a 60-year-old woman of Danish-Irish descent. She died in Brisbane from typical FFI after 13 months of worsening nocturnal insomnia, long bouts of daytime stupor, confusion, slurred speech, difficulty in walking, dementia and occasional jerks in her limbs. Her condition was linked to the death 14 years earlier of a son, one of her nine children.[10] The son had died in May 1978, aged only 20, after seven months of a rapidly worsening illness. This patient — the youngest-known person to die from FFI — first complained of headaches, memory loss and an unsteady walk. He deteriorated, soon slurring his speech and walking with difficulty. He was in a coma for the fortnight before his death. Strangely, insomnia was not remembered as a symptom by any family member and was not found in his medical records. The apparent lack of insomnia, despite the name of the disease, was also absent from the medical histories of two members of another FFI family.

Genetic screening is now available for members of families affected by GSS, FFI and familial CJD. In the FFI family from Brisbane, apparently unrelated to six other family cases then known in other countries, six of the 20-year-old man's eight siblings requested genetic testing. So did four of the seven surviving siblings of his mother. Of the boy's sisters and brothers tested, three sisters and two brothers, aged between 30 and 50, were found to have the FFI mutation. In addition, one of two children of one of those six adults was found with it. None of the four siblings of the mother was positive for the FFI mutation. The result is that six of the 12 family members identified to be at risk of FFI have the mutation. They will die of the disease unless something else kills them first.

Two members of a second Australian FFI family, the eighth known family in the world, were discovered in 1997.[11] Although of Irish extraction like the other Australian FFI family, there appears to be no common ancestry. The family came from Victoria and was remarkable in that one female member had been adopted and had no knowledge of her ancestry until she was admitted, dying, to a nursing home. Her daughter, who had recently turned 18 and was thus eligible to access her mother's birth registration records, did so. It was soon learned that the dying woman was one of six members of her family — her biological mother and brother, a maternal aunt and the aunt's two sons — who had died of confirmed or retrospectively determined FFI. The woman died aged 54, 21 months after the onset of her illness, without noticeable insomnia in the four months she spent in the neuropsychiatric unit of a Melbourne hospital.

Some elderly members of FFI families who do have the mutation appear to escape the disease. This is because FFI can have a very late onset, and so an individual may die of other age-related diseases first.

By the time molecular genetics became the vogue, Alfons Jakob's familial CJD family tree, which he identified in the 1920s, had spread through four generations. That family, the Backer family of Germany, was not alone. Seven decades later, by the early 1990s, that family had been joined by more than 100 others in which members had succumbed to familial CJD thanks to their inherited genetic mutation.

As far back as the late 1960s, large-scale epidemiological studies of the frequency and distribution of sporadic CJD had been conducted. Two of the biggest were carried out in France between 1968 and 1982, and in Britain between 1970 and 1979. The information gleaned gave a much greater insight into the occurrence of CJD, particularly in clusters.

While other epidemiological studies showed no significant clustering to indicate any environmental or other cause,[12] an exception occurred in Israel. When hospital records were checked and neurologists and EEG labs were visited for details of cases between 1963 and 1975, researchers discovered an extremely high rate of CJD among Libyan-born immigrants.[13]

In Czechoslovakia two small but apparently significant clusters were found in the rural areas of Orava and Lucenec in the 1970s and early 1980s. For a time those cases of CJD were thought to have resulted from the practice of the inhabitants of those areas of eating sheep eyeballs and brain that had only been lightly cooked. Orava in particular was known to be a scrapie-affected area. In Hungary, just over the border from one of the Czechoslovakian clusters, another interesting cluster of five CJD cases was identified in the 1980s. A second cluster of 10 cases was found near the Tsiza River in the middle of the country.

In 1983 Chilean researchers reported clusters which were later found to include six families with up to 17 affected family members.[14]

As TSEs came under more scrutiny through molecular genetic analysis, two siblings of Polish descent were found to have an unusual mutation in their PRNP genes. By 1990 this same mutation, called a codon 200 mutation, was found in individuals genetically tested in both the Czechoslovakian clusters. Here, then, was the cause of the clustering — an inherited mutation on the PRNP gene — not undercooked sheep's eyeballs.

By late 1990 investigators in Gajdusek's laboratory had found the same codon 200 mutation — which is not found in GSS or kuru victims — in seven Sephardic Jews. Four of them had been born in Libya but were living in Israel. Thus a codon 200 mutation was responsible not only for the Czech clusters but for the Libyan-born Jews as well.

Because this mutation had not been found in CJD patients of other diverse ethnic origins, scientists concluded that it was only one of the factors contributing to disease, probably one of several different mutations that triggered the normal PrP protein to convert itself into infectious amyloid or killer prion protein.[15]

By the early 1990s codon 200 mutations, evident in a sweep from Eastern Europe to the Mediterranean were clearly an inheritable form of CJD. Soon they were found in unrelated families in Japan and the United States.

By 1993 the basis of the Chilean cluster was reported — again a codon 200 mutation that had remarkably similar symptoms to sporadic CJD.[16] It was also identified in two people in Britain, one of whom was of Libyan Jewish ancestry.

In a 1987 review of the results of a 15-year French epidemiological study of CJD, Paul Brown and colleagues from the NIH proposed that person-to-person or environmental transmission of CJD was not the root of the problem. Instead it could be that the infectious agent was naturally present in humans and on some occasions resulted in disease because of mutation or trauma.[17]

From the early 1980s many surgeons, neurosurgeons in particular, had been horrified to discover that person-to-person CJD contamination had probably occurred much earlier than the 1974 report of the corneal transplant transmission in America. The 1435 cases referred to Gajdusek's laboratory between 1966 and 1978 resulted in the first definitive paper on patterns of worldwide occurrence and clustering of CJD cases. Colin Masters, the Australian pathologist who reviewed Jakob's original cases in Heidelberg, carried out the analysis. Masters was working with Gajdusek in the late 1970s and from the series of cases was able to find all sorts of interesting facts. But of special significance in the scientific paper that resulted was the inclusion of some of the eight defining cases of CJD described by the English doctor Sam Nevin in 1960. Masters found that three of the patients reported by Nevin in his seminal 1960 paper had been operated on by the same neurosurgeon, in the same neurosurgical unit in London, within eight months.[18]

These findings were investigated further in Britain in the early 1980s. At that time Alan Dickinson's study on the scrapie-infected hGH protocol in mice was underway in Edinburgh and fears of CJD contamination of the hGH supply had resulted in the funding of a five-year study of the incidence of CJD in England and Wales. Britain's MRC conducted the study between 1980 and 1984.[19] This was the same body that ran the Human Growth Hormone Program from 1959 to 1977.

The MRC's epidemiological study was conducted by Professor Bryan Matthews, who in the past had worked cooperatively with Gajdusek's laboratory. Matthews, by now professor of clinical neurology at the University of Oxford, was assisted by Scottish neurologist, Dr Robert Will. Will, 29 years old when he began the fieldwork from

Oxford, made some ironic and tragic retrospective findings during the study, which were published in a paper in 1982.

Will examined the case notes of patients treated at Nevin's own hospital, the Maida Vale Hospital for Nervous Diseases — long before it was known that CJD was infectious. In January 1952, two patients Nevin had described in a report in 1954 were admitted to the hospital suffering from rapidly progressive dementia. They died within a week of each other on January 12 and January 19, 1952. Records from the first patient only were retrieved, and these showed that he had two procedures carried out on his brain. The first was the drilling of burr holes for ventriculography into his skull on December 31, 1951. This allowed the injection of a dye that would show up abnormal shapes, like tumours, in the ventricular system, the connecting cavities of the brain.[20] In the second procedure, depth electrodes were inserted into his brain on January 10, 1952 — two days before his death from CJD.[21]

Another two of Nevin's many patients, their cases reported at length in his seminal paper of 1960,[22] had neurosurgical procedures in the same operating theatre as the first two patients. The second two patients underwent neurosurgery in late January 1952, within three weeks of the exploratory neurosurgery and death of the first patient "almost certainly using common instruments", Dr Will noted, and at least 15 years before it was known that rapidly progressive dementing illnesses could be infectious.

The first of the latter two patients was a formerly heavy-drinking engineer, aged 58, who had his own burr holes for ventriculography drilled on January 23, 1952. Seven days later, in a second neurosurgical procedure, a golf ball-sized benign tumour rising out of his dura mater was surgically removed. Although the engineer seemed to improve, he died of CJD in October 1953 — 21 months after his neurosurgery and 20 weeks after his symptoms began.[23]

The second patient was a 67-year-old retired engineer admitted to the Maida Vale Hospital on January 15, 1952. He had a brain abscess drained the next day. With probably the same theatre instruments used for the ventriculography on the other two patients, he had the abscess removed on February 29. He died of CJD in November 1953 — 14 weeks after his symptoms had begun and 18 months after his operation.[24]

Will also uncovered a third probable case of accidental transmission of CJD via surgical instruments. On February 3, 1956 at London's Brook Hospital, a 47-year-old housewife underwent brain surgery for a cortical undercut. This procedure appeared to cure her of her 10-year history of depression and obsessional neurosis, which included compulsive washing of her hands, repeated boiling of cooking utensils and milk straining, all part of a phobia that she might harm her family through food preparation. The operation was successful. But 17 months later symptoms like double vision and giddiness began and then worsened to severe memory loss, difficulty walking and muscle jerks. She died on September 12, 1957, 19 months after her neurosurgery.

Will's check of operating theatre records showed that the woman's cortical undercut operation took place on the same day as burr holes were drilled in the skull of another patient — a 61-year-old civil servant. The civil servant died the following day of CJD after an eight-week rapid progression of symptoms, which included delusions and the statement recorded by his doctors, "Let me arrange these things as the Queen Mother is coming today".[25]

A fourth probable case of CJD from surgical instruments — this time in France — was reported in 1980. The report came from a retrospective look at a case from 1965 in which a patient developed CJD two years after an operation in which the same instruments were probably used several days beforehand on a patient who died of CJD.[26]

The three cases of CJD following neurosurgery in England in 1952 and in 1956 and a fourth in France in the 1960s remain circumstantially probable. To be fully proved, the instruments used and tissue from the infected brains would need to have successfully induced disease in experimental inoculation in primates. This was the method used to prove the world's second case of iatrogenic or accidental transmission of CJD — via the depth electrodes used in Switzerland on the young epileptic patients whose deaths were reported in 1977.

The 1979 paper in which Colin Masters reviewed the 1435 cases that had been referred to Gajdusek's laboratory uncovered other fascinating facts on the worldwide occurrence of CJD. This included two cases in which a husband and wife both died of the disease. Health professionals, farmers, farmers' wives, physician's wives, and food handlers including housewives and raw meat handlers or butchers were among occupations affected that were of interest in the review.

In their 1982 paper, which revealed the accidental transmission via neurosurgery on Nevin's patients, Will and Matthews also revealed two more interesting findings. They found a tiny but remarkable cluster for such a rare disease in three people who lived within 250 metres of one another in Britain. The first, who died of CJD in 1965 and the second, who died in 1968 shared the same doctor, but the doctor's medical records were destroyed by the time these cases were found two decades later. A third person, a dentist, lived within sight of the homes of the first two patients. He died in 1980 having used his home as a surgery between 1950 and 1977. His records, however, were incomplete and did not refer to the first two patients.

Perhaps more interesting from the point of view that it may remain forever a mystery, is the patient who died of CJD in 1980 in southern England after social contact with two sisters and their cousin — all three of whom appeared to have died from a familial form of CJD. The familial disease claimed its victims after a long progression of symptoms between 1966 and 1970. One of the sisters was confirmed to have had CJD after her death but the other two were classified from their probable symptoms because they did not undergo autopsies. The fourth woman died in 1980. She was related to all three by marriage, knew one of the sisters and had met her socially and at family gatherings for 20 years. She last saw her in hospital five months before the sister's death.

CJD in a patient who merely had contact with cases of familial Creutzfeldt-Jakob disease but was not genetically related has been reported in Chile and France as well. In neither of those two cases did the spouse of the non-familial case have the disease, Will and Matthews found. As contact transmission between sporadic cases has never been reported, they found it "remarkable" that all reported possible "contact" transmissions have been with cases of familial CJD.[27]

In the early 1990s, researchers continued to reinforce what scrapie researchers had found 50 years before — that whatever caused TSE diseases was an extraordinarily resistant infectious agent. Using what was thought to be a fairly heat-resistant strain of scrapie in unmodified brain tissue, Paul Brown and colleagues in Gajdusek's laboratory tried various methods of inactivating scrapie by heat. Preparations of brain, and others of scrapie-associated fibrils (SAFs), were each given four separate treatments. One batch of each was mixed with formaldehyde and autoclaved for 30 minutes at 134 degrees Celsius. Another batch was subjected to dry heat in a furnace at 160 degrees Celsius for 10 minutes, and another batch for one hour. A fourth lot was left in the furnace at 360 degrees Celsius for an hour — a lengthy period at phenomenal heat.

Unexpectedly, while these treatments decreased the amount of infectivity (fewer mice injected with what remained after the treatments died of scrapie), the agent was not totally eliminated. Even the SAFs, although mostly bent from their normal, straight, rod-like appearance into wavy filaments, were not entirely destroyed. It raised "the disturbing question of whether even incineration can be guaranteed to inactivate the agent".[28]

In another experiment Brown decided to test whether burial underground had any degrading effect on the infectious agent. He took 100 millilitres of the clear fluid which remained after blending 14 scrapie-infected hamster brains in a saline solution and poured it on to dry topsoil. The resultant mulch was divided between two petri dishes, both with holes in their covers and one with a hole in the bottom as well. The sealed dishes were embedded in soil just under the upper levels of two small plastic flowerpots each filled with soil. The pots were then buried under a thin layer of mulch in Brown's backyard. It was September 1986, a time when the human hormone drug toll of CJD victims was still under 10 and the BSE epidemic was in such infancy that the drooling and staggering cow disease had not yet been given a name.

The pots, to the surprise of Brown's neighbours years later when the innocuous experimental site in his backyard was filmed, written about and flashed around the world via television satellite, remained buried in that backyard. Through freezing Washington winters and humid, sweltering summers, rain, snow, thaw and wind, the pots sat for three years.

In the February 21, 1991 issue of the *Lancet,* Brown and Gajdusek reported the extreme durability of the infectious agent. By this time the human hormone drug toll of CJD had climbed into the thirties and infected dura mater had claimed at least eight lives. BSE was well-known as "mad cow" disease and the epidemic, not yet at its peak, had appeared in thousands of British dairy herds.

Brown and Gajdusek found that while infectivity in the scrapie mulch topsoil had diminished during the burial period, it was *still there* three years later. Infectivity had leached into the soil only immediately underneath the petri dish with the hole in the bottom. And when the three-year-old soil had been filtered to remove bacteria and was injected into Syrian hamsters, the hamsters later developed scrapie. "Our data help to explain how, in Iceland, healthy flocks of sheep contracted scrapie after being brought to vacant farmland that had three years earlier been grazed by scrapie-affected flocks," Brown and Gajdusek wrote. "Other unconventional viruses, such as Creutzfeldt-Jakob agent, all of which are highly resistant to ordinary methods of disinfection, may also survive for a long time in contaminated environments."[29]

Brown and Gajdusek called for "the practice of ploughing-under carcasses of animals dying of scrapie or BSE, even with the addition of quicklime, [to] be abandoned" unless an autoclave was used to heat the remains of TSE infected animals under high pressure.[30] A group of vets present when Paul Brown previewed the contents of his paper at a conference in Brussels, several months prior to publication in the *Lancet* joked about how many cows they could bury before the paper came out.

By the early 1990s analysis of those large epidemiological studies of the 1970s and earlier had revealed extreme variations in the symptoms, duration and disease progression between CJD sufferers. Unlike kuru, which had a totally reliable onset and progression of symptoms lasting 18 months at most, CJD cases created a far more complex diagnostic picture. There were short sharp durations of illness of mere months. Others had sudden onsets that at first looked like MS or stroke. Others still had initial symptoms that mimicked Parkinsonism or amyotrophic lateral sclerosis (ALS — Lou Gehrig's disease), which can be differentiated by nothing but time and a post-mortem examination. Some CJD patients experienced initial non-specific symptoms that can happen to anyone — anxiety, weight loss, decreased appetite and insomnia — before more specific neurological symptoms took over. Others complained first of confusion, memory loss or uncharacteristic behaviour. Sometimes dementia was the first noticeable sign. Little wonder that CJD, an unusual and rare disease, is still misdiagnosed.

When Will and Matthews looked at sporadic cases of CJD in England and Wales during an earlier study between 1970 and 1979, they found six per cent of the patients had a mean disease duration of about 33 months — far longer than the average 12 month progression from initial symptoms to death. These British patients could be subtyped into three categories. In the first the CJD progression was slow and inexorable. The second had a slow progression of degenerative symptoms leading to a quick terminal period. The most rare was a third type with rapidly developing symptoms followed by a long terminal phase.[31]

Brown has stressed in papers over the years the need for post-mortem verification and transmission to laboratory animals, if possible, to confirm any CJD diagnosis — solely because the disease can be mistaken for a host of other strange-sounding chronic degenerative conditions. Without doubt the most common confusion is with Alzheimer's disease. Some forms of CJD, particularly familial, have symptoms lasting up to five years — extremely long for CJD. A 73-year-old American woman died in July 1982 after suffering from CJD and Alzheimer's simultaneously. It was proved when a post-mortem examination of her brain revealed not only the amyloid protein plaques of Alzheimer's disease (which are different from the plaques of CJD), but also spongiform change. A spider monkey and a chimpanzee injected with her brain tissue died of CJD. At least two other people are believed to have died suffering from both diseases.[32]

In another rare case, CJD killed a Boston neurosurgeon as well as several chimpanzees and squirrel monkeys that were later injected with samples of his brain and lung. A review of his case indicates he may also have been suffering simultaneously from Köhlmeier-Degos disease, a nasty, malignant, atrophic disease involving the central nervous system that also affects veins and skin. None of the chimps or monkeys developed the neurosurgeon's vascular or skin problems.[33]

In 1988 Paul Brown proposed that the newly emerged cases of CJD in growth hormone recipients came either from a single strain of the infective agent, distinct from kuru and sporadic CJD, or that the circumstances surrounding the infection may have held the clue. This was in the light of the very early sign of CJD in the 16-year-old growth hormone recipient who had died prematurely from pneumonia in 1979. According to Brown:

> The infective particle, which has long been known to be biologically 'sticky', may adhere to the hormone molecule during its extraction from the pituitary gland, and enter the CNS as a nefarious passenger complexed to hormone molecules heading for their receptors in the hypothalamus, with subsequent spread to the nearby basal ganglia and their cerebellar projection.[34]

Around the time in the early 1980s when Pat Merz and Robert Somerville found their abnormal fibrils (SAFs) in scrapie brains under an electron microscope, Prusiner was isolating what he termed prion rods. To many in the field, the fibrils and the rods were identical. SAFs were consistently found in all infected material that was examined under electron microscopes. Merz and colleagues proposed that perhaps the SAFs were the infectious agent itself, a possible new type of filamentous virus.

The question remains, however, whether SAFs and rods are both composed of PrP^{sc}, the killer form of normal prion protein (which appears to be necessary for normal transmission of messages between nerve cells) in the brain. Are the minute SAFs or rods not the infectious agent, but perhaps enormous amounts of the infectious unit aggregating into threads or rods, which are visible only under an electron microscope? Merz claimed the SAFs were the building blocks of amyloid plaques found in TSEs. Prusiner claimed that something else made the plaques, that the rods were the aggregate or build-up of the PrP that comes from a different source — not the infectious unit.

Later in the 1980s Harash Narang, a British-based clinical microbiologist who worked for a time in Gajdusek's laboratory, modified Merz's theory that the SAF could be the infectious agent. Narang and his co-workers proposed from their experiments that the SAF is merely the protein component of the infectious agent.[35]

Another theory proposed by Laura Manuelidis, professor of neuropathology at Yale University, and colleagues — was that TSEs were caused by a retrovirus, similar to HIV or at least something very similar to a virus.

Recently the proponents of the protein-only theory — which originated around 1967 with Tikvah Alper, and also British mathematician John Griffiths — have admitted that it can't account for all the strain variations in TSEs. There are more than 20 known in scrapie plus the three genetic subgroups of CJD (familial CJD, GSS and FFI), and probably kuru as well. The arguments over the cause of TSEs continue.

By 1991 when the first six hGH patients in Britain had died and Jenny Halford had been buried in the churchyard at Inkpen in Berkshire, genetic susceptibility was viewed as an additional marker for those accidentally contaminated with CJD. In London, John Collinge, by now head of the Prion Disease Group in the department of biochemistry and molecular genetics at St Mary's Hospital Medical School, suggested in the *Lancet* that a common PRNP gene variation called a codon 129 polymorphism, might be a susceptibility factor. Those with two of the variations who had been exposed to human hormone drugs or other forms of accidental transmission appeared more susceptible to contracting the disease.[36]

Collinge's susceptibility theory resulted from his study of DNA extracted from either blood or brain tissue from all six then-known British hGH CJD victims. They included Terrence Newman and Alison Lay as well as Jenny Halford, the only one of Australia's four hPG recipients to die overseas. Collinge used sequence analysis; which basically means he looked at the order in which the DNA was placed to see if it was arranged as a normal PRNP gene. Other researchers had used this technique in the quartet of human TSEs and found mutations that were common to cases of familial CJD, GSS and FFI. None of these mutations — many were identified later — were present in any cases of sporadic CJD.

What Collinge found was that, in four of the seven patients he tested, the ordering of the DNA was different to the majority of people at one point — codon 129 on the PRNP gene. Two protein sub-units, or amino acids, which are coded for by the DNA are valine and the other methionine. There are three combinations of coding for these amino acids that can be inherited. These are valine-valine (VV), methionine-methionine (MM) and valine-methionine (VM). Most people are what is called heterozygous, VM, at this position, but these four hGH recipients were uncommonly homozygous for the coding VV at codon 129. Only one of the six human hormone recipients who had died of CJD by the end of 1990 was homozygous for the alternative coupling MM. The remaining two hGH recipients were heterozygous at that position, having one gene each of methionine and valine, MV, as does the majority of the normal population.

The DNA results underpinned Collinge's proposition that valine homozygosity (VV) at codon 129 might predispose anyone exposed to accidental CJD contamination to contract the disease, more so than someone who did not have this mutation. This was also supported by findings of Paul Brown and British experts. They found that, of DNA tested from nine hGH recipients who died of CJD in France and

America, four had VV coding and four had MM coding. Only one had the normal VM coding.[37]

To help test a suggestion by Paul Brown that homozygosity for VV meant a person was more susceptible to accidental CJD infection, the Melbourne research scientist Lynette Dumble tracked down tissue belonging to three of the four hPG-treated women who died of CJD in Australia. Skin lesion tissue taken from Jan Blight and brain tissue retained from the autopsy of Jane Allender was airmailed to America in early 1993. DNA testing carried out at the NIH by Paul Brown and colleagues showed that both Jane Allender and Jan Blight were MM at codon 129. Jenny Halford had already been found to have VV coding in the earlier Collinge study in Britain.[38]

Brown was excited by these findings. They supported earlier findings from DNA tests on accidentally transmitted CJD cases including the two Swiss epilepsy patients, "Linda" the corneal graft recipient, dura mater graft and hGH recipients. In this study 93% of those tested were MM or VV. Of the 110 control subjects (people without CJD) only 49% had MM or VV coding.[39]

Later Paul Brown's hopes of identical genetic mutation in all four hPG CJD victims were dashed. In early 1994, retained liver biopsy tissue from Vonda Cummings, the fourth woman to die in Australia, was found with MV coding.

Basically what all these studies mean is that either MM or VV coding increases susceptibility to all forms of sporadic or accidentally transmitted CJD and kuru. It also appears to affect the age of onset in some GSS cases. And although MV coding is good news — it appears to protect people from developing TSE diseases, or it prolongs the incubation period in which symptoms are not present — it is not proof against the development of TSEs.

By the 1990s kuru, familial CJD, GSS and FFI were recognised as variants or strains of sporadic CJD. But another — as yet unrecognised — variant would soon enmesh politics, agriculture, economics and science in one unruly crisis. And it was already incubating in the brains of the susceptible — in Britain.

CHAPTER 16

Victims fight back

WHEN THE ROAR of the lawn mower stopped, Geraldine Brodrick surveyed her half acre of back garden with satisfaction. Since the collapse of her marriage in 1982, she had moved from Canberra to Brisbane and, following the divorce, to a large brick home built to her design in a thriving new development on the Gold Coast in Queensland. It had a large pool, a huge garden and plenty of native Australian gum trees providing shade from searing summer heat. Her youngest children were both in high school. Her eldest daughter, Belinda, was a nurse in Sydney and second daughter, Jacqueline, was completing a hairdressing apprenticeship.

As Geraldine went to pay Leo, the man who mowed her lawns, he asked if she'd seen a current affairs show on television the previous night, December 8, 1992. "No, as a matter of fact I was out," she said.

"Well, they didn't exactly mention you by name but they did mention the fact about a lady having nine babies. I can't think of anyone else I know. I think you should perhaps ring them."

"Why," asked Geraldine, puzzled by his peculiar and out-of-character evasiveness. "Can't you tell me?"

"No," he said, "but I think you should ring up and find out what it was all about."[1]

Mystified, Geraldine joined some friends for a weekly round of tennis. Some of them had seen the program and told her the subject: how everyone who had received the fertility drug hPG, as well as children who had taken hGH, were at risk of a fatal brain disease that took years to incubate and killed within 12 months of the symptoms appearing.

Geraldine subsequently rang the program's producer, who was staggered that, as the most famous recipient of human hormone therapy in the world, she had not been told of her risk of CJD. The producer gave Geraldine the CJD hotline number, just set up in the Department of

Health in Canberra. The number rang out several times without answer.
After the festivities of Christmas and the New Year, she rang the hotline
again. When it was answered Geraldine pointed out that she should be
on the list of recipients, considering her five separate courses of the
drug back in 1969 and 1970. The woman on the end of the phone said
someone would get back to her. No-one did.

Meanwhile in January 1993, after reading a government advertisement
seeking recipients of hPG and hGH in the high circulation *Australian
Women's Weekly* magazine, Muriel Cummings tried again to link her
daughter-in-law's fertility treatment to Vonda's untimely and horrible
death from CJD. She wrote to the Department of Health. The department contacted the Queen Elizabeth Hospital in Adelaide. This time
checks were made specifically for treatment under the AHPHP in the
hospital's department of obstetrics and gynaecology. Documents kept
separately in this department, not apparent when the Cummings' GP
made inquiries in 1991, confirmed Vonda Cummings had received hPG.
She had had two courses of the drug recorded from batch 44. As a
result, late on the afternoon of Friday January 29, 1993, a press release
was issued by the Federal Department of Health to announce the death
of a third hPG recipient on the AHPHP. Although Vonda's autopsy
report clearly listed CJD as the cause of death, her death certificate did
not. This meant that departmental checks on death certificates of human
hormone recipients had not identified Vonda. Her death from CJD had
remained hidden because of a technicality.

The announcement of Vonda's death was the ammunition Ted Allender and Noel Halford needed. Immediately they fired off an open letter
to the media demanding a meeting with the Minister for Health, and
foreshadowing a call for an inquiry into the whole program. Stephen
Cummings then contacted Ted Allender. Now there were three of them.
A series of regular broadcasts on ABC Radio in Adelaide kept the issue
alive.

In early March Allender and Halford flew to Canberra for a meeting
with Department of Health officials including the Commonwealth's
chief health officer, Dr Tony Adams, and Dr Robert Hall from the communicable diseases section. Efforts were under way to trace all recipients of hPG and hGH, despite an admittedly slow start. Calls for an
inquiry were backed by the Sydney-based Public Interest Advocacy

Centre (PIAC), an independent legal advocacy and policy centre which undertook work in areas of public interest. PIAC had been flooded with calls from angry hormone recipients desperate for information but stonewalled by bureaucrats manning the CJD hotline in Canberra.

Peter Costello, far more advanced in the opposition parliamentary Liberal party than he had been in 1991 when he asked the first questions about the AHPHP, was now the shadow Attorney-General. Should the government fall in the federal election that month, he was likely to be confirmed in the top law portfolio. He vowed to compensate the families of the CJD victims should he become Attorney-General.

But the Labor Government of Paul Keating was returned to power in March 1993. The hopes of Allender, Halford and Cummings for an independent inquiry and swift compensation crashed.

Meanwhile, unaware of all these events, in early 1993, Geraldine Brodrick received a letter from a Sydney gynaecologist who had been given the late Professor Carey's list of patients to contact about their risk of CJD. She listened as the doctor explained the small risk and the three confirmed deaths so far. There wasn't much she could do about it, so in characteristic fashion she just got busy. She worried in case someone ever suggested she was not capable of looking after her children, and occupied herself with a new job in the classic car insurance business.

Soon after, Geraldine Brodrick changed her will, just as she had when her pituitary tumour was discovered in 1975 and she was given two years to live. A practical businesswoman, she wanted her affairs in order ... just in case.

She did not learn for another three years that the departmental database section relating to children born after hPG treatment did not refer to her nine babies. Her doctor, she was informed by letter in 1996, had not provided the department with any details. Geraldine wondered what else had not been recorded.

On the other side of the world, the curve of the BSE epidemic appeared to have plateaued. The rate of confirmed cases fell for the first time. British authorities were citing an average of 890 confirmed cases of BSE reported each week for the first nine weeks of 1993. The 8099 suspected animal cases over that same period had fallen from the 8581 suspected cases reported in the same period in 1992.[2] And the Spongiform

Encephalopathy Advisory Committee (SEAC) found that the dairy farmer who died in 1992 had died of sporadic CJD, prompting the chief medical officer Dr Kenneth Calman to reiterate the "beef is safe" line. "I wish to emphasise that there is no scientific evidence of a causal link between BSE in cattle and CJD in humans," he said.[3]

The CJD Surveillance Unit reported a slight increase in deaths for the third successive year. Between May 1990 and April 1991, 32 cases had been reported. This rose to 37 for the year to April 1992 and to 48 by the end of April 1993. The head of the surveillance unit, Dr Robert Will, attributed the increase to more awareness and better reporting of the disease.

On April 30, 1993, just three months after Vonda Cummings was reported as the third Australian woman on the hPG program to die of CJD, another grim announcement was made — again late on a Friday afternoon. The two-page press release was faxed to media outlets around the country.

> The Commonwealth Department of Health, Housing, Local Government and Community Services has discovered that a fourth woman who was on the National Human Pituitary Hormone Program almost certainly died from the rare brain disorder Creutzfeldt-Jakob Disease. The woman from Western Australia died in 1989 aged 50 from what was originally described as a non-specific neurological disease.[4]

Jan Blight's death slotted neatly into the CJD death tally. Her death in 1989 meant an Australian woman had died each year for four consecutive years, beginning with Jane Allender in 1988. It brought into sharp relief the variations in incubation period for the disease. Although at 16 years, Jan Blight's was the longest, it still meant the average incubation period from infection to display of symptoms in hPG-treated women was about 14 years. It also meant that they were dying before the children they had so desperately wanted reached their teens.

Worldwide CJD deaths following hPG had been confirmed in only four women — all from Australia. Beryl Friel, the English woman who died of definite CJD in 1975, 15 years after giving birth to her daughter Jackie Adamson in 1960, cannot definitely be bracketed into this group.[5] Although she is believed to have received hPG, all hospital records have been destroyed, the hospital itself has closed, and the treating gynaecologist and hospital staff are all dead.

In May 1993, less than two months into the job, the Keating Government's new Federal Minister for Health, Graham Richardson, acted quickly and more decisively than his predecessor. Jan Blight's death announcement was the "trigger" Richardson said he needed to launch the inquiry that Ted Allender and Noel Halford had been fighting to initiate for nearly 18 months.[6] "I believe that the people who were treated while on the program and who are at risk of contracting this disease have a right to know how and on what basis the decisions to start and continue use of the product were taken."[7]

The role and actions of CSL, the government-owned laboratory that manufactured the drug, were not included in the terms of reference. CSL had been indemnified by the Federal Government; its public float on the stock market was due just before the inquiry's head, associate professor Margaret Allars, an administrative law expert from the University of Sydney, was due to report back to the Federal Government in 12 months time.

Noel Halford couldn't believe his fight for an inquiry had ended so quickly. Ted Allender was as usual extremely cynical about the timing of the inquiry, coming as it did on the eve of the issuing of writs by himself, Noel Halford and Stephen Cummings. The government had been warned the writs were about to be lodged. "The public relations performance of this whole ghastly mess has been appalling," Ted told his local newspaper, the Adelaide *Advertiser*, after Richardson's announcement.

The next day their writs, suing both the Commonwealth of Australia and CSL for damages for the wrongful deaths of their wives, were issued in the Victorian Supreme Court. Their then solicitor, David Rush of the firm Rennick Gaynor Kiddle Briggs, said the three men were "reluctant litigants", frustrated by the Federal Department of Health's lack of response to their submissions for compensation.[8,9]

For the first time since their wives died, one way or another, they felt their questions would finally be answered. The trio were soon to be joined by Lyle Blight, Jan's husband who lived in rural Western Australia, in their legal action. They all sat back and waited for the flaws in the AHPHP to be revealed. They were convinced they couldn't lose.

Around the world, law suits began following transmission accidents that had resulted in CJD. On March 8, 1993, the United States Court of Appeals upheld the Louisiana Court's decision in the case of Lyodura implant recipient Richard Nesom. The court still believed — despite the tendering of 36 reports of incubation periods of CJD from the *Morbidity and Mortality Weekly* — that 31 months was the longest known incubation period for dura mater-linked CJD. A rehearing of Nesom's case was refused on April 14, 1993.[10]

A product liability case launched by the family of Brian Bowler, the fourth known victim of CJD from a Lyodura graft, against the manufacturer, B Braun Melsungen, in London's High Court was settled on confidential grounds in December 1993.[11]

The damages case launched by Julia and William McKenzie, parents of Deborah, the first New Zealand victim of CJD from Wilhelmi-prepared hGH, was inching forward to a hearing in Mississippi in 1993. It was the first law suit in the world involving a former hGH recipient who had died of CJD. A three-year statute of limitations in Georgia, where at Emory University in Atlanta Dr Alfred Wilhelmi had made countless batches of both hGH and hPG, meant they were three years too late (following Deborah's death in 1987) to lodge a writ in that state. Lawyers for the McKenzies instead lodged a writ in the neighbouring state of Mississippi. Mississippi had a six-year statute of limitations for cases of personal injury and wrongful death. The writ was based on the tenuous grounds that glands were collected from around the country and therefore may have been collected from cadavers at the University of Mississippi.

In October 1993 the case was transferred but the time was always out. In February 1995 the case was dismissed on technical grounds. The court decided that neither the McKenzies, residents of New Zealand, nor Emory University, which manufactured the contaminated glands in Georgia, had any link with Mississippi. No-one in the case had any personal jurisdiction in the state of Mississippi, the court ruled.[12]

In September 1993, a woman who would become known only by the initials APQ joined a small but growing band of hPG and hGH recipients who sued in Australia. Like Ted Allender, Noel Halford, Stephen Cummings, Lyle Blight, and the family of "Stephen", Australia's only hGH-linked CJD patient to date, they sued the Commonwealth of Australia and CSL. But it was on the basis that the anxiety caused by being told they might one day contract CJD had caused them to suffer nervous shock. The symptoms were so severe, they argued, it was akin to post-traumatic disorder suffered by war veterans or witnesses to horrific accidents or events. This group would swell over the next three years to more than 130.

APQ had been given hPG intermittently for nearly five years before the AHPHP had shut down. In February 1985, admitted to hospital with tremendous pain from multiple ovarian cysts, one the size of an orange, APQ also discovered she was pregnant with triplets. When she had her first ultrasound scan, four sacs were detected in her uterus but only three had heartbeats. The pregnancy, tragically, was doomed due to the rare presence of a potentially fatal hydatidiform mole. The mole had begun as the fourth embryo, itself a result of hPG hyperstimulation, but had developed instead into a grape-like tissue that consumed the placenta around it.

In 1986 and 1988, after years on the adoption waiting list, APQ and her husband finally took home two babies. Finally they were parents. But APQ's life changed in December 1991. She was told by her gynaecologist that two women had died of Creutzfeldt-Jakob disease after treatment with hPG, the same fertility drug she had conceived on. A newspaper article had carried a story on it and although the risk of others contracting the disease was low, the doctor said all recipients were being advised now not to donate blood or organs.

APQ was worried. She changed her organ donor status on her drivers' licence and contacted a friend from the hormone program, who had not been warned by her doctor. Together they discussed the situation. With no mention by anyone of a lengthy incubation period, both concluded, pessimistically, that they would probably die of the disease.

APQ requested and got copies of her files from the fertility clinic, which included the batch numbers of her treatment. One of them was batch 128, later the subject of much controversy due to its initial contamination with hepatitis antibodies. It was reprocessed and cleared for distribution by CSL.[13]

During 1992 APQ went from being a formerly fit and healthy person to a woman plagued by sleeplessness and headaches from continual worry about her risk of CJD. She became severely depressed. Bouts of the flu, colds, sore throats and ear problems battered her immune system. She was perpetually tired. In July 1993 she was referred to a neurologist who said an EEG examination had shown "high anxiety".

APQ's unrelenting fatigue continued to the point where she could not walk across her lounge room without bumping into furniture.

Thereafter with her headaches, balance problems, CT and MRI scans that showed nothing, and continuing tiredness, almost everyone, including APQ and her GP, thought she might have CJD. Her forgetfulness worsened. She forgot to collect the children from school. She once forgot the route home from school. On one occasion she completed her weekly shopping twice, within an hour, at two different shopping centres.

APQ filed her writ on September 15, 1993. She thought she had CJD — "being in half panic mode anyway. I just didn't realise it would be so soon" — and decided to sue those she claimed were responsible.

Her CJD-like symptoms of 1993 were finally diagnosed in mid-1994 after a plethora of tests. The myriad problems — which expanded to include hair loss due to high levels of ACTH secretion brought on by stress, heart problems, high blood pressure, nightmares and an inability "to shake off the notion that I will die of CJD one day" — were eventually diagnosed as another rare combination. Her balance problems were due to labyrinthitis, an inner ear inflammation sometimes accompanied by vertigo. Drugs controlled her balance problem and high doses of anti-depressants controlled her severe depression. Chronic fatigue syndrome was responsible for most of her other problems.

APQ was one of only two volunteers to be the test case. Another 132 litigants would eventually ride on her back. She had the best case. She was treated late in the program when the CJD risk was known and — in 1982 when 500 glands were destroyed by CSL after the warning that one of them came from a CJD patient — specifically feared. She had no history of psychological or psychiatric problems before being told of her CJD risk, and she was now under treatment for related and ongoing extreme anxiety. She settled down for the long countdown to court.

The British Department of Health had not bothered to tell its own female fertility drug recipients of their CJD risk until late 1993. This was despite it knowing of the CJD risk to human hormone drug recipients since 1985, the avalanche of publicity over the "timebomb children" in 1991 and 1992, the Dumble–Klein letter to the *Lancet* in October 1992 and continuing publicity in Australia about the risk to its hPG recipients.

A storm over the use of hPG broke in Britain on September 2, 1993. On that day, a press conference announced that at least 300 British women were at risk of CJD after receiving hPG in the 1960s and 1970s. The announced hotline number was immediately deluged with thousands of calls from women who had received all kinds of fertility drugs, including hMG, the drug made from the urine of menopausal women.

"The information from Australia [that there were now four hPG deaths from CJD] has come to light only over the past year or so, and particularly in the past few months," said the chief medical officer, Kenneth Calman. "There is a balance between worrying individuals and giving information. We were anxious that we should have a help line available before we released this."

The announcement of the hotline sparked a run of publicity on CJD. Stories included fears that 12,000 Britons were at risk of CJD from dura mater grafts, fears about BSE risks in six-year-old frozen beef stockpiles and the claims by Jackie Adamson that her mother Beryl Friel's death from CJD had resulted from treatment in Swindon with hPG.

Two months later, in November 1993, a jury at the inquest into the death of Patrick Baldwin returned a verdict of medical misadventure. His was the first inquest held to determine the cause of CJD in a former hGH recipient. Apart from the tracing program initiated by Professor Michael Preece, head of the Institute for Child Health at the Great Ormond Street Hospital for Sick Children, the verdict was the first official legal acknowledgment that contaminated hGH had caused CJD.

In December 1993 Ted Allender was shocked to receive confirmation from an unexpected source that his suspicions — of being fobbed off, given wrong information and kept ignorant about the cause of his former wife's CJD — were true. It was just one line of evidence at a short but doomed Administrative Appeals Tribunal hearing in Sydney in which six of 100 human hormone recipients were appealing a ruling that prevented them getting access to hundreds of Federal Department of Health documents on the AHPHP. The evidence was that "the department was notified of the patient's [Jane Allender's] condition in April 1988…"

When he was told by this author about that one line of evidence, Allender was almost apoplectic with rage. All the frustration of his abortive attempts, following Jane's death, to establish a definitive link to her hPG injections rushing back. Within a few months, after the release of Dr Allars' *Report into the Use of Pituitary Derived Hormones in Australia and Creutzfeldt-Jakob Disease* in June 1994, he knew the full extent of how he was kept in the dark.

A week before Jane's graduation, on April 27, 1988, the executive secretary of HPAC, Mr A. Godek, was telephoned by the Flinders Medical Centre clinical pharmacist, Dr C. Alderman, and told of Jane's probable diagnosis of CJD. A cascade of paper and phone calls followed. HPAC had ostensibly terminated itself after its last meeting in February 1988, following the discontinuation of pituitary-derived hormone extracts. But Godek quickly found Jane Allender's file and informed the HPAC chairman, Leslie Lazarus, Mr Des Threlfall, from the pharmaceutical benefits branch of the Department of Health and Dr A. Ayres, the secretary of the department, about her illness.

By May 3, 1988 — the day after Jane's graduation, a group of senior Department of Health officers knew she was dying of probable CJD. So did the chairmen of the hPG and hGH subcommittees of HPAC. Two days later, Lazarus sent a memo to everyone on HPAC and its subcommittees, and some former members, as well as some other departmental officers — more than 20 people. Unlike the Allender family, these people were left in no doubt about any link to her fertility treatment. The memo was entitled "Possible C-J disease in a patient treated with hPG".[14]

The memo revealed that Jane's treating doctor, Professor Lloyd Cox, had told Professor Lazarus — before the memo was sent on May 5 — that Jane Allender had had six courses of hPG. Cox was present at the graduation ceremony when Jane Allender officially became an architect on May 2. But three days later, he told the Allars inquiry he was ill with heart problems and did not read the memo. Nor was he contacted about the condition of his former patient by either the Flinders Medical Centre or Queen Elizabeth Hospital.[15]

On May 6 everyone who had the Lazarus memo, was additionally sent the report of Dr Rick Burns, Jane Allender's treating neurologist. Later in May a handful of key doctors, including Lazarus and Cox were sent an update on her condition. In June 1988 — two months before Jane Allender died — the director of CSL wrote to the legal division of the Department of Health advising of the possibility of a future legal claim and seeking advice about a Commonwealth indemnity. And by

November 1988 — months before the diagnosis of CJD itself was confirmed to the Allender family — at least two of the more senior departmental officers had been informed that Jane Allender had died of confirmed CJD. This was the same month that Ted Allender had spoken to an anonymous departmental officer and been told there was no known case of CJD linked to fertility treatment in Australia.

By 1989, when Ted Allender had given up hope of his ever establishing a link between Jane's death and her fertility treatment, large groups of Australian and American pharmacists knew more than he did. Dr Alderman, the clinical pharmacist who had discovered the link, presented Jane's case in November 1989 at the Annual Meeting of the Society of Hospital Pharmacists, and again in the following month at the American Society of Hospital Pharmacists in Atlanta. Details of the case are also believed to have been presented at the Australian and New Zealand Society of Neuropathology meeting at the end of April 1989. Dr Alderman, according to the later Allars Report had raised the question of a report to the Adverse Drug Reactions Advisory Committee (ADRAC) with Lazarus. But reports must be made voluntarily by the treating doctor, although there was confusion about this. None were ever made for any of the hGH deaths.

CHAPTER 17

The French catastrophe

WHILE Australian human hormone recipients reeled under the announcements of two more deaths and the start of the Allars inquiry in 1993, a far worse scenario had already unfolded in France. French health authorities were already under a cloud from the 1991 revelations of a French doctor-turned-journalist Anne Marie Casteret. Her six-year investigation had uncovered the irrefutable fact that pooled French blood, collected before the Americans developed the first HIV antibody test in early 1985, and almost certainly contaminated with AIDS, had been distributed for months until it was all used up. The National Centre for Blood Transfusion did not alert its 163 transfusion centres, nor the thousands of haemophiliacs who depended on life-saving blood clotting factors, that it was not offering heat-treated blood products. This was despite knowledge that a small proportion of its blood donors were HIV carriers. Stocks of untreated blood worth an estimated US$10 million were not pulled from distribution to blood transfusion centres and haemophiliacs. This resulted in up to 5000 HIV infections from French blood transfusions and 1200 haemophiliacs given an almost certain death sentence.

What few knew was that a second scandal had occurred almost simultaneously in 1985. Coming so soon after the blood scandal, it would scorch the caring veneer of the medical profession again and lead to legitimate public concern about medical practice and ethics. On December 6, 1991 Ilyassil Benziane, the 15-year-old Moroccan boy who started hGH injections in 1983, died of CJD. His parents had already engaged a lawyer, Maître Giselle Mor, convinced their son's hGH therapy was the cause of his death. They thought they were alone in their misery and anger. In reality they were the vanguard in the fight for information that would follow.

An examining magistrate had already begun a time-consuming preliminary investigation, based on the claims of the Benzianes, directed at finding the identities of anyone responsible for the tragedy.

In February 1992 the *Le Monde* article on Jean-Philippe Mathieu and other media stories, alerted the public to deaths from hGH therapy. Just as it did after Casteret's sensational blood scandal revelations, the French Ministry of Health acted swiftly. It demanded reports on the national hGH program and CJD. The reports, delivered late in February and early March 1992 by two senior officials, revealed 10 French children were dead or dying of CJD.

The ministry then ordered an investigation by its Inspection Générale des Affaires Sociales (IGAS). Four investigators from IGAS, which controlled and evaluated all services, establishments and institutions controlled by the ministries of welfare, health and labour, uncovered a disturbing scenario behind the distribution of the miracle drug, hGH, in France. On Christmas Eve 1992, IGAS delivered its second devastating report on French medical authorities. Detailed in its 500 pages was a litany of administrative anomalies, weaknesses and malfunctions in the French hGH program. Frighteningly, the death toll had climbed to nearly 20 by this time. The IGAS report findings received enormous publicity under banner headlines including "the new contamination scandal".

Chief among the IGAS criticisms was the decision in 1985 to continue producing cadaver-derived hGH in the wake of the shutdown of programs elsewhere including the US, Britain, Australia, New Zealand, the Netherlands and Sweden. French optimism that additional purification and viral inactivation measures with an 8 molar solution of the chemical urea would render cadaver-derived hGH free from CJD has yet to be proven beyond any doubt. Although at the time this book was written no-one treated after June 1985 had contracted CJD, experiments in the interim had shown that 8 molar urea treatment greatly reduces the infectivity in pituitaries heavily contaminated with scrapie. But it does not necessarily eliminate it totally.[1,2] Confidence in the 8 molar urea treatment was bolstered by the French attitude to pre-1977 American hGH manufacturing methods (linked to the initial CJD deaths), that they were archaic. Even so, France was not alone in continuing with cadaver-derived hGH. Japan, Israel, Spain, Italy, West Germany and the Copenhagen-based pharmaceutical company Nordisk continued production for varying periods.

In testimony to a later CJD-related court case in England, Norwegian paediatric endocrinologist, Dr Olav Trygstad, the pioneer of human hormone drugs in his country and consultant to Nordisk, said CJD-infected pituitary glands were sent by Nordisk to the Pasteur Institute in Paris for testing in 1985. The action followed the news that CJD had claimed its first four hGH recipients. Using this "spiked sample" on a laboratory animal, the protocol for the production of Nordisk's Nanormon brand hGH was tested for its ability to remove the infectivity, just as Alan Dickinson had tested Lowry's protocol with scrapie in the early 1980s. In 1987, when the Nordisk test was completed, it was negative for CJD. The results were never published.[3]

Neither Nordisk nor Trygstad, who treated about 300 Norwegian hGH recipients with his own hGH, stopped using pituitary-derived hGH until 1987 — two years after the majority of user countries abandoned it. In Israel, endocrinologists in Tel Aviv claim to have used pituitary-derived hGH from Nordisk and Ares-Serono, which used a 6 molar urea treatment, until 1992.[4] Trygstad was confident that his extraction process allowed no infective material into the final product. He was also wary of using the newly available synthetic hGH because of reports of antibody development in up to 80 per cent of patients. French authorities shared his concern about the antibodies and used it to support the continued distribution of cadaver-derived hGH.

Just as no transfusion centre doctors, blood transfusion recipients or haemophiliacs were told there was a definite risk of AIDS contamination in blood, few of the hGH recipients or their parents who consented to their treatment were told there was a definite risk of CJD from cadaver-derived pituitaries. Association France Hypophyse had given that responsibility to treating doctors, but even the information given to them was minimal.[5] Jean-Bernard Mathieu, father of Jean-Philippe who died of CJD in 1993, recalls that his wife asked his son's treating doctor after the 1985 HIV scandal if there was any medical risk to his son from his hGH injections. The reply was no. The IGAS inspectors detailed in their report how no recall was ever made of the vials of hormone that were already packaged before the May 14, 1985 decision in France to continue production of pituitary-derived hGH. Prepackaged vials, which could not be treated with 8 molar urea, had already been sent to hospital pharmacies. Nor was there a recall of vials already collected by parents and kept refrigerated for future use on their children.

Administrative failures noted in the 1992 IGAS report included the fact that there was no licence to market cadaver-derived hGH for the first 15 years of the program.[6] It was a product that did not constitute a medicine but it was controlled — just like blood products — by a monopoly. That monopoly was Association France Hypophyse, a non-profit making group of paediatric endocrinologists, pharmacists, scientists and representatives of the ministry of health and the national health insurance fund. It had a triple role in the French hGH program. It was responsible for gland collection, not only in France but for those imported from eastern European countries. Association France Hypophyse also controlled the distribution of the hormone and coordinated the system under which the central pharmacy for the public hospitals processed and dispensed the hormone to hospital pharmacies or directly to Parisian patients. When supplies were short it bought commercial preparations of hGH more expensive than the French-manufactured hGH.

IGAS inspectors singled out two key findings: inadequate preparation of hGH by the Pasteur Institute and "manifestly insufficient" exclusion criteria for pituitary gland collection.[7] Their report highlighted the lack of thorough checks on pituitary glands and the fact that they were collected from hospitals with neurological and long-stay departments. Even though advice was sought after the scare from the 1979 rabies transmission through a donated cornea, and the Association France Hypophyse backed the advice from the Pasteur Institute's own Professor Luc Montagnier that strict exclusion criteria should apply to collected glands, the exclusion criteria were not adhered to.

This was revealed in 1983, in an earlier report by IGAS investigators. Nor were hospital authorities told that glands were collected by mortuary attendants who were paid FF30 for their efforts — a tip later bumped up to FF50.

Until 1985 at least, hGH was produced in a research laboratory — just like the labs used for making hGH in England by Hartree and Lowry. None of them had the status of a pharmaceutical establishment. The French lab also re-used chromatography columns between batches.[8]

An epidemiological survey of hGH recipients in France was conducted after the first CJD deaths in America in 1985. The survey found no hint of the disease[9] because it wasn't until 1989 that the first probable case of CJD in France emerged. A second case was discovered soon after and a new epidemiological survey was launched in June 1990. Carried out by the French Institute of Health and Medical Research and

Association France Hypophyse, that survey was completed in December 1990 but included patients who had been followed for longer. The results were published in 1992, by which time three children had died of CJD and seven more were suspected of dying from it.[10]

It was only after the escalating cases of CJD were aired in the media in early 1992, that French health officials issued their first communique, a bland statement, on the risks from hGH therapy and deaths to that point. This was three years after the disease hit young Nicolas Guillemet and Isabelle Norroy and seven years after the first four deaths had occurred in Britain and America.

The June communique followed a management meeting in April 1992 and the annual general meeting on May 9, 1992, of Association Grandir where the topic of French cases of CJD was first aired within the group. Association Grandir was a non-commercial group that grew to about 800 people after its establishment in 1979 by the head of Association France Hypophyse, Professor Jean-Claude Job. The association was a lobby group to obtain government sponsorship for treatment and a channel of information between doctors and parents, as well as between parents who had children with growth difficulties that were not restricted to hGH therapy.

Job, who generally held irregular meetings of the association at his office at the St Vincent de Paul Hospital in Paris, made his first wide dissemination of the knowledge to date on the contamination affair in the association's magazine, *Grandir* (Grow), published in November 1992. It was the first official information parents of children who received pituitary-derived hGH were given about CJD contamination. According to Giselle Mor, Ilyassil Benziane's original lawyer, information when it was released was biased and directed at minimising responsibility.[11] Parents affected by CJD grew wary, and lost any trust in Association Grandir.

The IGAS report of December 1992 drew attention to the appalling fact that the French led the world in the toll of hGH recipients who had died of CJD — two of them had not even lived to their teens. It also refocused attention on the CJD legacy of human hormones.

By 1993 it was apparent that all the French CJD cases had been treated between January 1984 and June 1985, and that incubation periods were shorter in France than anywhere else.[12] This, it was suggested in an article in the journal *Science,* could have been due to either bad luck or a much higher infectivity titre present in glands processed in France, many of which were exported from hospitals and morgues in Bulgaria and Hungary.[13] In addition French batches contained an average of about 1500 glands while those in America sometimes contained thousands and it would have been easier on one view to have heavier contamination in the smaller batches.

France, when it added its 8 molar urea purification step, also switched to the Lowry method of producing hGH from frozen glands. According to Lowry, who manufactured hGH in Britain between 1975 and 1981, the French problems might have arisen from several possibilities. These included that the infectivity of one batch of glands used may have been too high for their method of purification to handle, leading to the final material being significantly contaminated, or that an error in the production of hGH had contaminated the final material.[14]

In the summer of 1993, spurred by the amount of information contained in the IGAS report and an interview with the parents of Ilyassil Benziane, the investigating magistrate Marie-Odile Bertella-Geoffroy instigated investigations into named people on charges of involuntary homicide. A conviction on this charge could mean up to three years in jail or a fine of up to FF300,000. Penalties are heavier for deliberate breaches of precautions leading to manslaughter.

The persons named, amid more world media and scientific attention, on the charges of involuntary homicide were Jean-Claude Job, paediatrician and president of Association France Hypophyse and Fernand Dray, a retired biochemist formerly head of the Urea Laboratory of the Pasteur Institute.[15] By October 1993, Henri Cerceau, the former director of the Pharmacie Centrale des Hospitaux de Paris — the public hospitals' national pharmacy centre, had been added as a named person in the investigation. Later three more people were named: Dr Elisabeth Mugnier, who was responsible for pituitary collection in France; Jacques Dangoumau, director of pharmacy and drugs at the Ministry of Health; and Marc Mollet, the scientific director of the Pharmacie Centrale.

Echoes of the French HIV blood contamination scandal could hardly be forgotten. The news of the investigation into the role of Job and Dray broke only days after the jailing of a senior scientist at the National

Centre of Blood Transfusion, for failing to halt the distribution of HIV-contaminated clotting agents for haemophiliacs which had followed similar convictions of two French physicians the previous year.[16] Both the blood and the hGH scandals dated back to mid-1985. Both involved arms of the Pasteur Institute and, according to some, boiled down in part to the same factor — money. All the families involved in both scandals wanted vengeance, someone to blame for the infection of their family member and the decisions that led to the death — no matter how long it took.

In 1993 Job, after his name was splashed prominently across French newspapers, was adamant that all stocks of hGH existing after June 1985 were re-treated or destroyed. This claim was contrary to the IGAS finding that some stocks were not re-treated or destroyed, a fact later confirmed by the investigating magistrate.

IGAS had also blamed the "current dramatic situation" on "negligence", "lack of perception" and "stubbornness" by Association France Hypophyse, which misinterpreted the withdrawal of cadaver-derived hGH by other countries as a marketing ploy by Kabi of Sweden to generate sales of synthetic hGH.[17]

Cerceau, the director of the central pharmacy, had also insisted that from June 1985 his office had delivered only urea-treated hormone. Later, Bertella-Geoffroy's investigation would allegedly reveal the fact that two lots of already-packaged hGH (that was impossible to treat) were not dispatched until June 11, 1985. A third lot was marketed from July 29 to October 9, 1985 and a fourth lot was made available to stunted children from October 25, 1985 to early 1986.[18] Much later in another shattering expose, the French journalist, Casteret, revealed that Bertella-Geoffroy had consulted a chartered accountant about the cost of the four lots totalling 30 grams of untreated hormone, which represented 20,000 ampoules of hGH. The earning shortfall from the first two lots, alone, would have been more than FF5 million, it was claimed.[19]

France, alone, continued to have double the world tally of hGH recipient deaths from CJD — all of them linked to the troubling January 1984 to June 1985 period when about 1000 of the 1700-odd pituitary-derived hGH patients were under treatment. It was a dominant lead that would not be relinquished in the years to come.

While IGAS investigators pored over documents involved in both the blood and hGH scandals in the early 1990s, a clutch of hGH recipients were dead or dying of CJD. One of them, Benedicte Delbrel changed from a vibrant young woman on the threshold of her adult life, to a stumbling, mumbling and unquestionably sick young woman. When Benedicte was a cute 11-year-old, the darling of the class but still dressing in the clothes of a 10-year-old, she told her mother, Francine, that the boys at school called her "gadget". Her teacher had dubbed her "the flea". During a visit to the doctor for a vaccination, Francine Delbrel mentioned Benedicte's shortness, compared to her classmates, and was told about hGH. She was reassured that the "hormone" was natural and prepared by the world famous Pasteur Institute. Benedicte was examined and found to have a "bone age" slightly behind children her own age. From 1983 she began a course of hGH injections.

The therapy continued until 1986 — a year after the majority of countries around the world had banned cadaver-derived hGH. Her injections, collected from the Central Pharmacy in Paris in a three-month refrigerated supply of ampoules — sometimes with another child's name on it due to shortages — had caused her to grow barely four centimetres. Neither she nor her parents were aware of the reports in the medical literature of the demise of Nicolas Guillemet or Isabelle Norroy who died of CJD before reaching their teens, or of older teenagers like Jean-Philippe Mathieu.

In 1989, when Nicolas Guillemet had begun staggering, Benedicte Delbrel had entered university. But she soon became depressed, was prescribed drops by a psychiatrist who advised her to continue her studies lest she feel a failure. By the European summer of 1990, she had developed an active social life but fainted several times, once on a bus, which worried her mother. In September 1990 during a family gathering at the beach, Benedicte, always sporty, while skylarking fell from the top of a three-metre wooden dinosaur. She complained about her balance and laughed about walking home one night like a drunk and bumping into someone, even though she'd only had orange juice.

Gradually, Benedicte's symptoms worsened. Typing essays on a computer became impossible when her hand flew uncontrollably back into her face. After sessions with her psychiatrist, she put it down to nerves, to the fact that her parents were moving for the fifteenth time because of her father's job in the French Navy, and that she would be living away from them for the first time. Several rounds of medical tests had already revealed nothing, and trips to a number of neurologists, again found nothing abnormal. Benedicte's memory worsened and she hurt herself falling in the bathroom. Despite her mother's concern, she continued to drive her car.

In a moving account of her daughter's last year, *Pour Benedicte,* Francine Delbrel relates some unbelievable conversations with psychiatrists, one of whom suggested she, herself, should consult another of his colleagues to help her accept that her daughter was ill. The same psychiatrist told Benedicte that the reason she fell one day and knocked her head against the central heating in his waiting room was because she was punishing her body for having been so good. And he made her repeat the statement. "When she falls, Madame, you mustn't interfere," Francine Delbrel recounts of the psychiatrist's advice in her book. "You must above all pretend you didn't see anything and you don't pay any importance to it." When she asked the psychiatrist whether he thought he could successfully treat her daughter, Francine Delbrel was told: "If I didn't believe it, I wouldn't do this job, Madame".[20]

Later, with her brother Xavier who was studying medicine, Benedicte consulted a neurologist, Dr Y, who recommended MRI scanning and a lumbar puncture. Filling in her hospital forms, she included her previous hormone treatment. Dr Y, too hastily, concluded that Benedicte had MS and started her on a strong dose of drugs before the final results came back. He was wrong. Dr Y then told Francine Delbrel to take her daughter to a psychiatrist, considering her previous depression, as he could not find any medical cause for her symptoms. Dr Y was not aware of the growing toll of hGH recipients dying of a disease that normally killed about 55 elderly French people per year. Clearly the death of Ilyassil Benziane had not filtered through from the endocrinology to the neurology community in France.

Having heard of good results from a psychiatrist, Dr K, Benedicte and her mother consulted him in desperation. Their first consultation was reminiscent of the Kafka novels that all French schoolchildren study. France Delbrel recounts.

The psychiatrist spoke first to Benedicte.

"There was nothing on the MRI. Are you happy or disappointed?"

Benedicte turns to me, her eyes wide open: He's crazy!

"And you Madame, your husband is not here at this interview. Don't you find that symptomatic?"

"My husband is in Brest, he can't be everywhere!"

"And you, Mademoiselle, you must have suffered during your youth to have an absent father, mustn't you? A father in the Navy, it must've been difficult to accept for a little girl!"

Benedicte starts crying.

"But you are crazy! Completely crazy! You want to make my father responsible for my disease? You are a monster. It's his job, my father, to travel, his job …"

Afterwards the psychiatrist gave Francine Delbrel his conclusions, which he told her separately from her daughter: "An interesting case, this young lady … And the fact that she reacts so violently when I talk about her father … That's symptomatic … A badly accepted Oedipus, that's for sure … We are on the right track, but there's a lot of work to be done! It's rare to put the finger right on it as soon as the first meeting."

Benedicte continued to deteriorate. Two small car crashes did not change the psychiatrist's view that she should be encouraged to keep driving. She stuttered in phone calls to her mother and complained of double vision. With broken teeth and covered in marks from her numerous falls she finally returned to her parents' home to rest. Finding it hard to walk unaided, Benedicte often clung to her mother for support. This behaviour, the psychiatrist told Francine Delbrel, was her daughter trying to take her "hostage" and must be discouraged. A neck collar, bought to support Benedicte's flopping head, was "theatre" according to the psychiatrist (the Delbrel family had by now nicknamed him "Sigmund"), and was an attempt by Benedicte to get attention.

On December 29, 1992, a week after the devastating IGAS report was released, Benedicte was admitted to hospital. There she was denied any form of contact with family or friends in a form of extreme treatment designed to give her the will to walk again, and to behave normally. In early January, after comments by family members in the wake of the IGAS report, Francine Delbrel reminded the hospital authorities that Benedicte was a growth hormone recipient, a fact already stressed by Benedicte and her brother Xavier on her admission.

Francine Delbrel's sister had a consultation with "Sigmund" after a television report had alerted the family to the link between CJD and hGH. When questioned, Sigmund said he knew about CJD from books. When she told him that 15 children were apparently dead from the disease after their hGH was contaminated and that Benedicte showed symptoms of the disease, he snarled at her. "Of course not, Madame! The neurologists must know about it, you imagine … Benedicte has seen three, Madame, three! The case of your niece is not very usual, of course, luckily for us, but I have already seen similar cases, a bit less acute, with people full of sexual taboos … I must say that on that topic, your family is quite a specimen …"[21]

A week later the Delbrel family knew the worst when called to the centre where Benedicte had received most of her hormone vials. Her problem was not, and never had been, psychological. She was going to die. On January 26, 1993, surrounded by 60 friends and family, Benedicte was taken on a stretcher to the holy shrine at Lourdes where they all prayed for a miracle that never came. Her illness followed the usual course until her death on May 4. She had just turned 21.

A victory, of sorts, resulted for the families of the dead with the announcement in November 1993 of FF2 million in compensation for each CJD patient and their family from Ministry of Health funds. These were calculated on the scale of compensation paid to haemophiliacs and transfusion recipients infected with HIV. The Association Grandir engineered compensation from the government for future cases — providing FF1 billion for up to a staggering 500 potential victims who may be stricken well into the twenty-first century — received mixed reactions. They ranged from allegations that it was "hush" money for hGH recipients and their families, to feelings of solidarity generated by the families who had agitated for it. On any view it was an acknowledgment that the French Government did not exercise enough control over the national hGH program.[22]

By 1994 the death toll from CJD in France was 30 and rising rapidly. According to Paul Brown, virologist, epidemiologist and avowed Francophile who conducted a 15-year epidemiological study on sporadic CJD in France between 1968 and 1982: "The French did not recognise a case [of hGH-related CJD] until about '89. Around '86 or so, a paper came out, a very self-congratulatory paper saying this is what we did. We haven't had any cases die so good for us. One of the more embarrassing papers ever written, as far as I can tell, because within a few years they started having an avalanche of cases. It's up to 41 [in 1996] — and counting. It's probably because they took glands from a lot of neurology patients because that's where the autopsies included the brain. Very shrewd from the point of view of getting pituitaries but in retrospect not very smart from the point of view of risk of contamination. The risk in France of getting CJD if you were treated with growth hormone is running about two and a half to three per cent," he says. "Very bad odds."[23]

CHAPTER 18

An independent inquiry

O N JUNE 28, 1994 in a large meeting room in Parliament House in Canberra, a sombre group of officials faced a crowd of journalists. Flanking Dr Margaret Allars before the assembled media was the Chief Medical Officer, Dr Tony Adams, and the Federal Minister for Health, Dr Carmen Lawrence. They confirmed what had long been suspected in the confusing aftermath of human hormone-linked CJD deaths. The AHPHP was flawed. None of the treatments had ever officially left trial status.

In addition, laws had been bent, ethics ignored, rules stretched, corners cut, red tape avoided and dead bodies had been unlawfully raided for pituitary glands. Doctors with dual roles — administering the program and treating patients — had a clear conflict of interest, were unregulated by any other body and had even breached their own strict treatment guidelines to provide hPG and hGH for experimental research.

These were the disquieting findings of the Allars report into the use of pituitary derived hormones in Australia and Creutzfeldt-Jakob disease, the inquiry that had been established a year earlier in the wake of the federal election and the announcement of a fourth Australian CJD death on the program. When the report was tabled in parliament earlier that day Lawrence had described the results as "very disturbing — both for governments and for the medical community". "Frankly," she added, "patients deserve better from the people in whom they place trust for their health".[1]

Associate Professor Allars had produced a report of 815 pages that was critical, particularly of HPAC, which monitored the program, and of CSL, which had been indemnified by the Commonwealth against any legal action. Under eight terms of reference — which included scientific knowledge of risks and benefits of human hormone treatment, information given to and informed consent of patients, manufacture and collection of pituitaries and departmental response — Allars and her small team had received written submissions or personally interviewed 100 hPG or hGH recipients. In addition to interviewing scientific and administrative officers of the Department of Health, CSIRO and CSL, the inquiry team interviewed 20 treating specialists, six other doctors, 11 pathologists, five nurses, two counsellors and six mortuary attendants.

Questionnaires were filled out by others in these occupations. Most of the living HPAC members were also interviewed. A mammoth list of written submissions was received from public interest and professional groups, health and support organisations, recipient support groups, royal colleges, health services, hospitals, and pathology institutions. Based also to a large extent on minutes from AHPHP committee meetings, the report ripped a hole in the bright picture built up over many years of miracle drugs that gave life to childless couples and precious height to stunted children. It also gashed the reputations of key doctors involved.

HPAC head Professor Leslie Lazarus told this author several days before the report was tabled that he would "never" comment on its findings. The report attributed over-enthusiasm by doctors as the motive for their crossing the boundaries of ethics and regulations, causing them to experiment with drugs on patients — sometimes without their knowledge or consent. Doctors were particularly piqued with these criticisms.

They say that these criticisms are made in hindsight, and that the vast realms of acquired knowledge are being attributed to specialists in widely disparate medical disciplines at a time when the concept of informed consent of patients for treatment did not really exist.

Of major interest in the report were the references to hormones supplied as research allocations — for experiments — in contravention of HPAC guidelines. Several decisions by both the hGH subcommittee and the FSH subcommittee of HPAC that were "open to criticism on ethical grounds", according to Allars. The scheme under which a lower dosage of hGH was given to patients in some states than in other states was singled out. By comparing the minimum effective dosage "this scheme stepped across the line between making clinical observations and conducting a research study".[2]

Some allocations of pituitary hormones for research were made directly from CSL, bypassing HPAC altogether before 1978. Other allocations, in particular three lots of 50 ampoules, came from the apparently lethal batch 25, the only batch recorded as being the source of hPG given to Jan Blight, the second Australian woman to die of CJD after treatment on the AHPHP.[3]

Tony Adams admitted at the press conference what most later treating doctors on the program did not appear to realise: that no clear demarcation was ever drawn between the initial "clinical trials" of human hormone drugs and a regulated transfer of the treatment to routine therapy. In Australia, such therapy had merely evolved from one to the other. Adams also described as "horrendous" the proposal under which experimental hGH had been approved by HPAC to be used in the Malnourished Aboriginal Children Project in 1974.[4]

Under the proposed eight-week project, three groups of malnourished Aboriginal children were to be compared: one group given hGH, insulin and a "standard diet"; another group were to get glucagon instead of hGH; and a third "control" group was to receive only glucose. The researcher had submitted a protocol and advised that prior approval had been obtained from the Department of Aboriginal Affairs and the National Health and Medical Research Council. A Melbourne endocrinologist and member of the hGH subcommittee, Dr Henry Burger, wrote to Lazarus in November 1974 reporting his discussion of the project with the researcher. He was "satisfied in regard to the aims of the study and the numbers of children involved".[5]

But a week later, according to the Allars report, reservations were expressed at a meeting of the hGH subcommittee. Despite this, it eventually agreed to recommend the project. In her report, Allars said the merits of the project to a "particularly vulnerable" group already disadvantaged by "Aboriginality, age and socioeconomic position" received scant attention in the minutes of HPAC. The project did not go ahead after the researcher, now dead, left the hospital at which he was working. The Allars report cited it as an example of the lack of concern by HPAC to ensure that project reports were completed. Basically, once HPAC gave its approval for research allocations outside normal guidelines, it exercised no further control over the use of the drug.[6]

These and other instances of human experimentation with AHPHP drugs received wide media coverage, as did the findings of the whole report. Other experimentation included hPG stimulation tests, which if they worked the first time and the woman became pregnant, were never recorded on the program database. Nor were records kept of women who failed to respond to stimulation tests.

Normal control volunteers, used to compare results against patients needing treatment, are impossible to trace. One doctor told the Allars inquiry his controls were ovulatory women, normal men, men with sperm disorders, patients lying around the hospital for elective surgery or those in traction, confined for months to bed with broken limbs. In the 1960s doctors often used themselves and colleagues and laboratory staff as normal volunteers. Professor Henry Burger told the inquiry that hGH produced in Melbourne together with some hGH obtained from Dr Alfred Wilhelmi in Georgia was used in one study. In such studies the normal controls can only be identified from their initials in the research paper.[7] Allars could not assess the extent of unofficial treatment during either the 18-year course of the AHPHP or in the earlier unregulated period from the early 1960s, on the evidence she had.

In 1972 the HPAC was asked for hormone for a study of the length of time the body takes to process, then store or eliminate, gonadotrophins. Approval was given retrospectively after the hormone was supplied. Only later was it revealed that 40 pituitaries from batch 25, Jan Blight's batch, had been used to measure the metabolic clearance rate of fertility-related hormones in a series of "normal and anovulatory women". In 1973 a further supply of that batch was approved. In 1975 the researchers published the results of the study on 10 normal men, three normal women and 12 women with ovulatory disorders, all of whom gave consent for the treatment.[8] But it was later reported to the CJD task force by one of the treating doctors that a total of 31 people were treated in that experiment. Ten of them received hPG, of which one man and one woman were normal.[9]

This gives a small indication of the number of people who are at the same risk of CJD as anyone treated with human hormone drugs. These "normal" patients are not among the government's official list of 1400-odd hPG recipients, 62 of whom were men. Allars also reported that two people received doses from batch 19, a batch of such low potency that the results were deemed not worth reporting. Other experiments relevant to the terms of reference of the Allars inquiry included research allocations of hormone for use on hypoglycaemic babies. The effect of hGH on patients with kidney failure and kidney and liver disease, a metabolic clearance rate study using hPG, a new treatment regimen for ovulation induction using clomiphene citrate *after* hPG, and the hyperstimulation of ovaries for IVF research known as the "egg project", were also among experimental uses of human hormone drugs.[10]

One woman who contacted this author in 1993 claimed to have received prolactin injections to stimulate lactation following the birth of a child at Hornsby Hospital. Her treating doctor had since died.

Some research projects were applied for by senior researchers — who sometimes held the dual role of HPAC member as well — when the study was actually to be performed by a more junior doctor, Allars found. In one instance a member of HPAC and a colleague made an application on behalf of someone else.[11] And on another occasion, Allars found that the rejection by the Australian Drug Evaluation Committee (ADEC) of a general marketing application by a European manufacturer of commercial hGH had occurred in 1980 after advice from an "external evaluator" — Professor Lazarus.

In Australia, between at least 1974 and 1982, hPG was used in contravention of AHPHP guidelines to stimulate egg production in patients undergoing the new reproductive technology — in-vitro fertilisation (IVF).[12] This HPAC-approved research allocation of hPG from CSL was also supplemented by other stocks of hPG still available in Melbourne from Professor James Brown, the pioneer of hPG production in Australia. More than 50 women were treated on an IVF program at the Royal Women's Hospital in Melbourne between 1972 and 1973 with Brown-manufactured hPG. From 1974 CSL stock was also used, some of it beyond its shelf life and hardly potent.[13]

While women from all over Australia were treated with hPG on what was the world's largest hPG treatment program, it is estimated that more than 100 Australian women not registered as part of the AHPHP were given hPG injections to stimulate egg production until at least 1982. One experimental IVF regimen, the "egg project", ran from 1974 to 1976 and involved about 23 women. The deliberate hyperstimulation of 14 of these women to recover eggs for IVF was reported in 1976.[14] Records of women given hPG for stimulation were scant, scattered or not kept at all.

By the mid-1970s, CSL-manufactured hPG was also used under criteria other than the AHPHP guidelines, which stated that women given the drug should be anovulatory and have failed to respond to clomiphene citrate first. Also outside the guidelines was the use from 1976 of hPG for patients who were ovulating normally but had cervical mucous problems due to clomiphene treatment. This was really hPG treatment being used for research purposes, Allars found.[15]

> On balance it appears that hPG produced by CSL and by Professor Brown were used in the IVF program at Royal Women's Hospital [in Melbourne], but there are no records indicating which was used in treatment of each patient. Those [doctors] involved in the use of hPG in IVF programs prior to 1977 were unable to provide the inquiry with an account of their use of hPG which was consistent or as accurate as might be expected.[16]

Between 1977 and 1978, leftover hPG from the AHPHP was "liberated … available in an ad hoc way" for IVF patients in Melbourne.[17] This was despite the fact that all unused hPG was supposed to be returned to CSL.

It was a surprise to many reading the comprehensive Allars report to see another side of the AHPHP. Success stories on growing children and "good news" about high multiple births for childless couples had been the only public knowledge of the program. Even the Brodrick nontuplets were perceived at the time by members of the public to be, on the face of it, a tragedy unrelated to complicated fluctuating potencies and dosages of early-era fertility drugs. The births of triplets, quadruplets and quintuplets featured in women's magazines and newspapers in the late 1960s and 1970s emphasised the success stories. But up to 1974, for instance, the drug failed in more than half of the 390 women treated.[18]

Between the shutdown of the AHPHP and the availability in Australia of synthetic hGH in 1986, some media stories extolled the benefits of hGH therapy. The tone was that it was being denied to children because of a slim risk of CJD that doctors thought was unlikely to occur in Australia because of the different production methods used.[19] The majority of relationships between the parents of hGH recipients and their treating endocrinologists were happy. The doctors were generally frank about the risks of antibodies or poor response to the treatment. In any case, there was nothing to replace hGH.

But the opposite was the norm for many female hPG recipients, it appears. In the more enlightened times of the 1990s, many of these women look back with regret and sometimes bitterness at the patronising attitudes of some doctors of whom some felt they could not ask questions. Some doctors relied on their nursing staff to deal with patient concerns and to dispense information about the treatment. Despite the alternative, albeit expensive hMG, which was not government-sponsored, few were offered it by their doctors. Many were treated with hPG as the inevitable next — and last — opportunity for them to ovulate and conceive.[20] The Allars report found that it was the common law duty of doctors to inform patients of any risks in treatment received. Doctors should have disclosed that there were alternatives to hPG. These included hMG, no treatment at all, waiting, or adoption.

A 1968 paper by Adelaide gynaecologist and long-term FSH sub-committee member, Professor Lloyd Cox and colleagues, reported that they had "lost two promising cases from treatment because they were offered a child by adoption before successive ovulations occurred".[21]

In addition, some recipients were not told the source of the drug, a gruesome issue for a number of them who made oral submissions to the inquiry and one which would have ruled out continued treatment on hPG. Others, particularly childless women, admit they were desperate for treatment and would have tried anything, regardless of its source. Some treating doctors told the inquiry that the majority of their patients were so desperate to have children they would have accepted almost any risk. Some women also acknowledged that the social pressure to have children, especially in the 1960s, was great.

"Had I known that my patients could have had 1 in 400 chance of developing Creutzfeldt-Jakob disease I am quite sure they would have gone ahead with treatment ... They would go to no end of trouble a lot of these people," one gynaecologist said. Another said: "Their infertility was such a problem ... if I told them they could die they still would have treatment." The Allars report found that the source of the drugs should have been disclosed to patients.

With both hGH and hPG doctors sometimes shared some batches between patients. When hGH was in short supply the ampoules, specifically allocated for one patient and recorded against that person's name, were given to one or more other patients until supplies returned to normal. Thus it was difficult to pinpoint who had received what from particular batches over the many years hGH recipients were treated. Some women given hPG were never recorded as being on the AHPHP because their doctors, in the hope of helping them more quickly, cut cumbersome bureaucratic red tape by giving the next new patient hPG left over from the allocation of the previous patient who had become pregnant. Stimulation tests were made possible by left-over hPG or ampoules that were beyond the normal shelf life of two years.

One of the biggest and most worrying risks relating to hPG, due to wide fluctuations in response between individuals and differences in potency of the drug itself, was hyperstimulation, of which several horror stories are related in the Allars report. This was a potentially fatal side-effect that was not fully appreciated by some patients. One Sydney woman, who developed 19 ovarian cysts during her treatment, was admitted to hospital and could not bear anyone walking into her room due to the pain this induced in her acutely sensitive and stretched ovaries. Perinatal death was "directly related" to hyperstimulation, Dr James Evans, a member of the FSH subcommittee told the Allars inquiry.[22]

The obvious hyperstimulation that produced Geraldine Brodrick's nontuplets resulted in a survey on perinatal deaths on the AHPHP. By April 1978 the FSH subcommittee recognised that twin pregnancies had resulted in a high perinatal mortality rate, and that perinatal mortality rates generally in multiple pregnancies were, in one report, at an unacceptable high of 35.7 per cent. This was far higher than in the normal population where the mortality rate in single pregnancies was seven per cent.[23] At its October 1978 meeting, when the FSH subcommittee noted that the perinatal mortality rate in its latest report was 62 per cent of all pregnancies, it was decided that Evans would draft a questionnaire. This was sent in 1979 to doctors who had reported "stillborn", "neonatal death" or "congenital anomaly" on their patients' treatment forms. The results were not discussed by the committee until early in 1981, when it was noted that the majority of the deaths were in the "pre-viable multiple pregnancy group".[24]

At least three maternal deaths were also reported in FSH subcommittee minutes quoted in the Allars report. One of them was listed under "complications of pregnancy" in its June 1979 meeting minutes. It is not clear whether this death was included in the three deaths mentioned briefly in the minutes of the FSH subcommittee in August 1984, the only other time the subject was discussed. When he was interviewed by the Allars inquiry, Evans said that one woman had died of septicaemia and the other specific causes were not recorded, but that no-one in Australia had died after hyperstimulation.[25]

None of these deaths, nor those of Jane Allender, Jan Blight, Jenny Halford or Vonda Cummings, were reported to the Adverse Drug Reactions Advisory Committee (ADRAC).

Regarding exclusion criteria of pituitary glands, the Allars inquiry found that in general HPAC revised the exclusion criteria in "a reactive and slow fashion as possible sources of infection came to light".[26] For instance HIV was only considered for exclusion in December 1984. The collection instructions excluding patients with HIV were only issued in June 1985 as the AHPHP was being shut down. Earlier, Creutzfeldt-Jakob disease was only included specifically (and in brackets) under pre-senile dementia in 1983.[27]

Even when exclusion criteria were revised, they were never effectively communicated to pathologists and mortuary attendants. CSL representatives, who collected filled bottles of unidentified pituitary glands every few months from morgues, paid for the service but failed to provide copies of the infrequently updated exclusion criteria. In 1983 a collection of glands at the Flinders Medical Centre in Adelaide was destroyed after it became known that a gland from a hepatitis sufferer was included. Afterwards, the collection of glands from bodies in which the presence or absence of hepatitis was unknown was encouraged. This was because testing for the virus antigen occurred on arrival at CSL.[28]

One of the key findings in Allars' report was that the removal of pituitary glands was largely illegal. Although it was thought by most participants in the AHPHP that tissue removed could be taken "for therapeutic purposes, medical purposes, or scientific purposes" during an autopsy, authorised consent was actually conditional on the pituitary gland being necessary for diagnosing the cause of death. The Allars inquiry found that the removal of glands was solely for the supply to CSL and therefore unlawful under uniform human tissue legislation enacted in each state in the late 1970s and early 1980s. Before that time there were no records to indicate that anyone had sought permission from relatives of the dead for the removal of pituitaries under either common law or early human tissue legislation.

Importantly, Allars found that although the doctors and other experts on HPAC and its subcommittees were qualified to provide advice in clinical and research areas, their knowledge did not extend to unconventional slow viruses. They were not equipped to serve as a regulator of themselves.[29] Despite a request by the chairman of HPAC, Professor Lazarus, for departmental resources to conduct a tracing and epidemiological study of recipients no assistance was given.

The Allars Report found the Department of Health had had a "moral duty" to inform human hormone recipients of the risk of CJD in 1985 when the AHPHP was suspended. Those recipients had a fundamental right to know, and just because some patients did not request information, it did not mean they should have been "left in the dark". When the department was forced, after continuing publicity to begin tracing in earnest in 1992, Allars found that departmental officers were unnecessarily and unduly guarded in their restricted responses to requests for information. They were "adversely affect by the fear" of acting in breach of Section 135A of the National Health Act, which imposes penalties as steep as jail sentences for disclosing medical information to third parties. Doctors, she said, had been left to their own devices in tracing former patients with no help from the department and no extra resources. Lawrence told parliament:

> We must learn from the mistakes of the past: give support to the victims, and ensure that new medical treatments and procedures continue to be the subject of the most rigorous scrutiny and monitoring so such tragedies do not occur again. This is particularly critical in these times, when medical advances are moving at such an incredible pace.

Five months later Lawrence announced a $10 million package, which included funds for Australian research, a national support group, medical costs for people who developed CJD and a $5 million counselling trust account. Lawrence admitted that the findings in the Allars report had shown that the government and bureaucrats who approved the setting up of the AHPHP in the 1960s were clearly wrong "to put doctors in charge of the program". That was why the present government felt "a sense of moral responsibility" now. She also revealed publicly that legal advice had been taken and that no disciplinary action could be taken against doctors responsible for the AHPHP. The only remedy lay in civil court proceedings or action by state medical boards.

That the doctors administering the program would not be held accountable for the anxiety and death that had ensued provoked immediate outcry from many still bitter human hormone recipients. Peter Costello, Jenny Halford's neighbour, the man who first raised the issue in Federal Parliament in 1991 and who had risen again in rank to become Deputy Leader of the Opposition said that it was "beyond belief" that "apparently no-one is responsible".[30] In one extreme response, an hPG recipient, who described herself as "a laboratory rat", said the government's counselling and medical package was "like saying to a rapist that you will give him compensation to counsel his victim".[31]

The Federal Government had also granted CSL a blanket indemnity to cover damages claims before its privatisation and listing as a public company in mid-1994. The scope of the indemnity was believed to have been unprecedented in the assets sales of former government-run institutions. As well as human hormone drugs, the indemnity covered the blood protein known as albumin used in the treatment of shock victims. Between 1961 and 1968 CSL processed more than 200,000 kilograms of human placentas to extract albumin before switching to the less costly method of extracting it from blood plasma.

Just before Christmas in 1994 Ted Allender, Noel Halford, Stephen Cummings and Lyle Blight settled their claims for compensation with the Federal Government — 19 months after their writs were lodged. The confidential settlements contained no admission of liability and covered all expenses, legal costs and loss of future support of each woman.[32]

Two months later came the shock announcement that all Australian growth hormone recipients had dreaded. The government announced "Stephen", the 27-year-old man who died after strange neurological symptoms in Westmead Hospital in 1991, had possibly died from CJD. He had received hGH from at least "a dozen" batches of the hormone, which heightened the anxiety of those already worried about their CJD risk. Until that announcement, in February 1995, Australia had been in the apparently freak situation of having four gonadotrophin deaths from CJD and none from hGH, which had killed, by then, more than 70 hGH recipients overseas.

Then in August 1995, in what some of the human hormone recipient population regard as the sixth victim of the AHPHP, an Adelaide woman, and mother of three children, committed suicide following a long period of depression and anxiety. The woman, a state coordinator for the local CJD support group, had been very concerned that her identity — as a person at risk of CJD — might have been publicly revealed when a letter containing her name and address was tabled during a Senate committee hearing in June 1995. She contacted various people about her concern at this apparent invasion of privacy — including friends, several members of the Senate, Ted Allender and other recipients of hPG.

On the morning of her death, the woman visited her lawyer, Sean Millard, of the now re-named Rennick Briggs, and gave him every piece of correspondence she had received from the time she learned of her risk of CJD. The woman was one of the more than 130 human hormone recipients suing the Federal Government and CSL for damages for nervous shock. Apart from APQ, who had become the test case, this woman was the only other volunteer to be the test case.

On the afternoon of August 15, she addressed a meeting of the National Pituitary Hormones Advisory Council, chaired by Associate Professor Margaret Allars, regarding her allegation of invaded privacy. She left a copy of the letter she presented for this author, Ted Allender and another hormone recipient with whom she had constant contact. That night, after refusing to return home to Adelaide she checked into a Melbourne hotel, attached a belt of divers' weights around her neck and climbed into a full bath. A forensic pathologist later found her death was consistent with drowning.

Confusion surrounded her wishes regarding an autopsy. Eventually, at the Coroner's discretion and after advice from several sources, no autopsy was performed. This was not due to any concerns expressed by mortuary staff at the Victorian Institute of Forensic Medicine. Rather, it stemmed from the advice of a neuropathologist that if the woman was suffering from early symptoms of CJD (which she did not tell anyone about) then an autopsy was unlikely to reveal damage to the brain at such an early stage.

The woman had been under the care of a psychiatrist since 1992 and had been prescribed sleeping tablets and Valium. The Coroner, Ms Jacinta Heffey, found the woman had died by her own hand after a significant period of depression and anxiety. Her preoccupation with her risk of contracting CJD was "heightened by her sensitivity to any publication of her being in the risk group". That she would commit suicide after the tabling of her personal details in the Senate committee hearing could not have been reasonably anticipated by anyone.[33]

A small group of recipients of pituitary fractions including prolactin, thyroid-stimulating hormone (TSH) and luteinising hormone (LH) have never been warned officially that they carry a risk of CJD. Until 1985, America's NHPP distributed prolactin, LH, FSH and hGH for clinical use in America only, due to limited supplies, under Investigational New Drug applications. The hormones were also used by scientists overseas for laboratory research. About 5000 awards of these hormones were made each year.[34]

In annual reports of the NPA, America's original hormone collection organisation, research projects were listed along with awards of glands to hundreds of investigators and the number of medical journal articles attributed to NPA gland research each year. According to one report, techniques developed with research allocations of both FSH and LH were used to study male infertility. And "forty researchers will receive clinical grade follicle stimulating hormone and/or luteinising hormone for investigation in 1969".[35] Clinical grade hGH had also been used on severely burned patients. Pituitary-derived hGH and TSH were used in experiments on the obese in America.[36]

In 1976 more American projects for studies on boys and women were approved by the NPA. These included projects "to determine the metabolic clearance and excretion of hFSH given to hypopituitary males" and "to study further a female with isolated FSH deficiency. An attempt would be made to saturate the antibodies and then permit stimulation of the ovary by hFSH".[37]

In late 1989, with the American death toll from CJD in hGH recipients still seven, and news just to hand of the deaths of Jane Allender and the Brazilian hGH recipient, American experts on the Public Health Service Interagency Coordinating Committee on Human Growth Hormone discussed, at a regular meeting, the use of pituitary-derived LH and FSH in America. Dr Judith Fradkin, from the National Institute for Diabetes and Digestive and Kidney Diseases, had reviewed the use of those hormones and found that, unlike children who were named in the applications for hGH, none of the LH or FSH recipients were identified in applications for use. These patients, who can never be traced, received the hormones for a few months only with "only a handful" having treatment for up to six months.[38]

In Britain in 1977 up to 30 ampoules of clinical LH, one of two hormones necessary to complete ovulation, were released by the MRC to two of the pioneers of IVF treatment, Drs Patrick Steptoe and David Edwards. Late that year, the MRC's Steering Committee for Human Pituitary Collection was told that two ampoules of LH had been used on patients but had not resulted in ovulation.[39] At the same meeting, it was noted that a request by one doctor for ampouled prolactin had been granted.[40]

In 1980, the head of Britain's National Institute for Biological Standards and Control, Dr Derek Bangham, wrote to the World Health Organisation (WHO), supporting a call by Professor Leslie Lazarus, the head of HPAC, for an international meeting for human hormone program representatives. Lazarus, even before the 1982 disaster with the 500 dumped pituitary glands that followed the inclusion of a gland from a CJD case, wanted to discuss various aspects of gland production including specific legislation and screening for hepatitis antigens.[41] Dr Bangham's supporting letter confirmed the use of other pituitary hormones on humans. It stated:

> There is certainly a great need for discussion and guidance on manufacture and control of preparations of growth hormone, FSH, LH and TSH for administration to man.[42]

None of the recipients of these stimulation tests, IVF trials or other pituitary fraction experiments have been traced and told they are at risk of CJD. No-one knows who they are.

Another, bigger and also hidden risk group for CJD are elite athletes and bodybuilders. They have obtained hGH on the black market or through prescribing doctors in various countries to build muscle, reduce body fat and avoid dope detection tests.

The use of hGH by anyone but growth retarded children was unapproved worldwide. Trials for other uses of hGH have since occurred, including on non-growth deficient but merely short children. These have been possible due to the wide availability of commercially prepared synthetic hGH. From 1985 onwards, as synthetic hGH became available, warnings were sounded from sporting and medical quarters about a potential rise in abuse of the drug by athletes desperate for any edge on international competitors. But it had been going on for years.

In South Africa, the former director of the national health laboratory service Professor Lionel Smith was aware that "some of my colleagues were giving prescriptions to body builders … It happens all over the world. Since body building has been a thing and hGH has been on the market they have been using it for body building".[43]

The professor of endocrinology at the University of Cape Town and Groote Schour Hospital, Professor François Bonnici, recalls body-builders beginning to contact South African doctors for supplies around the late 1970s and early 1980s. "In the early 1980s I visited about 10 main gyms in the city of Cape Town when we started doing some studies on athletes regarding the effects of steroids on insulin resistance. One unit at that time cost around R25. I know from anecdotal isolated reports that hGH reached this country without import permits."[44]

Once the production of human-derived hGH was stopped in the USA and by commercial manufacturers such as Kabi and Ares-Serono from mid-1985 onwards, the USA-based Genentech brought out the first of several commercial preparations of synthetic hGH. It was approved from September 1985 by the US Food and Drug Administration (FDA) under "compassionate use" as an investigational drug.

By 1986 Elizabeth Rappaport, a medical officer with the FDA's division of metabolism and endocrine drug products, was reported to concede there would probably be abuse of the hormone by athletes. "It depends on how long and how much they take," she said. "Acutely, if you give large doses to adults, they may develop glucose intolerance; it may unmask frank diabetes. Over the long term, an adult who takes large doses of the hormone can develop acromegaly."[45]

Acromegaly is gigantism, an often painful and disfiguring condition in which the organs, bones and facial features overgrow due to excessive secretion or use of growth hormone. Toes and finger bones thicken and enlarge, coarse skin results, menstrual problems and loss of libido occur and the life span can be shortened due to the development of diabetes or heart problems.

In a 1986 review of hGH treatment in Canada, an estimate was made of how many people worldwide had received pituitary-derived hGH to that time. The quoted figure was at least 50,000. It included not only growth-retarded children, but girls with Turner's syndrome, of which short stature is a feature, and physically normal but merely short children in highly-controversial experiments. "In addition, the illicit distribution and sale of GH has become popular among body builders."[46]

Warnings about abuse of hGH in the new synthetic era of hGH production also came from Australia in March 1986 and later, when successive Olympic bids were put in for both Melbourne and Sydney.

The Allars inquiry received no evidence that any Australian doctor provided hGH to an athlete. However, it was aware from departmental correspondence of an attempt to trial it on athletes. In Australia, doctors' approvals for the importation of commercial hGH were granted by the Therapeutic Goods Branch of the Federal Department of Health under what as known as the Individual Patient Use Scheme. Strict conditions regarding full permission and responsibility for the experimental nature of the drug applied.

In 1984, a year before the shutdown of most human hormone programs worldwide and when pituitary-derived hGH was recognised to be unable to meet the needs of hGH-deficient children, a doctor in NSW asked to be able to import commercial hGH. She wanted to conduct a clinical trial involving athlete patients — and also herself. She said that some of her patients who were athletes and had been bringing hGH into Australia from the USA wanted to know whether they needed permission to do so, according to a TGB memo.[47] The application was refused after it was pointed out that, in addition to the scarcity of the hormone for growth deficient children, the risks, which included antibody development and contraction of "some viral or exotic disease" such as AIDS, were too great to give gGH to healthy adults merely for sporting purposes.[48]

In March 1986 a review of growth hormone by Canberra-based sports drug expert, Steve Haynes, said sports use of hGH was anecdotal but undoubted as a tool to cheat competition doping controls. He cited a passage from the *Underground Steroid Handbook,* first published in 1981. "GH use is the biggest gamble that an athlete can take, as the side effects are irreversible. Even with all that, we love the stuff."[49] In 1993, as chief executive of the Australian Sports Drug Agency, Haynes agreed that "thousands" of body builders, many more than those who were treated with human hormone drugs, were at risk of CJD from abuse of hGH in the 1970s and 1980s before synthetic hGH became available.[50]

The CJD task force of the Federal Department of Health incorporated any hammer, discus or shot-put thrower, sprinter, power lifter or weight lifter who used the drug into the list of those at risk who should be warned not to donate organs, tissue or blood. These athletes would also be eligible for anxiety counselling, along with approved hGH and hPG recipients. It is believed none ever applied.

In New Zealand, on parental consent forms given to prospective hGH recipients in 1988 following a scare about reports of leukaemia in hGH patients, athletes were singled out in the background information section. "Athletes have been known to take large doses of growth hormone and this may cause hypertension and diabetes. This does not occur with the doses used for growth stimulation in children and the practice of taking excess growth hormone is frowned upon by medical authorities."

Sport and bodybuilding magazines are littered with references to the benefits and sometimes the hazards of hGH, particularly in combination with anabolic steroids. This dual drug taking is known as stacking. Stacked with steroids, hGH is thought to aid faster healing or prevent common tearing injuries in connective tissue and cartilage — injuries that often result from over-use of steroid-bulked muscles. There is no hard evidence that hGH actually has this function. But taken on its own hGH can be a powerful psychological stimulant during competition, when steroid detection in random urine tests results in instant disqualification and varying periods of banning from competitive sport. There is no test for naturally occurring hGH. It is secreted due to various stimuli at differing levels throughout each day. Any test that does not involve some sort of chemical marker added by the manufacturer would result in multiple testing of athletes throughout one day. This would not only be inconvenient but a gross invasion of privacy.

Cynics pointed out that in the run-up to the Barcelona Olympics in 1992, note had been taken of the fact that among the nine top athletes of the Santa Monica Track Club in California who had competed in the previous World Championships in Tokyo, seven had had braces on their teeth at some stage. The point was made in a magazine article by former Australian Olympic hockey player, Dr Ric Charlesworth to illustrate that anecdotal evidence of acromegaly, which can cause crooked teeth in elongated jaws, was under close scrutiny.[51] Charlesworth also noted that Seoul triple gold-medal winner Florence Griffith-Joyner retired the same day that out-of-competition dope testing was introduced, just five weeks after the end of the Seoul Olympics. In 1989 Griffith-Joyner emphatically denied sensational allegations made by fellow athlete Darrell Robinson, whose story was paid for by the mass-circulation German magazine *Stern,* that she had bought hGH from him six months before her gold medal feats in Korea.[52]

The Canadian sprinter, Ben Johnson, spectacularly stripped of one of the most sought-after of Olympic gold medals in track and field — the 100 metres sprint final at the Seoul Olympics in 1988 — certainly took hGH in his lead-up training.

In Canada, the 1989 Commission of Inquiry into the Use of Drugs and Banned Practices Intended to Increase Athletic Performance, which was established in the wake of the Ben Johnson scandal, pointed to the use of hGH by sprinters, bodybuilders, weight lifters and inter-collegiate football players — all of whom obtained their supplies on the black market. The commission heard that in mid-1988 Johnson, who had had successive hamstring injuries, spent C$10,000 on 10 bottles of growth hormone. Part of it was to have been purchased on the black market by Toronto bodybuilder, Steve Brisbois but Brisbois failed to deliver and the hGH was eventually bought from other sources by Johnson's personal physician, Dr Astaphan, who testified at the commission and personally administered the injections.[53]

Canadian sprinter Angella Issajenko eventually developed diabetes, which she blamed on her use of growth hormone, the inquiry report also stated.[54] And Lyle Alzado, a former Los Angeles Raiders defensive lineman who died in 1992 from a rare form of brain cancer, blamed it on his long-term abuse of both steroids and hGH. hGH, he told the *New York Times* and *Sports Illustrated* magazine in 1991, had become the drug of choice for athletes in the 1990s. For one four-month supply he had paid US$4000 on the black market.

Manufacturers of hGH and doctors involved in administering it for its only legitimate medical use — the treatment of pituitary dwarves — doubt that anyone buying hGH on the black market is getting what they pay for. Not only is its distribution monitored closely by manufacturers, but its administration is tightly regulated by treating doctors (although some of these, it is admitted, may unethically prescribe the drug. One such doctor in America used his medical licence to buy large supplies of hGH and then established a marketing chain to distribute it without a prescription.)[55]

Between October 1985 and December 1988 at least 115 vials of synthetic hGH were confiscated by US authorities on 13 occasions. Earlier, in both 1983 and 1985, three vials of Asellecrin, manufactured by Serono, were confiscated. In 1985, after the banning of all pituitary-derived hGH in America, 28 vials of pituitary-derived Crescormon, manufactured by Kabi, were seized from the black market.[56] By 1989 a US Senate committee, which recommended studying the abuse of anabolic steroids and hGH in sport, had reported that synthetic hGH was being abused by athletes who obtained the drugs on the black market through other athletes or gymnasiums. "Justice officials estimate that human growth hormones are selling on the black market for $500 to $1500 per unit."[57] Many American states enacted legislation to outlaw the distribution and possession of hGH by the late 1980s.

In Australia in the early 1980s, a white American marine stationed at the US Embassy in Canberra was involved in distributing an unknown quantity of performance-enhancing drugs, including hGH. The marine, a champion bodybuilder, left Australia in 1984, well before synthetic hGH was available. His drugs were mailed to him at the embassy and were not detected by Customs inspections. Evidence about the marine was given to confidential hearings of an Australian Senate inquiry into drugs in sport in the late 1980s. Subsequent checks with US officials confirmed that the named marine had served officially in Australia.[58]

All hGH clients of the US marine, and anyone who was or is a recipient of cadaver-derived hGH are at the same risk of contracting Creutzfeldt-Jakob disease, as any legitimate child hGH or adult hPG recipient. It just hasn't been publicised widely.

In 1992 the journal *Clinical Pediatrics* reported that a survey of adolescent use of hGH in two suburban mid-western schools in the state of Arkansas had revealed that five per cent of the 224 males in grade 10 were either using the drug then or had been since about age 14. Another 31 per cent of boys knew of others using the substance. Only one girl from the 208 females surveyed was using the drug.[59]

More alarmingly, two Austrian doctors warned of the manufacture and use of cadaver-derived hGH in the former Soviet Union in a letter to *The Lancet* in March 1993. Citing one of their own studies on the effects of synthetic hGH on hormonal and physical parameters in power athletes, endocrinologists Roman Deyssig and Herwig Frisch said performance "cannot be improved in trained power athletes or in untrained subjects by administration of growth hormone". They were particularly worried, having obtained an ampoule of the drug which they claimed, after testing, was low in potency and not pure hGH — much like hGH prepared in the early 1970s before purification methods were expanded and improved. In view of its consistency, it was unlikely, the doctors concluded, that it was treated with anything to rid it of the CJD agent. "Because this type of growth hormone is used in other countries (anecdotally we know of use by weight lifters and body builders in Germany, Poland, Italy, and Austria)," more information should be given to potential users. This should include the potential risk from CJD and the further possibility of transmission via tissue or organ donations, they warned.[60]

CHAPTER 19

Blood:
Another route of infection?

TRANSFUSIONS OF BLOOD and blood products save lives. Whole blood replaces massive blood loss, particularly in traumatic accidents. Packed red blood cells provide vital oxygen properties for patients undergoing radiation therapy that has killed off many of their own red blood cells. White blood cells fight infections, and platelets, the third type of cellular component in the blood, build a plug at the site of bleeding and begin clotting. Plasma transfusions replace the fluid lost when blood drains from the body.

Other blood components — fractions — also save lives. Albumin, derived from either human placentas or blood, provides essential protein needed for body function, especially in shock and burn patients. Immunoglobulins protect the immunosuppressed — AIDS and organ transplant patients in particular — who have little or no immunity to fight infectious diseases. And the clotting agents, Factor VIII and Factor IX, provide vital coagulation for sufferers of the hereditary disease haemophilia.

But just as the transfusions prolong life, they can also harbour death. Blood-borne viruses such as HIV, which causes AIDS, hepatitis B, which can cause cirrhosis of the liver, and hepatitis C, which can result in liver cancer, have been passed from donor to recipient in a multitude of cases. Generally, however, the benefits outweigh the risk. Certainly death may follow quickly without one. Patients can now donate their own blood before operations in some hospitals. But no supply of blood, donated voluntarily or for money, is guaranteed to be safe. Modern screening tests are helpful but not foolproof. There is no totally reliable test, screening or otherwise, to confirm CJD during incubation.

People who have later died of CJD are known to have made blood donations before the disease was evident. For instance Jenny Halford and Vonda Cummings were regular donors. Patrick Baldwin gave blood through the Royal Navy. Theoretical blood transmission risk from CJD "merits continuing interest", according to NIH neuroscientist, Paul Brown. "The numerical danger would dwarf other forms [of accidentally transmitted CJD] because of the hundreds of thousands of people who get donated blood each year".[1] It has also repeatedly been shown to be infectious during the incubation period and clinical phase of CJD in experimentally infected animals.[2]

Experiments on animals in the 1980s showed CJD transmission via buffy coat. This is the lighter, fluffy blood component of white blood cells and platelets which remains on top when whole blood is separated by centrifugation and the heavier red and other blood cells sink to the bottom. Another experiment in the 1980s documented the passage of CJD from urine — a feat even the author of the experiment could not reproduce — which resulted in speculation about laboratory contamination.[3,4] Only patchy blood transmission of CJD in animals such as mice, hamsters and guinea pigs has been managed, and then in just four laboratories around the world.

No case of CJD has ever been reported among patients with diseases like haemophilia, sickle cell disease or the hereditary blood disorder, thalassalmia.

Proven cases have never been reported in those who, before some synthetic products became available, needed repeated transfusions of whole blood, blood derivatives or blood components including plasma, leucocytes, albumin, interferon, immunoglobulin, and clotting factors VIII and IX throughout their lives. There is no concrete proof that blood donation is a viable route for CJD in humans. A few cases of what have been labelled sporadic cases of CJD have followed transfusions of blood or blood products. But these appear, to date, to have been unlucky coincidences.

The public health risk of CJD transmission through blood products is a possibility usually greeted with horror. Horror that it might happen and dismay at the expense of tracing blood records back to donors from patients who die of CJD years after a transfusion. The frequently quoted line used by British politicians on the risk of transmission to humans of BSE is also used by health authorities in many countries in relation to blood: there is no evidence, no "clinical proof", that blood can transmit CJD between humans. But researchers argue that CJD transmission via blood would be a peripheral contamination, typical of CJD in human hormone recipients and kuru victims. It would result in initial balance and incoordination symptoms typical of those cases — not the dementia and mental deterioration of early stage sporadic CJD that afflicts mainly elderly patients.[5]

In British case control studies covering the years 1980–84 and 1990–92, no significant difference was found between people who had died of CJD after blood transfusions and age-and-sex matched control groups. Those who died of CJD largely had mental deterioration, typical of sporadic CJD, as an initial symptom. The CJD Surveillance Unit (CJDSU) report, published in the *Lancet* in January 1993, did attach the rider that although blood was not a major risk factor for CJD, isolated cases could arise from transfusions.

As that report was published, so was an article by Melbourne research scientists Drs Lynette Dumble and Renate Klein, in a bimonthly magazine for GPs in Australia. They argued again that human hormone drug recipients should be traced to warn them not to spread the disease inadvertently via organs or blood donations.[6]

After the announcement of Vonda Cummings' death in early 1993, Dumble and Klein sent another letter to the *Lancet*. It was published under the headline, "Transmission of Creutzfeldt-Jakob disease by blood transfusion".[7] In the letter the two women reported the deaths from CJD of four Australian women aged in their fifties or sixties. They died between 1992 and early 1993, five or more years after blood transfusions. All had the cerebellar symptoms typical of peripheral contamination of CJD in kuru and human hormone recipients — balance and muscle jerkings with no dementia. Although this letter is usually cited when CJD and blood are mentioned in the same breath in scientific literature, critics point to its anecdotal nature and the absence of any comparable information on age-and-sex matched control patients. Australia's National Blood Transfusion Service did not investigate whether the four women had received blood donations from human hormone recipients, stating that there was still no demonstrated evidence of transmission via blood.[8]

In 1993 German researchers published the results of their efforts to trace the recipients of a 65-year-old blood donor who died of CJD in 1991. They found almost three-quarters of the 35 patients who had probably received the 55 units of blood he had donated between 1971 and 1991. None had any sign of CJD up to 22 years after receiving blood from that donor.[9]

In March 1995 — only a month after the announcement of the 1991 death in Sydney's Westmead Hospital of "Stephen", the 27-year-old hGH recipient and Australia's fifth probable CJD victim — Australian human hormone recipients were left reeling by another revelation. For the past two years a list of all their names had been provided to blood and tissue banks and organ transplant coordinators nationally. The number of agencies sent the list by the Pituitary Hormones Task Force of the Federal Department of Health since March 1993 totalled 31.

The existence of the list became public in January 1993. Sue Byrne, a Melbourne mother of six and one of the women who had gone public with her fears of contracting CJD after Dumble and Klein had written to the *Lancet,* was now the national coordinator of the CJD Support Group Network Inc. In the course of a conversation about exclusion criteria for blood donors at risk of CJD, Marion Dunlop, then head of the CJD Task Force, told Byrne: "Don't you know that the blood banks have a list of recipients' names and that you *cannot* donate blood?" The matter had been referred to obliquely in the Allars Report, but recipients had not realised its significance.[10] The list detailed name, date of birth, type of treatment and sex. It warned authorities against human hormone recipients. Should they attempt to donate blood, tissue or organs, they were automatically rejected as a precaution against the spread of CJD.

Victorian hPG recipient, Gina Stachlewski made sure it was known. She complained to the Privacy Commissioner, and sent letters of protest to politicians and various media organisations that her medical details had been given without her consent to these donor organisations.[11] Others who had received human hormone injections were not as angry as Stachlewski was, although they were surprised they had not been told earlier about the list. With no screening test, some thought an automatic exclusion such as that provided by the list, was a sensible move in the early days of the department's concerted effort to trace recipients. The list, which remains in existence, is the only list kept by the Australian Red Cross that it has not generated itself. It is believed to be unique in the world.

Two months after Gina Stachlewski's complaint was made public, Australia's first international workshop on CJD was held in Melbourne, organised by Professor Colin Masters, by then the head of the pathology department at the University of Melbourne.

One of the invited speakers, Paul Brown, revealed that potential contamination of blood by CJD was clearly a question that was not going to go away "and it's a matter of great concern to blood banks".[12] Like others before him, he isolated white blood cells as the problem — not red cells or plasma because they contain no DNA. The chances of accidental transmission to recipients of blood derivatives like Factor VIII, albumin and gammaglobulin were reduced after blood separation techniques, but perhaps not entirely removed.

Brown had barely returned home to Bethesda, Maryland, when Canada made its largest ever blood product recall. Carried out by the Canadian Red Cross (CRC), it was precautionary and unprecedented and carried out swiftly against the backdrop of what was known nationally as Canada's "tainted blood scandal".

Like France's problems with HIV-contaminated blood, Canada had its own blood disaster in which 43 per cent of the country's 2300 haemophiliacs contracted HIV in the early to mid-1980s. Once news of deaths and court cases on medically acquired AIDS emerged, the government established a Commission of Inquiry on the Blood System in Canada under Ontario Court of Appeal judge, Justice Harold Krever.

The commission, which received massive publicity, had been underway for a year when a Canadian haematologist working in America testified on July 11, 1995 that potential CJD contamination of blood was like a second AIDS scenario, 10 years on.

Looking directly at the judge, Dr Nathan Kobrinsky, the former director of the Haemophilia Program at the Health Sciences Centre in Winnipeg, said: "I would hope that we are not facing Krever Part 2 a decade from now."[13] His concern arose from the lack of a screening test for CJD in blood products and the fact that albumin, a blood derivative, was used as a stabilising factor in new recombinant Factor VIII used widely by haemophiliacs. While that type of Factor VIII was synthetic, it was suspended in albumin which, as a component of blood, posed a small risk of CJD transmission. The use of albumin in the preparation of Factor VIII should be stopped, not least for the CJD risk factor. In his 10-chapter interim report tabled in early 1995, Krever described CJD, in the context of his brief to recommend changes to the blood system, as one of the potential threats of the future. The disease, he said "emphasises the need to have continuing surveillance mechanisms to identify ... new risks to the blood supply".[14]

Kobrinsky's evidence was published in the Canadian media on July 11, 1995. That day, a Vancouver woman notified the CRC that her father had recently died of CJD and had been a blood donor. His records were immediately checked and revealed that he had made 21 donations since 1989, the most recent being six weeks earlier.

Within 24 hours of the Vancouver woman's call, the CRC ordered the removal of stocks of fresh blood components including red cells, platelets and fresh frozen plasma. They also ordered the quarantining of another clotting agent, Factor I, and intravenous immunoglobulin, used for organ transplants and immune deficiencies, pending recall and destruction. However, albumin was in such critical supply that it was not withdrawn until replacement stocks arrived. Potential recipients were advised of the theoretical risks and advised to postpone any elective surgery in which this blood component was likely to be used.

Criticism before and during the Krever hearings had caused the CRC to act quickly and decisively despite the massive cost of importing replacement blood components and the resultant shortages of some products. "The proof [of CJD transmission] won't come until you get the first case, and I certainly don't intend to have that kind of proof," said Dr Bert Aye, director of the Red Cross blood transfusion service at the time.[15] On July 13, as a further precaution, the Canadian Red Cross ordered the withdrawal of donated plasma from the daughter of the Vancouver CJD victim — a decision later seen as unnecessary. She was banned from future blood donation.[16]

The blood recalls were made in conjunction with the North Carolina-based pharmaceutical company, Bayer Inc, the main fractionation partner of the Canadian Red Cross. Within a week — on July 18, 1995 — a similar but much smaller precautionary recall began when the CRC was told a Toronto donor had been diagnosed with probable CJD. The man had given blood five times between 1984 and 1995. His most recent donation had been shipped to Bayer for fractionation into red cells, platelets and plasma on February 7, 1995.[17] Blood products imported into Canada as replacements for those destroyed from the Vancouver donor covered this recall.

A huge amount of blood products were included in the larger recall. They totalled 3,865,780 units of Factor VIII, 5496 vials of intravenous immunoglobulin (IVIg) for patients who were deficient in gammaglobulin or with auto-immune disorders, and 60,000 litres of albumin products including 10,557 vials of 25 per cent albumin and 8,352 vials of five per cent albumin.[18] The recall decisions, which also included the donations of three adult children of the two CJD donors, meant that the CRC wrote off more than $4.5 million worth of blood products. Through blood brokers in America, it bought about $12 million worth of replacement blood products from virtually every licensed company in the US.[19,20] Buying all but 11,500 of the 58,000 vials of blood products through brokers had added more than C$1.8 million to the bill.[21]

The Canadian Haemophilia Society dubbed the recalls a knee-jerk reaction to media reports in the absence of the solid policy on CJD and blood that it had called for months earlier.[22] The society criticised the CRC for its lack of policy, its inability to effect a total recall and leaving the legal liability on the use of albumin to hospitals.

Hospitals were advised in strong terms to notify their patients and stress the lack of clear data on transmission via blood. Updated blood donor questionnaires were distributed on July 31, 1995, to pinpoint among potential donors any recipients of tissue transplants such as corneas or dura mater or infertile adults who had been injected with human pituitary gonadotrophin. In America, to that point, nine recalls of blood had occurred, from donors found later to have CJD.[23]

Elsewhere in the world, the European Association of Plasma Products Industry recommended no withdrawals or "lookback" procedures when CJD donors were identified. Switzerland, Austria, Germany and Britain followed these guidelines and also a 1995 European Union statement that no recall was necessary due to lack of proof of risk of CJD transmission. However, Pharmacia's policy in Sweden was to withdraw all implicated products. In France, Pasteur Merieux, which had about eight per cent of the world albumin market, had the same policy. Already under pressure from French health authorities alarmed at the growing toll of CJD-infected hGH recipients, it had been screening donors of the seven million placentas it collected annually from 44 countries. These placentas had been used to manufacture its supplies of albumin since late 1993.[24] In 1994 several blood donors had developed CJD in France and both their blood and the blood of their relatives was recalled, according to a letter of August 7, 1995 tendered at the Krever Commission from a Dr Burnouf to Bert Aye of the CRC.

By November 1995 — a year after two blood recalls from US CJD donors and after several calls by the Canadian Haemophilia Society for a policy on CJD and blood — the Federal Bureau of Biologics, the division of Health Canada that regulates the Canadian blood supply, devised a policy for excluding those at risk of CJD from donating blood. It was similar to that in force in Australia[25] and the United States. Similar exclusion criteria have since been recommended to all member countries of the World Health Organisation.[26]

On March 14, 1996 Ben Roth, 69, a vehicle inspector for both the Canadian and British armies, died from CJD in Holy Cross Hospital, Calgary. Roth had received a transfusion during triple bypass surgery in August 1994.[27] He was one of more than 1,000 people in the province of Alberta who had been informed by letter the previous year that they could be at risk of CJD because they had received blood from the Vancouver donor who sparked the first huge blood recall.[28] However, doctors later decided that the incubation time was not long enough for the CJD agent to proliferate and cause the disease in its usual slow fashion. Owing also to Roth's age, it was considered a coincidental case of sporadic CJD.

While the Canadian recalls were occurring in the northern summer of 1995, away from the media spotlight, French doctors raised a possible new mode of CJD transmission — liver transplantation. A 57-year-old French woman died of CJD two years after receiving a new liver and the blood derivative albumin during the operation. While the liver donor had no history of neurological disease, one of the multiple donors of the pooled albumin, a male, died of CJD three years after donation. The woman was homozygous for valine at codon 129 while the liver donor was homozygous for methionine. This meant that both were at apparent higher susceptibility to contracting CJD. A "random association of two very rare conditions remains the most likely possibility", according to doctors who alerted the medical world to the case in July 1995 in the *Journal of Neuropathology and Experimental Neurology* and later in the *Annals of Neurology*.[29] It was reported in the mainstream media as well.

However, among the interesting factors they noted was that the

woman developed the cerebellar symptoms of CJD most often associated with peripheral transmission — balance problems, kuru-type
plaques, deposits of protein and the absence of any genetic markers for
familial forms of CJD. Even though she may have died of sporadic
CJD, her initial symptoms mimicked those of former human hormone
recipients. What weighed against it being anything more than coincidence was the very short incubation time of the disease — if, indeed, it
was transmitted during the woman's operation. Peripheral transmission
can take from several years to up to four decades to manifest itself, as
in the youngest kuru child who died at age five, and the youngest
French hGH victims who died aged 10 and 11.

Later in 1995 doctors from the Department of Medicine at the University of Southern California, Los Angeles, published a sensible
reminder for all those concerned about CJD from pooled plasma derivatives. In all the 14-odd years since haemophiliacs, for instance, had
been at risk of HIV from supplies of Factor VIII, there had not been a
single case of CJD in a regular recipient of plasma derivatives.[30] This
remains the case.

However, the French doctors replied in a letter to the *Lancet* editor in
February 1996 that the 57-year-old French woman who died two years
after her liver transplant not only received albumin in her transplant, but
during the grafting procedure she had also been given transfusions of
blood, plasma and immunoglobulins. Like pituitary-derived hormones,
these were made from the pooled donations of many, many blood
donors.[31]

Among those who considered the French liver transplant case was
Paul Brown, who thought it unlikely that the albumin was the source of
the woman's CJD. He placed it in his "interesting case file".[32]

In the late 1980s in Tokyo, a team of doctors at the Kitzsato University
School of Medicine followed the case of a 10-week premature birth of
a baby boy to a woman dying of what appeared to be a long-duration
CJD. They began a series of experiments. Specimens from the blood,
placenta and umbilical cord blood were collected from the woman.
Four days after the baby's birth, a sample of breast milk was also taken
and was injected with the other substances into laboratory mice. In February 1992, the doctors reported that the woman's brain, placenta and
umbilical cord leucocytes, and colostrum were all infected with CJD.

Given that none of the children among the 3000-odd documented kuru victims from Papua New Guinea had contracted the disease from their pre-symptomatic or dying mothers, this was a controversial finding.[33] Also, the boy remains healthy more than 10 years later.

Peripheral injection of CJD-infected brain tissue into experimental animals has never had a uniformly successful transmission rate. It has been irregular at best and, while it shows the potential for transmission through blood, the evidence remains inconclusive when applying it to human-to-human transfusion. If it does occur in humans, it is so rare that it has not been detected beyond a small number of anecdotal cases. Genetic susceptibility may also play a role. However, a recent comprehensive scientific article on CJD blood transfusion risk, states the obvious. "The absence of evidence is not evidence of the absence of transmission of CJD through blood …" [34]

In Britain, Paul Andrews, the young man who gave up his promising marketing career when he learned he could carry the lethal legacy of CJD from his hGH treatments, assumed the role of spokesperson for fellow recipients. When women were identified as being at risk from their fertility treatments in Britain in September 1993, he was approached for comment from the media. Handsome, articulate and intelligent, he was the central character in a documentary aired in October 1994 by the influential Granada TV "World in Action" program.

Andrews was immensely angered by Britain's then Secretary of State for Health, Virginia Bottomley, who repeatedly refused to order an inquiry into the affair of contaminated hGH.

Later, after the inquest on Stuart Smith in October 1994, Smith's parents, Tony and Isobel, repeated their son's plea for justice in the hope that no-one else would suffer as he had done. Andrews added his voice to this plea. Smith had been the twelfth hGH recipient to succumb to CJD in Britain. Sadly, he had recognised his own symptoms while watching a television program.

Meanwhile at the beginning of 1994, Barham Khan, a 26-year-old European sales executive with a textile company in Leeds, had his life before him. He socialised in his shiny red Volkswagen, given to him by his doting parents Ashraf and Parveen on his graduation from Leeds University with a degree in textile engineering. Bonny, as he was known, flew regularly between cities on the Continent for his job. He always returned with an ornament for his mother. He lifted weights kept in his bedroom to maintain body strength in his svelte 165-centimetre frame — his height achieved solely through years of hGH injections from the ages of nine to 17.

In September 1994, after a mild cold, Bonny began to lose his balance. Then his memory began to fail. Watching television on the night of October 10, he saw Paul Andrews on Granada's "World in Action" program and diagnosed himself — much as Stuart Smith had done two years earlier. After a visit to Sheffield Hospital he knew the worst. Bonny Khan was the fourteenth British hGH recipient to contract CJD. It devastated his older brother and sister, while his parents blamed themselves for sanctioning the hormone injections, which they had not known had come from corpses. "I'm losing my son for a few inches. It's a terrible price to pay," Ashraf Khan said bitterly in January 1995.[35] He and Parveen, both Muslims, went to mosques, had prayers said for Bonny, even sacrificed a goat in the hope that a miracle would happen and their boy, the keen athlete with the room full of sporting trophies, would re-emerge from his dying shell.

By this time Bonny's limbs had wasted and twitched continually. He had no strength to operate the television remote control. Because of his double vision the TV was hazy anyway. He was the first hGH CJD victim to grant a press interview. "Would like to be around to get the bastards that gave me this," he slurred optimistically to a reporter in January 1995 about the upcoming trial in London's High Court in which the families of CJD victims were seeking damages — and answers — in the wake of the government's refusal to hold an inquiry into the scandal. "Somebody messed up man! People should know what went wrong," said Bonny who died three months later in a hospice, 12 months before the trial was scheduled to begin.[36]

When the trial did start, a still bitter Ashraf Khan, a retired British Rail clerk, was there most days to observe. "They didn't just kill my son," he nodded to the closed court door, his finger stabbing the air, "they killed the whole family."

In stark and, seemingly unique contrast was Donald Spear, a 32-year-old motorcycle courier who grew to be the same height as Bonny Khan. Spear's CJD symptoms appeared in early 1995 with dizziness and strange sensations. He contacted doctors at Great Ormond Street Hospital for Sick Children, and a series of tests were performed. Asked to return with his girlfriend after the test results came through, he was told he had less than a year to live.

Only the second living CJD victim to speak publicly about his condition, Spear was actually the seventeenth British hGH recipient to contract CJD. In an interview published in September 1995, during which his body trembled and he sometimes forgot words, he said he was glad he had lived until then at a normal height. This was preferable, he thought, to living a full life span at the 132-centimetre height his parents were told would be all he could achieve when he began hGH injections in 1971. Spear was walking with a stick by the time of the September interview and had married his girlfriend. "I am happier being tall and dying … If I had known then what I know now, I would still have had it," he said, not expecting to see Christmas 1995.[37]

Determined not to let anger and bitterness mar his last months, he told a friend who was a tattooist to practise new lettering on his arm. "I'm going to be dead — it won't matter if you get it wrong," he told his friend. On his inner left arm were left the words "Immortal So Far."

Meanwhile, the first hint of a larger impending catastrophe was the suggestion by doctors in England that odd neurological symptoms observed in an 18-year-old boy might be CJD. In March 1995 specialists at the CJDSU in Edinburgh reviewed a brain biopsy from the boy. Although it failed to reveal any spongiform change that indicated CJD, prion protein accumulation in the brain biopsy was identified, and information was collected from his family just in case. Five months later, in August 1995, the same specialists reviewed another biopsy — again in a teenager. This time the victim was a girl and the tiny section of her brain showed the typical spongiform changes of CJD. Although it wasn't appreciated at the time, the sliver of frontal lobe brain tissue also featured kuru-type plaques — the aggregates of protein that were a feature of many kuru brain specimens.

The medical histories and clinical symptoms of both teenagers were collected, as in all cases investigated by the CJDSU, which has a strict confidentiality policy. It never reveals the identities of its patients — even if the families of the patients later speak to the media.[38] Both young people biopsied had an unusual presentation of symptoms for any type of CJD. Their initial symptoms included psychiatric treatment for depression, progressive balance problems and mental deterioration.

By this time BSE had officially claimed more than 150,000 cattle in Britain.[39] Already, great media attention had been paid to the deaths of Peter Warhurst, a 61-year-old dairy farmer from Manchester who had owned a BSE-affected herd, and Duncan Templeman, a 65-year-old from Weston Farm near Crewkerne in Somerset, whose cattle had been slaughtered due to BSE.[40] Richard Lacey, professor of clinical microbiology at the University of Leeds, continued his attack on the government for its repeated assurances that there was no link between BSE and CJD in humans. He accused officials of a massive cover-up and claimed that two CJD deaths in farmers "are simply not explicable on the grounds of probability".

In September 1995 the *Lancet* reported the death, from sporadic CJD, of a third dairy farmer in the space of two years. This death provoked even more condemnation from food safety critics of the government. For most of his working life, this farmer, aged 54, had worked among a herd of cattle in which three BSE-affected cattle had been reported in 1988, 1991 and 1992. He had assisted with calving but had not been involved with any surgical procedure on cattle and it was thought unlikely that he had tasted cattle feed as some farmers did. He was homozygous for valine (VV) at codon 129. His death, when reported in the September 30, 1995 issue of the *Lancet,* was described by doctors at the CJDSU and the Bristol Hospital where he was examined, as "clearly a matter of concern".[41]

An accompanying letter in the *Lancet* from members of an EU-funded CJD surveillance program presented comparable data on definite or probable CJD cases in people employed on farms in four countries in 1994. This data, from Germany, the Netherlands, France and Italy, where there was a negligible rate of BSE compared with Britain, helped place the British farmer deaths in perspective. There were five in France, two in Germany and three in Italy — compared with the three that had caused such consternation in England.[42]

October 1995 was a dreadful month on the BSE front. In early October Gwendoline Lawrence, 64, a farmer's wife, died of CJD. None of her husband Jim's dairy or beef cows on their farm near Wrexham, South Wales, had been affected by BSE.[43] She was regarded as a sporadic case and would be one of two farmers' wives to die of CJD in 1996. The CJDSU's annual report, tabled in Parliament, showed that 55 Britons had died of CJD in the previous year — double the figure of

1985. However, the report concluded, again, that this was probably due to improved diagnosis rather than any link to the consumption of BSE-infected meat products.[44]

But another bombshell followed. It was the probable diagnosis of CJD in a fourth farmer, this time from north Wales, who had had cases of BSE among his beef herd. A confidential report on the matter to all members of the Spongiform Encephalopathy Advisory Committee (SEAC) was mistakenly sent to a private fax number in the north of England and leaked to the press.[45] The report included an extract of a deliberately cautious statement drafted for SEAC members that was only for use should news of the fourth farmer's death leak out. It stated:

> Three previous CJD cases have been confirmed in dairy farmers whose herds had had cases of BSE. The committee concluded that it was difficult to explain this as simply a chance phenomenon. There is a statistical excess of cases in cattle farmers compared with the general population but the absolute risk, even for cattle farmers, is extremely low at about 2 cases per million per year.

A SEAC member was reported saying the committee did not want to spread alarm when it was not known exactly what was happening.

Britain's Agriculture Minister, Douglas Hogg, was also forced in October 1995 to announce that government veterinary surgeons had discovered four cases of slaughterhouses failing to remove spinal cord, in contravention of the specified bovine offal (SBO) ban put in place in 1989.[46] This seemed particularly ominous in light of a letter the same month to the *Lancet* editor that revealed the diagnosis of CJD in the two teenagers, the youngest victims of this disease on record in Britain.

One of the teenagers was Stephen Churchill, whose parents Dorothy and Dave Churchill of Devizes in Wiltshire, had already spoken to the media, questioning the cause of their son's death at age 19 in May 1995. Stephen had no family history of dementing or ataxic illness causing balance problems, no dura mater graft, no human hormone drugs or neurosurgery. The previous year, due to depression, Stephen had visited a psychiatrist and told him he thought he had "gone nutty". He had a six-month history of memory problems, a decline in school performance that had led to him leaving suddenly and a strange incident in which he was one of the drivers in a head-on collision for which no cause could be found. (No-one was seriously injured.)[47]

As he declined, Stephen Churchill began having hallucinations and difficulty with simple tasks like unlocking a door or eating a boiled egg. He developed an excessive fear of water and sharp objects, and refused to shave his face or wash. As his balance worsened he had a seizure and was referred to a neurologist in Bath who found slurred speech, occasional myoclonic jerks in his limbs and an abnormal EEG reading. Frequently he would scream and appear frightened for no apparent reason. A brain biopsy was performed in London, which raised the possibility of CJD before Stephen died in a nursing home.

By this time, Collinge, Prusiner and other researchers around the world had discovered more than 14 different gene mutations that were associated with TSEs.[48] (By late 1997, 20 TSE mutations had been identified.) Stephen Churchill had none of these mutations. But like most of those who develop non-inherited CJD-type illnesses, he had apparent susceptibility. He was homozygous for methionine — MM — at codon 129. Of note in the autopsy report, apart from the conclusive spongiform change in his brain, was the mention of "scattered amyloid plaques" in his cerebellum.

The other teenage case reported in the *Lancet,* was the 16-year-old girl who had undergone the brain biopsy in August 1995. This had followed a 12-month history of slurred speech, balance problems and clumsiness. Like Stephen Churchill, this unidentified girl had no medical history that put her in the risk group for accidentally transmitted CJD. A Muslim of Turkish-Cypriot parentage, she had been born in Britain but had visited Turkey and Cyprus many times during her childhood. Doctors from Guy's Hospital in London reported that she had eaten cow brain in Cyprus in 1989, a place where BSE had not been known. Generally, while in Britain, she ate lamb and occasionally corned beef or beef burgers. The biopsy of one of her frontal lobes showed spongiform change and "numerous plaques".[49]

Doctors from the department of neurology at Guy's Hospital and King's College Hospital in London said the case "inevitably prompts discussion of a possible link between her illness and the recent epidemic of bovine spongiform encephalopathy (BSE)". However, since there were four other reports of CJD in teenagers in other parts of the world before the 1985 start of the BSE epidemic, these two British teenage cases might be coincidental, they concluded.[50]

In the latter half of 1995, scientists and doctors in Britain and France had become very concerned at the increasing incidences of CJD on

several fronts. In France the death toll from hGH injections administered to short children in the trouble period between January 1984 and
June 1985 had topped 34 with more cases suspected.[51]

And Dr Robert Will, head of the CJDSU, was worried. The Scottish
neurologist, who had researched the CJD transmitted between neurosurgery patients of Sam Nevin in London in the 1950s, had been sent an
unprecedented number of referrals of suspected CJD in younger
people. After the 16-year-old girl's biopsy proved positive for CJD,
more cases had been referred to his unit: two in September, two in
October, one in November and one in December. A comparative difference between the teenagers of 1995 and teenagers with CJD in the pre-
BSE era was crucial for CJDSU investigators in finding out why young
people seemed suddenly to be affected in bigger numbers than normal
in Britain. In addition, an intriguing 1980 case of neurological disease
in a 16-year-old was unearthed in late 1995 by a neurology student who
had been seconded to the CJDSU.

Will remembered interviewing the 16-year-old girl's neurologist.
The girl's case had been difficult. Originally thought to have died of
CJD, which was listed on her death certificate despite her extreme
youth, the diagnosis after her autopsy was later changed. In a hunt that
took months, her neuropathological slides were obtained to double
check the pattern of her brain damage. It was necessary to compare her
brain damage with that in the cases of the 16-year-old Muslim girl who
had undergone the biopsy, Stephen Churchill, and the six subsequent
referrals in young people to the end of 1995.

A doctor at the Lancashire Centre for Medical Studies based at the
Royal Preston Hospital, wrote to the *Lancet* in November 1995 with his
theory that farmers may have contracted CJD through the previously
unconsidered and admittedly difficult to prove route of the olfactory
sensory nerve. Sense of smell is transmitted to the brain via this nerve
and "it is possible that farmer might have been exposed to the disease,
not through contact with cattle, but by breathing the dust from feed containing prion", the doctor warned.[52] Also in November 1995, one of the
largest cattle breeders in the west of England was found guilty of falsi-
fying cattle documents to assert that they had come from BSE-free
herds when they had not. Fined £30,000, he was ordered also to pay
more than £18,000 in costs and was described in court as having
"betrayed the farming community and put a substantial industry in
jeopardy".[53]

This court case followed claims that some farmers were illegally burying BSE-affected carcasses to save money after the July 1995 government edict that cow's heads be added to the SBO ban. This meant the farmers faced extra charges from slaughtermen. Burying the carcasses helped farmers keep their herds' precious BSE-free status for export. And, it was argued, the BSE-free requirement — increased from two to six years by the European Union anxious to prevent the importation of BSE in its herds — was an added burden on farmers. Public confidence in government declarations was eroded with each addition to the SBO ban. Eventually most of the edible portions of calves aged under 30 months old were added to this list. They had previously been exempt from any offal ban.

Sustained controversy erupted in early December 1995 when the *Sunday Times* newspaper surveyed 50 scientists knowledgeable about BSE and found that one in three of them now believed consumers could die from CJD after eating beef products. Some scientists had given up eating beef products. Prominent among them was Professor Sir Bernard Tomlinson, a retired neuropathologist who had changed his mind, he said, about the danger to humans from beef products. He would not eat beefburgers again "under any circumstances" because the risk of BSE infection passing to humans from organs and offal in meat pies was too great to be discounted.[54] Others, including Helen Grant, the retired neuropathologist who had successfully campaigned to have cattle brains removed from human consumption in 1989, claimed not to have eaten beef products since the first BSE scares in the late 1980s.

Media reports claimed that up to one quarter of Britons had given up eating beef. Meat sales plummeted by 15 per cent, not helped by estimates aired in November on the "World in Action" program that up to 600 BSE-infected cows were being eaten each week because they were slaughtered for meat before the symptoms of BSE had emerged.

In the wake of hundreds of schools removing beef from their menus, the government accused parents and schools of over-reacting. The then Prime Minister, John Major, felt compelled on December 7 to offer reassurance by repeating the oft-quoted line from scientific advisers that there was no evidence that BSE was transmissible to humans.[55] And they were right. But there was no evidence that it was not, either. The next day, the chairman of SEAC, John Pattison, professor of microbiology and dean of London's University College medical school, was quoted:

> It is not possible at the moment to give you the scientific proof that there
> is not any connection between BSE and human disease, but all the infor-
> mation we have suggests that this is the case ... There is no reason to
> panic. If the committee thought for a moment that there was any evidence
> that BSE could be transmitted to humans we would say so. We are under
> no pressure to say beef is safe. In fact we are constantly being pressed to
> say beef is not safe.[56]

As the year ended, the spectre of CJD in humans from BSE-infected
beef products hung over the British population. It was fuelled by media
reports of an increasing incidence of CJD in the general population (due
probably to more awareness of the disease and better diagnosis). As
well, there were the strange incidences of CJD deaths in the two
teenagers, four farmers and the farmer's wife — all in less than two
months. Each government attempt at reassurance that beef was "safe"
to eat was met with more and more scepticism by the public, which had
a far different interpretation of the word "safe" than did government
officials, who knew there was a silent "remote risk" built into the definition.

Then a second young person died of CJD. The post-mortem examination of the brain showed the same strange but uniform spread of kuru-
type or amyloid plaques dotted throughout the spongiform holes as
affected Stephen Churchill and the 16-year-old Muslim girl, who was
still alive. To rule out previous young cases of CJD having been misdiagnosed, details of suspect but unconfirmed cases of a similar but
non-transmissible infectious disease related to the measles virus —
subacute sclerosing panencephalitis (SSPE) — were reviewed by the
CJDSU in cooperation with Britain's SSPE register. No CJD cases were
identified.

By December 1995 John Collinge, who had carried out the DNA
analysis on Stephen Churchill and the young Muslim girl, had been
referred a third case in a young person, this time in a 28-year-old married woman. None of the three had any known mutations, a fact that
particularly worried Collinge. Beef sales, which had fallen by 15 per
cent in December, recovered partially in the New Year. No-one knew it
at the time, but it was the lull before the storm.

CHAPTER 20

A new CJD strain

IN JANUARY 1996 when Dr James Ironside emerged from the autopsy change room in Edinburgh's Royal Infirmary, he looked more like a futuristic astronaut than the white-coated pathologist made famous in the 1980s television series, "Quincy MD". Times had changed drastically since Gajdusek's hasty butchery with the carving knife in the howling New Guinea gale of May 1957. Modern, aseptic practices and an acute awareness of the potentially highly infectious nature of CJD in anyone referred to the CJDSU had resulted in the latest in high-tech precautions during autopsies.

As the neuropathologist attached to the CJDSU, Ironside's post-mortem examination garb included a green paper gown, full head plastic visor goggles, and gum boots with his name handwritten on the inside to distinguish them from others, which were in a neat line in the change room. Inadvertent splashes aside, the most important defence against cuts — and the most likely route of any infection — were gloves. It was mandatory to wear three pairs. The first pair was rubber. The second pair was made of high-tech fine chain mail. Over the top of those Ironside pulled on a second pair of rubber gloves. None was puncture-proof. But when he removed the top of a skull with his hand-saw, the metal lining of the chain mail protected against accidental "inoculation" of brain tissue from sharp, protruding pieces of bone. His instruments were restricted to CJD autopsies only and were kept in a separate autopsy room dedicated to infectious viral diseases such as AIDS and hepatitis. Inside that room, Ironside was to conduct full autopsies on two women who had been brought in by undertakers early that morning.

The tall, softly spoken Scot went over the case notes with two experienced mortuary technicians. He had already discussed both cases with the head of the CJDSU, consultant neurologist Robert Will. Will, in turn, had been briefed by the treating neurologists of both women who suspected that their patients, despite their youth, had died of a rapid degenerative illness like CJD. The younger of the two women on the morgue slab was Scottish and only 29. Ironside thought it sad that someone so young had possibly died from such a horrible disease. Any young person who died was a tragedy, but CJD was such a terrible way to go, he felt. A diagnosis of CJD was less certain in the other woman. From northern England, she was 41, only a few months older than Ironside himself.

Both women had experienced strange neurological symptoms before their deaths. The full autopsies conducted on both of them were not revealing in themselves, until their brains could be examined in detail after being allowed to set in formalin for several weeks. Different areas of the brains were later sliced into tiny slivers and mounted on slides to be examined under a powerful microscope. What Ironside saw through that microscope was familiar. It was an additional element in his gradual realisation that something new and frightening was emerging in some of the recent cases referred to the unit.

By December 1995 there had been a noticeable change in the yearly pattern of referrals to the CJDSU. Robert Will recalled:

> There seemed to be an excess of younger patients being referred, not teenagers, but in the younger age group, say twenties, thirties and forties ... We started getting worried and we were talking about it. 'What's going on? There's been another young case referred. That's very peculiar.' So we started to keep lists of these cases and they got a bit longer in January.[1]

Will and Ironside conferred with Dr Martin Zeidler, the neurology registrar attached to the CJDSU, who travelled all over Britain interviewing suspected CJD patients and their families for essential medical histories. As the lists lengthened they discussed the topic back and forth for months when their schedules allowed them to gather in the CJDSU's coffee room. Will remembers saying to Zeidler: "This is extraordinary. We seem to have identified *another* young patient. What on earth does this mean?"

In late January, Will was asked to give his opinion on a young man with strange symptoms. The patient had slurred speech and was "wobbly" on his legs. He had been depressed and anxious for some time. Will, always keen to examine puzzling cases of dementia, thought the symptoms were "peculiar" but otherwise had no idea what was wrong. He advised the boy's neurologist to re-admit him to hospital in another month when he'd take another look and decide what to do.

Meanwhile the BSE epidemic in cattle had slowed. By January 1996 only 170 new cases were being reported each week, just a few in a herd, and well down from the peak of more than 1000 reported cases a week in January 1993. Professor Richard Lacey predicted his "worst case scenario" on BSE infection in humans: between 500 and 500,000 Britons would die of CJD into the next century. By early January 1996 more than 2000 schools had reportedly taken beef off their menus, following the declarations of eminent British scientists that they and their families had sworn off hamburgers, sausages and pies. The giant fast food chain McDonald's was noticing a preference for chicken in its English outlets, despite advertising and product recognition firmly pointing to Big Macs and cheeseburgers as among the most popular orders around the world.

Infectivity experiments had shown that just one gram of scrapie-infected feed was enough to cause BSE in a cow. If those like Lacey were right, just how much would it take to infect a human being? Britain's then Secretary of State for Health, Stephen Dorrell, just kept saying there was "no conceivable risk" in eating British beef.

In February 1996, three weeks after he had performed the back-to-back autopsies on the two women, Ironside sat before a high-tech microscope that was capable of holding more than one slide at a time for easy comparison. Hundreds of slides from the cerebellum, basal ganglia, both hemispheres of the brain and the brain stem of each of the two women lay before him. He looked first at the slides of the brain of the 29-year-old Scottish woman. The spongiform change was obvious. But so were clumps of protein. Lots of them. These amyloid or kuru-type PrP plaques were dotted fairly evenly over each slide. This was strange, Ironside thought. He'd never seen so much protein in the CJD and related disease brain specimens he had studied since joining the CJDSU six years earlier.

Ironside switched to slides of the Englishwoman. Before him was exactly the same spongiform. And the same uniform spread of amyloid plaques. He could have been looking at the first brain. Just to make sure, he looked back to the first one to double-check. His eyes moved back to the second brain slide again. He felt a bit strange. There was no doubt. Ironside asked his senior colleague in the neuropathology department at Western General Hospital, Dr Jeanne Bell, to review the slides "just to make sure, obviously, that I wasn't somehow imagining it. I was astonished that two cases from two different parts of the country could be so similar and yet so different from other cases".[2]

Ironside was reminded of the damage found in the brains of Stephen Churchill and the still-living 16-year-old Muslim girl and the earlier reviews of their biopsies at the CJDSU. He hadn't appreciated the significance of the plaques at the time. Plaques were also found in the brain of the second young person who had died in December 1995. Now, Ironside's examination of the spread of plaques and the distinctive spongiform ring around many of them in the brains of the Scottish woman and the older English woman showed them to be virtually identical. And once tissue samples were obtained from the doctors of both the Muslim girl and Stephen Churchill, it was obvious that something unheralded had surfaced in the world of TSEs.

When Bell agreed with Ironside's findings, it was clear that five cases of CJD had emerged in a short space of time in people much younger than the average age at which sporadic CJD presented itself. The distinctive and new pattern of brain damage was something neither Ironside nor Will could explain. As usual, they talked it over with other unit members including Ken Sutherland, who, by statistical computer analysis, was able to measure the type and location of brain damage in all referred cases. Sutherland had devised a sophisticated computer program that measured the amount and position of spongiform change by virtually counting cells and amounts of plaque in a given area of the brain. With this important new technique, Sutherland was also able to compare the brain damage with other familial TSEs including familial CJD, GSS and FFI.

The new case of CJD in a young patient in January was replicated in February. Both those latest cases had been autopsied and found to have the same strange, floral pattern of plaques and spongiform. Now there were six cases.

In the meantime, to check that the brain damage in the young cases was not merely some function of their age, the new cases had to be systematically compared with the patterns of brain damage in other young people who had died of CJD. A time-consuming hunt had been under way for slides or tissue from other reported cases of CJD in young people around the world. The comparison was necessary to distinguish anything startlingly different about the British cases. The crux of the search was to locate any of this seemingly new and uniform spread of plaques in the brains of young people who had died well before the BSE epidemic emerged in 1985.

Ironside and his secretary worked hard to trace those medical records. It meant finding the hospital that had kept tissue samples, contacting the pathologist concerned and asking him to forward any available slides. When the slides arrived they were compared with slides of the newest "young cases" under the CJDSU's powerful microscopes. Those microscopes were kept in constant use. It took weeks to compare the hundreds and hundreds of slides of different sections of the brain. Sometimes Ironside, Jeanne Bell and the computer image analyser, Ken Sutherland, studied slides simultaneously under a microscope with three eyepieces.

Technical staff also assessed the immunocytic chemistry with which they stained the slides. This particular stain, used with new-generation antibodies to the PrP protein, showed the PrP as dark brown patches on what appeared to be a sea of holes. All the new cases had much more brown staining than any of the experts had seen before.

Up to 1985, only nine cases of CJD had ever been reported in people under 30.[3] By 1996 the number in the under-35 age group had cannoned up to 35 cases worldwide, with four of these cases occurring in teenagers. One of these was an American boy, called Jack, who developed CJD at 16. A keen athlete and honour student, he became confused in June 1976, swimming the wrong way in a race and unable to find the locker room afterwards. He wore his clothes to bed, his underwear over his pyjamas and dressed for school on weekends. Six months later he was unable to recognise the theory of a right angle triangle despite winning a prize in geometry the previous year.

By February 1977 he knew something was terribly wrong — "why can't I do anything" he had asked his parents — and could not name his sisters or brothers. He developed jerks, became incontinent, had difficulty swallowing, could not walk properly and was continuously agitated. He died of pneumonia in October 1978. CJD was confirmed when his body was exhumed[4] and the infection transmitted to experimental animals.

Other young CJD cases included a French girl of 19 who died in the early 1980s, identified from Dr Paul Brown's epidemiological back track through CJD cases in France.[5] Another case was identified in a British-born girl in Canada who contracted the disease at 14. Her case was published in 1988. In another paper on the incidence of CJD in Warsaw, Poland, over 15 years from the 1970s (reported only in 1991) three young patients, aged 19, 22 and 27 were included.[6]

By mid-February, at least 10 historic cases of young people with CJD had been reviewed alongside the two women from Ironside's January autopsies, the Muslim girl of 16, Stephen Churchill and two other newly confirmed cases. Ken Sutherland's computer-based image analysis confirmed what the CJDSU doctors were beginning to accept — there was something outstandingly different in the new cases, compared with the historic cases.

Not only were these new CJD patients young, they had unusual clinical features. Symptoms began with depression, and the evolution of the disease was around 18 months or longer. Image analysis showed far more spongiform change than even young kuru cases reported from the 1950s and 1960s. And few of the earlier cases of CJD in young people had plaques. The six young Britons identified by February 1996 had plaques "everywhere", according to Will. The plaques, which Stanley Prusiner had dubbed prion protein, were surrounded by a rim of spongiform change which gave it a flower-like appearance.

The next question the experienced team at the CJDSU had to answer was unavoidable. Could it have been caused by infection from BSE? A critical piece of the jigsaw at the time was whether this new type of brain damage was occurring in countries other than Britain. CJD monitors in another five countries — France, Germany, Italy, the Netherlands and Slovakia — had been contacted in January. Each European surveillance centre was asked to send details of any CJD patients aged under 40. By the time the answers arrived back in February, seven such cases had been identified in Britain. But only in one case in France was there even a remote similarity to the cases appearing so rapidly in Britain. At that stage there were no neuropathological details available in the French case.

Everyone at the CJDSU knew — Ken Sutherland recalls them talking of little else — that they were in the midst of a worrying yet exciting development. Why so many cases of CJD in young Britons — and why now? All other possibilities had to be ruled out before this apparent variant of CJD in young people could be deemed "new". And rather than exhilaration at their apparent discovery, a feeling of dread stole over Ironside and Will. They had kept open minds on the possibility of BSE jumping the species barrier to humans. They had written papers and given lectures on the fact that, up to this point, there had been nothing to indicate that BSE had or could affect humans. Was that argument about to be proved wrong?

They tried to remain logical. Scrapie had existed for hundreds of years and had provided no proven link to disease in humans. Even in scrapie-free Australia and New Zealand, there were comparable annual rates of CJD of about one per million just as there were in countries badly affected by scrapie. Another possibility was that these cases could have been a random convergence of hereditary cases. Plaques are commonly found in GSS patients.

Coincidentally, in January 1996, a local newspaper reported the death from GSS of Sue Smits, a 45-year-old grandmother from Brough, near Hull on Britain's north-east coast. Her three sisters, all from Rotherham, had already died of the same inherited disease.[7] Could these six cases in young people be a chance random convergence of GSS cases? Even some familial CJD cases of long duration had begun when the patients were in their 20s.

To rule out any hereditary component in the new pattern of cases, a total sequencing of the PRNP gene in each patient was undertaken by Kathy Estibeiro, a molecular biologist at the CJDSU. She began in late January. "It took a long time to find all that information," Ironside recalled. "The gradual realisation that something was changing created a feeling of sinking apprehension. Obviously the reason the CJD Surveillance Unit was set up was to monitor any potential effect BSE might have on human health. In a way we were fulfilling our remit."[8]

A seventh case emerged, then an eighth. All were confirmed as CJD either through autopsy or biopsy before death. At a scheduled meeting of SEAC in January, Will had mentioned the apparently consistent pattern of pathology that was emerging in a growing number of cases. A common picture was appearing to Will and his colleagues — early psychiatric symptoms, deteriorating balance and a relatively long duration of illness compared with general cases of CJD. John Collinge, the newest and youngest member of SEAC, was astounded to learn of five cases — only three of which he had known about and performed the

DNA tests upon. "For me that was the turning point," Collinge recalled. "At three cases I was extremely worried. At five we had to conclude something extraordinary was happening. A new risk factor was what we had to conclude. Whether it was BSE or not was something else. We had to think again whether there was sufficient protection for public health."[9]

Collinge requested a statistical analysis of the cases, aware that the SBO ban had not been totally enforced. He stuck his neck out at the meeting. "We can't ignore this," he told the others. "These are very unusual cases that have a kuru-like flavour and this could well indicate a link with BSE." By February's SEAC meeting Will reported that the number of cases had grown. SEAC members wanted to know much more and a briefing on all cases was requested for the next meeting in early March. By the end of February two more suspected cases of CJD in deteriorating patients were referred to the unit.

In the meantime, as deaths in young people occurred, their families — like Dorothy and Dave Churchill — intermittently called for a public inquiry into claims of a link between young CJD deaths and infection from BSE-contaminated meat products. Claims of a link by family members were usually accompanied by widespread publicity generated by at least ten competitive national daily newspapers, other Sunday papers, radio, television and county and suburban papers. Sometimes it was hard to tell whether the victim whose family was making allegations against the government's handling of the BSE epidemic was in fact one of these new-looking cases of CJD. Certainly, some cases in which the families went public were not in the category of this new and atypical type of CJD.

However, if families did not come forward publicly there was no other information available to the general public. The CJDSU's strict confidentiality policy, while frustrating for journalists, was essential so the unit could maintain the trust of families with whom it was dealing and build a clear picture of the extent of these new variant cases. Examining the brain after an autopsy remains the only way to confirm CJD of any sort. The CJDSU was always careful to have full family agreement on biopsy or autopsy and, where possible, it kept families informed of developments.

By March 6, Kathy Estibeiro had completed sequencing of the PRNP gene in four of the newest confirmed cases. None of the 20 known gene

mutations associated with TSEs had been found. The only genetic com-
monality was homozygosity for methionine (MM) at codon 129 — a
genetic variant in about 50 per cent of the population and thought to be
no more than a predisposing factor to contracting TSEs.

The unit used a methodical questionnaire to detail medical histories
and lifelong dietary habits from the families of the victims. In seven of
the eight confirmed cases, the questionnaire could pinpoint no history
of exposure to accidental routes of CJD transmission. The victims were
of different ages at the onset of disease and none had any occupational
link. There was not one factor, apart from their youth and the fact that
they all lived somewhere in Britain, which distinguished this cluster of
CJD victims from anyone in the normal population. That's when Will
realised they had discovered a scientific phenomenon with no adequate
explanation.[10]

On Friday March 8, 1996 Ironside, who had worked feverishly for
weeks assembling his data, flew with Will from chilly Edinburgh to a
slightly warmer London. There they briefed SEAC about the eight confirmed cases and another two suspected cases in the referrals to the
CJDSU over the preceding 12 months. Will admitted to the meeting that
it was possible the cases were "causally linked to BSE because we have
no other adequate explanation".

With both slides and overheads to illustrate his case, Ironside took
over and held the committee spellbound for 25 minutes. He showed the
qualitative changes in the brains of the unfortunate victims — the clut-
ter of the PrP plaques and the massive spongiform change surrounding
those plaques. These were quite different from the sight under microscopes of sporadic CJD or accidental transmission of the disease via
dura mater grafts or human hormone drugs.

Ironside also had Ken Sutherland's graphs showing where the brain
damage was most obvious, and how it was different to other forms of
CJD. The new variant brains had aggregated protein plaques and massive spongiform change in the deep grey matter of the brain, the basal
ganglia and the thalamus. The cerebellum, which controls motor function, was also severely affected by spongiform change. In sporadic CJD
spongiform change generally occurs in the cerebrum, which is where
plaques, if any, are also found. Accidentally transmitted CJD through
human hormone drugs produces a few plaques in the cerebellum, if any.
Sporadic CJD cases rarely produce plaques at all.

Jeffrey Almond, a virologist, professor of microbiology at the University of Reading, and a member of SEAC, well remembers the briefing by Will and Ironside. There were nearly 20 people in the room. Everyone was tense. He agreed later that what they were told left the entire meeting "gobsmacked", himself included.[11] Like the other members of SEAC, Almond had just turned a corner in scientific history. What the committee did after this information sank in would have a profound effect — on the British Government, the multi-million pound beef industry and on science itself.

Ironside looked around at the 12 virologists, epidemiologists, neurologists and veterinary specialists among the members of SEAC in the silence that followed. He thought to himself: "This is a momentous occasion".[12]

The SEAC meeting then focused on the possibility that these cases could represent a new inheritable variant of CJD, like GSS or FFI, or even a mutation that was another type of sporadic CJD. But that was immediately ruled out by the molecular genetic results. All the negatives — the lack of plaques in the historic young cases, the initial psychiatric symptoms, the length of the disease course — were pointed out by Will. What unusual factors had been present in Britain that were not present anywhere else in the world? There was only one "plausible explanation", everything else considered. It had to be linked to BSE. Both diseases were from the same unique family, although in cattle there were no plaques and the disease was confined mainly to the brain stem where the spinal cord and brain joined at the base of the neck.

Ironside's neuropathology reinforced Collinge's fears that a new risk factor had emerged and he urged a review of the measures in place to protect public health. The members, who by no means agreed that BSE was a likely cause, did, however, agree that it was vital that the news about this apparent new variant of CJD be released as soon as possible.

Initially Will argued that this should be done in the conventional tradition — via an announcement through a reputable medical journal. Others disagreed because of the length of time it might take to be peer-reviewed and published. Will recalled: "A lot of people thought it was very important that it should enter the public domain before the paper was published because it was a matter of great public health importance … it would be wrong to keep it hidden until a paper was eventually published."

They realised that accusations of attempting to hide the information would be made anyway. No one expected the political ramifications that followed.

On Sunday March 10, Will wrote a draft of a paper for the *Lancet*. In it he briefly documented the eight confirmed cases of the new variant. He knew an announcement was to be made soon, but he did not know when or by whom. In the week that followed and on the recommendation of the SEAC meeting, Ironside consulted senior neuropathologists, who agreed they had never seen anything like the brain damage obvious in the group of new patients.

Meanwhile, Will rang Paul Brown in Gajdusek's laboratory at the NIH. Will asked him if plaques had been mentioned in any of the neuropathology reports in the historic young cases of CJD that were known in North America. The answer came back in 24 hours. No.

That same week the doctors received the finished analysis of the slides found on the 16-year-old girl whose case dated back to 1980. The newer techniques in staining had confirmed that she had, in fact, died of sporadic CJD. And she had no plaques. This was a crucial finding because she represented a very young case that had occurred well before the BSE epidemic began in 1985. It also suggested that age was not a critical factor.

While all the information on the new variant was accumulating over January and February, Will saw the demented young man who had been referred to him in January for a second time during the week of the SEAC meeting. Only 31, he had deteriorated markedly. He had developed jerks in his limbs and had become very confused, although he could still talk. Will immediately recognised in him a possible case of the new variant of CJD and recommended a biopsy.

On Thursday, March 14, Will drove to England to seek an opinion on recent developments from a colleague. In his car by the River Thames, he contacted the CJDSU lab on his mobile phone for any results on the young man's biopsy. The biopsy, he was told, had shown spongiform change and many plaques. This was a ninth case, which was followed that week by a tenth confirmed case. As far as Will was concerned, the issue was cemented. There was unquestionably a human BSE problem.

BSE-contaminated beef products — anything containing the specified offal of cattle brain, spinal cord, spleen, intestines, thymus and tonsil — were incriminated. They were not taken out of the human diet until 1989 at the earliest. Consumers could have been exposed to them from the early 1980s, or earlier, well before the first known group of cows succumbed to BSE in 1985. All Will knew was that if a new type of CJD had appeared and it was linked to BSE, the infection was not recent. It had occurred five, 10, or maybe 15 years earlier as the infection slowly made its way to the victim's central nervous system, ate tiny holes in his or her brain and laid down the consistent pattern of plaques.

By March 1996 almost 160,000 cows on more than one in five of Britain's 136,000 farms had been reported with BSE, the majority of cases still in dairy herds. Outbreaks, many of them thought to be under-reported, had occurred in Switzerland, Ireland, Portugal, France, Germany, Italy, Oman, Canada, Denmark and the Falkland Islands. On Saturday March 16, an emergency session of SEAC wrestled with the official wording of a statement on the new variant that probably had an incubation period of five to 15 years between infection and death. Collinge and his colleagues had worked night and day to rule out any of the known mutations in these 10 new variant cases. Their existence suggested that something new in CJD that had emerged in mid-1995 had its roots in exposure to infection in the mid to late 1980s. It had to be BSE.

On March 17, Robert Will flew to the Netherlands, en route to Paris for a CJD conference. In Rotterdam he visited Professor Albert Hofman, with whom he jointly ran the European surveillance project, to tell him about the puzzling new cases. Pacing the floor of his rooms at the Erasmus University Hospital, Hofman was seriously concerned. He declared that a scientific paper on the subject should be published as soon as possible. Will showed him his draft before catching a train to Paris.

On Monday March 18, 1996, after James Ironside had delivered a paper to the CJD conference on neuropathology — none of it referring to the new variant — Will received a message to call the Ministry of Health in London. During a break in the conference, he called back, to be told there would soon be an announcement on a link between BSE and the new variant. Will knew he had a great deal of work to do, not least to notify the families of the cases of which nine were now confirmed — two in Scotland, one in Northern Ireland, one in Wales and the remainder in England. Will cancelled his scheduled delivery of a paper that afternoon on CJD epidemiology in Britain. To the bafflement of other international delegates, he abruptly left the meeting. Ironside had already left. In the British Airways lounge at Orly Airport, Will returned the call of a neuropathologist, who confirmed England's tenth case of what would become known officially as the new variant (nvCJD). The SEAC members met late into the Monday night in London finalising their report to the government. They had agonised, according to their chairman, John Pattison, over the possibility of an alternative explanation to BSE. There wasn't one.

Will returned to London, and the following day, Tuesday March 19, met with an eminent neurologist in London to discuss the best method of informing all of Britain's neurologists of the ramifications of nvCJD. He also attended the SEAC meeting that afternoon and night at the Department of Health. He flew home late to Edinburgh, where a message awaited him from BBC Radio 4 in London requesting an interview about an announcement the next day on BSE and CJD. So reporters already knew something was up. Earlier that day, the Prime Minister, John Major, had summoned the Secretary of State for Health, Stephen Dorrell, and the agriculture minister, Douglas Hogg, to a crisis meeting. Despite later reports of scepticism from some Cabinet ministers and a push to keep the matter under wraps, the three men agreed that a ministerial statement would be made to the House of Commons the following day.

Early on Wednesday March 20, Will and Zeidler frantically contacted the neurologists of as many of the 10 nvCJD victims as possible. In turn the neurologists contacted families of almost all the patients to warn them of the coming announcement of a circumstantial link between the CJD and BSE. Later that day Will and Ironside caught the lunchtime British Airways flight to London. Ironside joked later that it was a test of his resolve when he ate the mince pie put before him on the very day of the historic announcement of a link between a new form of CJD and BSE. Neither he nor Will had given up beef products. Theories varied on whether BSE or CJD or scrapie infection was passed on through a single, very infected dose or perhaps an accumulation of minimally infective doses. Will was inclined to agree with the general truth of most infectious diseases: that one critical dose creates the infection. Will and Ironside tucked into their airline meal with gusto.

At 3.30 p.m. they witnessed the bombshell in the House of Commons on a TV monitor. The reversal of at least eight years worth of denials on human risk of BSE rocked not just Britain, but the rest of the world — including most tourists to Britain over the past two decades. No doubt every immigrant, emigrant and expatriate thought back to how many beef products they had eaten in Britain, the land of roast beef and York-shire pudding. Those sausages at a BBQ, the mince pie at the football, the take-away hamburger any time. How many beef stock cubes had been added to their soups over the years? Which cow parts went into the human diet? Lots, as it emerged. Beef products were not wasted. They were in everything from serum in vaccines to cosmetics. Gelatine, lard, suet, beef extract granules or liquids, sauce mixes, dried sauce bases, many packaged and canned foods including baby food, and manufac-tured beef products containing mechanically recovered meat (including pies, pâtés, consommés, and stock cubes, and not necessarily only beef stock cubes) contained some part of a cow. For the British beef indus-try, the announcement meant one thing: immediate and irreversible crisis.

Dorrell told the House of Commons after announcing the link:

> There remains no scientific proof that BSE can be transmitted to man by beef but the [SEAC] committee have concluded that the most likely explanation at present is that these cases are linked to exposure to BSE.

The government was treated to an instant and inevitable avalanche of criticism. What Collinge later recalled as strange was the natural assumption by the media that Dorrell's announcement was some kind of conspiracy; that if this is what the government was willing to tell people, then the truth must be so much worse. "But Dorrell," Collinge maintained later, "read out word for word exactly what we had prepared in the SEAC statement."

Accusations flew from the opposition Labour Party as well as the government's chief critics on BSE, Richard Lacey, Stephen Dealler and Helen Grant. It was deemed too little too late in almost everything. The government was at fault in failing to conduct vital experiments with pri-mates. It had also failed to police the SBO ban on the most infective parts of cattle entering the human diet. And it had probably exacerbated the BSE epidemic by not properly compensating farmers for the full value of each stricken beast from 1988 onwards. With the announcement of a £4.5 million grant for further research, Dorrell attempted to dilute the growing damage. Despite the circumstantial link and no other obvious explanation, he continued to say that nonetheless "there is no scientific proof" of BSE infection passing to humans. He even mooted the slaughter of the entire British herd of more than 12 million cattle, worth £1.8 billion in beef sales each year, as a last ditch effort to eradicate BSE if nvCJD cases soared. It was a throw-away claim that would never be seriously contemplated by a government hoping for re-election the following year.

At 4.30 p.m. that afternoon Will and Ironside were among the group of advisers and government officials assembled for the subsequent press conference. There Pattison, the SEAC chairman, admitted that one extreme of the cluster of nvCJD cases was the risk of an epidemic. However, it would take close monitoring over the next two years to reveal the answers. Will told journalists that the "new phenomenon" was "reason for major concern".

Scientists advising the government had expected — despite the hollow reassurances of government spokespeople that since the 1989 SBO ban British beef had been perfectly safe to eat — that consumer concern and economic repercussions would follow Dorrell's announcement. But the wider political fallout surprised them. At the CJDSU in Edinburgh they watched in amazement as a worldwide ban on British beef exports was imposed by the European Union (EU) within days of the March 20 announcement. Within a week bans on British beef extended from Portugal to Finland, and from Singapore to South Africa, Britain's largest export market outside the EU.

The European Union did not limit the ban to beef, also including beef products used to make tallow, gelatine and pharmaceutical items like gel-covered drug capsules. In Australia, after frantic shelf-searching for imported food products containing British beef, five items were banned on March 29, 1996: Tesco's meat gravy granules and Scotch Broth Soup; Baxter's Scottish Haggis and Highland Broth Soup; and, surprisingly, Bender and Cassell's Cream of Broccoli Soup. Many packaged or canned supermarket items in Britain contained beef products. Unless they contained a special symbol on labelling that marked it "suitable for vegetarians" the chances were high that it contained a beef product of some sort.

Stephen Dealler, then consultant medical microbiologist at Burnley General Hospital, immediately warned that children should not be fed beef. SEAC soon advised, however, that there was no need for this precaution now that the SBO ban had been fully enforced. The chief medical officer, Sir Kenneth Calman said there was no need for beef products to be removed from supermarkets and that he would personally continue eating beef as part of a varied and balanced diet.

Lacey, who had refused to eat British beef since 1989, accused the government of putting public health behind the financial interests of farmers.

Beef sales, already down following the pronouncements of eminent scientists that they no longer ate meat, plummeted. The former agriculture minister John Gummer's 1990 publicity stunt, in which he fed his four-year-old daughter Cordelia a beefburger to demonstrate how "perfectly safe" they were, "was distasteful at the time and could now be seen as misleading as well", thundered an editorial on March 21 in *The Times* newspaper.

Catastrophe in the British beef industry followed the March 20 announcement. The government shied away from the drastic complete cull of all British cattle, opting instead for a compulsory cull of all cattle over 30 months old. But it was so slow in starting the cull, designed along with other political measures to restore confidence in British beef among export countries, that by early May some farmers had begun to process the animals themselves. To some the cull was merely another ploy, a cosmetic solution of officialdom to cover up the true extent of the epidemic. BSE rarely showed before 30 months and critics yelled that the root of the problem was not being tackled. Initial attempts to lift the international ban on tallow, semen and cattle embryos failed. Douglas Hogg, the agriculture minister, was criticised all over Europe for his handling of the crisis. Two British farmers committed suicide in despair at their economic future.

One vegetarian company in Australia quickly announced a new addition to their top selling UK range of beef alternatives called "Not Roast Beef". Booksellers reported a surge in sales of vegetarian books while books with meat in the title sold less well.

Theories about why nvCJD affected only younger people abounded. Dr John Wilson, a consultant neurologist from the Great Ormond Street

Hospital for Sick Children in London suggested that young people might have had greater exposure to beef products because of their taste for fast foods, including beefburgers.

Consumers reportedly spurned beef in the early period after the March 20 announcement. They turned briefly to buffalo, crocodile, kangaroo and emu after reports that sheep, pigs and other animals had also been fed the protein supplements that had allegedly infected the cows. McDonald's, Wimpy and Burger King, three of the largest fast food outlets in Britain, abandoned beef for a time — McDonald's eventually returning to British beef in June 1997. British Airways initially shied away from British beef too, due to "customer concern" only. Even Marks & Spencer, the most British of British stores, dropped British beef products outside Britain for a period.

Twenty tonnes of British beef sat on the docks at Cape Town for weeks throughout April while South Africa debated what to do in the wake of the scare and sent veterinarians to London to assess the situation. Butchers all over England displayed large signs in shop windows claiming they sold either non-British beef or meat products made locally or on the premises from locally reared BSE-free cattle. Some clung to pronouncements by Douglas Hogg that British beef was safe to eat and left neat piles of newspaper stories on the safety of British beef on their counters.

Every comment made by officials in the years preceding March 20 was thrown back at them by the media. These included several from the chief veterinary officer, Keith Meldrum. One classic example was his 1994 statement: "To hint or suggest that BSE could enter the human food chain is totally and completely irresponsible." Then on March 25, 1996, a letter from a reader in Kent to the *Independent* newspaper stated:

> Is the legacy of 17 years of Tory Government to be the death of up to half a million people because they thought it more important not to offend the farming lobby than to safeguard the health of the nation?

Such rhetorical questions went unanswered.

On April 6, Robert Will and his colleagues described the first 10 cases of nvCJD in a revised article in the *Lancet*.[13] In some instances the families of nvCJD victims had already gone to the media distressed that

BSE-infected beef products could have been responsible. All 10 nvCJD victims had initial psychiatric symptoms progressing to balance problems and dementia. The majority also suffered from myoclonic jerks.

Although as usual, none were named, it was later clear from the public comments of their families that the three dead men in the article were Stephen Churchill, who died aged 19 in May 1995; Maurice Callaghan, who died aged 29 in Belfast in November 1995, 10 days before the birth of his second daughter; and Peter Hall. Hall died just days before his twenty-first birthday, emaciated and unresponsive in Durham in northern England in February 1996. Reported by newspapers as a childhood lover of beefburgers, he had become a vegetarian at 18. His symptoms had begun with depression 13 months before his death. The 31-year-old male, whose biopsy had proved positive in March was still alive at the time his and the other nine cases were reported in the *Lancet*.

Fears about CJD contamination extended to the burial of Maurice Callaghan. According to his relatives, someone had given orders for the grave to be dug to lower than the usual depth and heavily limed. Zeidler from the CJDSU eventually had to collect the brain himself, in January 1996, two months after Callaghan's autopsy on November 5, when couriers refused to deliver it to Edinburgh. At his later inquest, in October 1996, the Belfast coroner found after expert testimony from Ironside that Callaghan had died probably as a result of eating BSE-infected meat — one of the first admissions in law of a link between CJD and BSE.[14]

The families of three of the five women who had died of nvCJD had also spoken out by the time Will's article was published in the *Lancet*. Michelle Bowen, 29, a former butcher's shop assistant, was delivered of her third child by caesarean section while in a terminal coma in the Manchester Royal Infirmary in November 1995. The older woman autopsied by Ironside in January 1996 was identified publicly by her husband as Ann Richardson, a 41-year-old mother of one and health care assistant from Huyton, Merseyside.

One case of degeneration that had initially baffled doctors in London until a biopsy in September 1995 had shown the pathological signs of CJD, was that of 29-year-old Anna Pearson. A married solicitor with no children, she died in February 1996 in the Kent and Canterbury Hospital after a 10-month illness that began with forgetfulness. A month later her memory had worsened with added confusion and dis-orientation. A non-smoker with no history of drug abuse or risk factors for CJD, she later developed childlike behaviour, poor short-term recollection, hallucinations, jerks in her limbs and inability to walk. Her mother, Karen Grice, blamed the fast food her daughter ate as a student in London for the onset of her CJD.[15,16]

In mid-April 1996 America's television talk show queen, Oprah Win-frey, had a dramatic effect on US cattle futures markets when she declared she had been "stopped cold from eating another burger" by statements from her studio guests on a show relating to BSE and the beef industry. Her guests included a vegetarian activist, Howard Lyman, who told of the cannibalisation of American cattle being fed rendered down parts of dead and downer cows as a protein supplement. Another was Beryl Rimmer, whose granddaughter, Victoria, had con-tracted what she claimed was CJD at 16, despite an inconclusive brain biopsy. She was convinced that Victoria, then 18 and in a coma ever since the biopsy procedure two years earlier, had contracted the disease from eating beef.[17] An American guest, Linda Marker, claimed her mother, who had recently died of CJD, had been infected from BSE-contaminated beef eaten in Britain in 1986. Within days, US beef con-tracts were in major decline. Cattleman later launched a multi-million dollar law suit against the show. BSE and the beef crisis dominated front and inside pages of most British daily newspapers for months.

As the political fallout from the new variant CJD announcement inten-sified, a spectacular arrest occurred across the Atlantic. On April 4, as Paul Brown and Carleton Gajdusek, who had just returned from a con-ference in Geneva, arrived in separate cars at Gajdusek's house in Mid-dletown, Maryland, a group of armed FBI agents sprang out of the shrubbery pointing guns. Gajdusek, now 72 and twice as big as in his kuru days, with a shocked Brown as witness, was arrested on charges of paedophilia relating to two of his adopted sons. One, a 23-year-old college student, claimed Gajdusek had molested him after his arrival in Maryland from Micronesia in 1987, when he was aged 17, until 1991. Another child, a minor and one of four living at Gajdusek's house when he was arrested, also told FBI investigators of alleged abuse. He and the other minors, one of them a girl, were put into foster care. The charges laid related only to the 23-year-old Micronesian man.

Gajdusek was kept in custody overnight and released the next day on

US$350,000 bail raised by a group of three friends, including the prominent AIDS researcher, Dr Robert Gallo and his wife Mary Jane, and Brown, who posted more than $250,000 of the bail money.

The prosecution claimed to have taped a telephone call in which Gajdusek was alleged to have made certain admissions to the 23-year-old. Gajdusek's friends rallied, claiming the charges were the result of America's fascination with child sexual abuse following several high profile court cases. They alleged the young man was cooperating because authorities had offered to continue paying for his education in America. Brown told newspapers that if the phone tape was not fabricated then it was a "set-up" in which "the FBI got to a boy and got him to call Carleton and get Carleton to implicate himself".[18] Gajdusek was himself later quoted as saying that he was a paedophile "as much as Jesus Christ and Mother Teresa, who also are unmarried and love children".[19]

The investigation into Gajdusek's activities, of which he had been aware for some months, followed the referral of some of his candid but not personally explicit journal entries about his travels to an American Senate investigator in 1995. Contained in the journals — long published by the NIH — were references to young boys he befriended and Polynesian cultural ideas on childhood sex and institutional homosexual practices in boys and men he had discovered on his South Pacific patrols. The FBI was called in.[20]

Gajdusek, who took leave from the NIH and vacillated, according to friends, between fighting the charge and committing suicide, was supported by a large group of friends and well-wishers, including almost all of his former adopted children. They had used their education well. One was a United Nations diplomat, another a doctor. Another was a cabinet minister in Micronesia. Another was the curator of a museum. Seven of his children were interviewed in the early days after the arrest, attesting to the warmth and generosity of the man they knew as "father". None of them could believe he had molested anyone.

Gajdusek had already signalled his retirement as chief of the Laboratory for Central Nervous System Studies at the National Institute of Neurological Disorders and Stroke at Bethesda and began winding up his massive collection of data, photographs, films, slides and specimens, accumulated since his return to the NIH in 1958. Whatever happened at the pending trial, his career in America was over.

More nvCJD cases emerged. By May 1996 the toll had risen to 12 confirmed cases, — one identified, after a brain biopsy, in press reports as 29-year-old father of two Barry Baker from the Ashford, Kent area where the first cow was diagnosed with CJD in 1985. The other was from outside Britain. A 26-year-old mechanic, known only as Henri, from Lyons in France, had been on holiday abroad once, to Spain and had been operated on twice as a baby for congenital glaucoma. Henri had the same CJD pattern as the Britons.[21] Meanwhile transmission experiments on animals still showed one strain of BSE, not the varied strains some experts expected if the disease had originated from scrapie. Even sheep were deliberately injected with BSE and their brains showed typical BSE changes.

In August 1996 further bad news emerged when SEAC confirmed that in preliminary results of a study of more than 600 cattle, a small degree of maternal transmission of BSE had been found. Translated outside study conditions, researchers from the epidemiology department of the Central Veterinary Laboratory in Weybridge, Surrey, estimated that about one per cent of cows born to BSE-infected mothers will die themselves from the disease.[22]

Later in 1996, the results of a transmission study of BSE into the brains of macaque monkeys in Paris was published in *Nature*. The results of this study (which were reviewed by Ironside) showed that changes in the grey matter of the brains were very similar to those in nvCJD, with many "florid" plaques. It provided further support for the suggestion that nvCJD was due to the BSE agent in humans.[23]

In September 1996, 10 years after Mike Harrington first published the results of his spot test on irregular proteins found in the spinal fluid of most CJD victims, a simplified, cheaper and quicker refinement was announced. This new generation test, published in the *New England Journal of Medicine,* revealed that an abnormal indicator protein dubbed 14-3-3 appeared in small test amounts of spinal fluid in TSE-affected people and animals, but not in healthy controls. A decade after its effectiveness was demonstrated as an additional diagnostic tool for CJD, Harrington, in collaboration with Clarence Gibbs and Paul Brown at Gajdusek's lab in Maryland, identified an antibody that dramatically simplified the tests. The antibody stuck to the indicator protein found in spinal fluid, which in turn indicated damage to the brain. Although still unable to screen healthy populations, the test had a 96 per cent accuracy rate after trials on humans, chimpanzees, sheep and cattle.

In October 1996, John Collinge published in *Nature* what was heralded as the first direct scientific link between BSE and nvCJD.[24] He and colleagues, including Ironside, found a molecular pattern, or signature, in the brains of mice, a macaque monkey and domestic cats deliberately or accidentally infected with BSE. A similar flower shape of protein deposit was evident, particularly in the basal ganglia, and its pattern of distribution was similar to that seen in the same area of the brain of nvCJD patients. The molecular marker evident in the nvCJD and animal transmissions was not found in other types of CJD. Although not proof itself, it was another link in the circumstantial chain that indicated BSE caused nvCJD.

Meanwhile all the prophecies were re-run by the media, particularly Richard Lacey's 1990 prediction that the first cases of BSE in humans would emerge in 1996. As 1996 became 1997, all eyes turned to special experimental mice, deliberately infected with BSE and nvCJD whose brains — once they died — would reveal the definitive proof of whether BSE was the cause of nvCJD.

CHAPTER 21

British victims:
Their day in court

THE MAIN GOTHIC-STYLE BUILDING of the Royal Courts of Justice lies at one of the boundaries to the City of London's square mile, just where The Strand becomes Fleet Street. No filming is allowed inside the huge building with its annexes, stained-glass windows and grand entrance hall. It was designed last century and opened by Queen Victoria in 1882 after a competition between 11 architects who wanted to build cathedrals but built a temple to the law instead. And as the death toll from nvCJD inched upwards and the beef crisis spilled into European Union politics, it was here that the first phase of the British court case into hGH recipient CJD deaths began — the first litigation of its type anywhere to reach court.

Just before the appointed starting time of 2 p.m. on April 16, 1996, 20 reporters from radio, TV, newspapers and court reporting services had lined up for the eight available media seats in Court 76 of the Queen's Bench division of the High Court. It was the biggest court room in the labyrinthine three-storey group of court buildings. The rest of the seating was reserved for the 28 members of the families who were suing the British Government for its role in subsidising, manufacturing and distributing the hGH which had killed — by then — 16 former child recipients in England and Scotland.

Ranged around the large modern courtroom, with its bookcase-lined walls and sockets for laptop computers on which real-time transcripts could be read as the case progressed, were also thousands and thousands of pages of documents. They covered the 26 years of the Human Growth Hormone Program (HGHP), which began in 1959 and was run consecutively by the Medical Research Council (MRC) and the Department of Health and Social Services (DHSS). In the colours of the Union Jack, the rows and rows of ring binder folders used by the plaintiffs were red and those of the government were blue. Witnesses and the judge, Mr Justice Morland, leafed through folders bound in white, stacked neatly on individual three-tiered carousels.

Unlike the experience in Australia, the British program formally moved from an experimental clinical trial to a limited and named-patient basis of treatment in 1977. As the case unfolded, it would become apparent that 1977 was a crucial year for other reasons.

Any hope by the plaintiffs for wide publicity to stir sympathy for the deaths was doused within an hour of the start of the marathon opening submissions for the plaintiffs, which lasted six days. All news was over-taken with the announcement from Buckingham Palace that after nearly 10 years of marriage the estranged Duke and Duchess of York were to divorce.

Justin Fenwick, QC, a former equerry to the Duke of Edinburgh, led the formidable government legal team of at least seven barristers, solic-itors and paralegals. At the start of the case Fenwick announced that — for the purposes of the case only — the government would admit that the hGH it had manufactured and distributed to 1908 children between 1959 and 1985 had resulted in the deaths of 20-year-old Terrence Newman and 15 others from CJD. A murmur passed through those assembled in the family area. This was an admission they had been waiting to hear for four years.

The only reason they were in court at all was because the government would not grant an inquiry into the HGHP, nor had it acknowledged lia-bility for the contaminated hGH. Those families who were eligible for legal aid sued. This negligence trial was the result. Written evidence from 13 expert witnesses, two of whom did not testify, formed the basis of the inquiry-within-the-trial that it effectively became. It was the equivalent of Australia's Allars inquiry, except that it cost the British Government a lot more money.

Mavis Lay, the mother of Alison, the first hGH victim to die, was there. Maureen Newman represented her son Terrence. Noel Baldwin, father of the navy engineer Patrick Baldwin who had died leaving two little daughters, spent six hours on a train every day travelling from Gains-borough to London and back to listen to every word of evidence he and others had agitated for so long to hear. Sitting next to Baldwin almost every day was Paul Andrews, the only "well-but-worried" hGH recipient litigant to regularly attend the trial. Andrews knew that the start of part two of the litigation — damages sought by the recipients of either hGH or the fertility drug hPG who had not contracted CJD but were fearful of doing so — hinged directly on a successful plaintiff outcome to this trial. Deliberately unemployed for the duration of the trial, he wanted to hear as much of the evidence as possible, having personally rattled the cage for so long.

Tony and Isobel Smith, parents of recipient Stuart Smith, were there for half the case. So were Barham Khan's parents, his mother Parveen's colourful saris swishing as she walked the width of the court to take her seat each morning. Donald Spear's brother, Peter, and his wife, Peta, attended several times.

Robert Owen, QC, his well-modulated tones hardly ever varying unless it was to laugh politely when the judge made an amusing aside, led the Celtic, and almost exclusively Welsh, plaintiff team. Welsh-born himself, he was experienced in medical negligence cases and would soon become the chairman of the Bar Council of England and Wales. Owen selected the statements of only two parents to read to Justice Morland on the opening day. The first was from Mavis Lay whose daughter Alison's death in February 1985 forced the shutdown of the British hGH program following the first three deaths in America.

The second statement was emotionally draining for the rapt listeners. Holding the court spellbound, Owen read several long excerpts from the diary of Donald Hefferon, who chronicled the last months of his beloved son, Saul Hefferon-Waldon.

Saul died aged 20 in April 1988 — about the time that in Adelaide, the family of Jane Allender was told there was no hope for her. Unlike the Lays and others who had no idea what was wrong, the Hefferons suspected Saul's initial lassitude and deteriorating neurological symptoms in late 1987 were signs of CJD. They had been sent a letter in May 1985 outlining why Saul's treatment with pituitary hGH had been stopped. By that time his hundreds of hGH injections had resulted in him growing to only 152 centimetres, or five feet. After initial admission to Addenbrooke's Hospital at Cambridge, Saul had been cared for at home. By March 1988 he had trouble seeing faces on television, ate little and could not manage to drink through a straw.

"Now his poor little legs are so bent at the knees with feet turned in and muscles wasted on his legs," his father wrote on March 19, 1988.

"I wish, oh I wish he could have had some professional manipulation/muscle therapy after leaving Addenbrooke's ... I wonder if he would have had so little care if he had been a professional footballer, sportsman or university 'blue'. He wants so badly to try and move his limbs."

On March 30 Hefferon lamented in his diary, "It is nearly three weeks since the community physio said she would come, had also promised him a walking support frame, no use now, but a pity to raise his and our hopes."

But it was the day before Saul's death that the anguish of a family watching a death from horrific CJD was vividly conjured: "We changed his T-shirt and turned him and laid his hips on a large soft [rubber] Sorbo ring. His upper limbs were so limp, his bones projecting and so loose inside his body I was afraid his limbs would tear. He groaned very loudly two or three times. We could not tell if it was cramp or pain in his knee and ankle joints, or his poor blackened heels, or even the burn on his shoulder. Poor little chap. It has been such a tough road. He has struggled and fought all the way through, never giving in — and met our fear and concern and care with love and humour ..."

"Saul is breathing very fast and laboured. Poor lad soaked in sweat. Eyes open, very tense ... Can't really believe it. He was so little and strong and humorous and full of life. My poor young man never had a chance."

But as the last of that diary entry was read aloud, most people in the court behind Robert Owen had been distracted by the dramatic and puzzling appearance of a clutch of extremely well-dressed women. They all wore hats, one of them a huge black and white creation that would not have disgraced its wearer at any of the world's great horse racing carnivals. Followed by five men in barristers' robes, they stood silently, obscuring the view of the court from the public gallery in front of Donald Hefferon, Noel and Janet Baldwin and Ashraf and Parveen Khan.

It was so out of place in relation to what was being heard that even the judge appeared uncomfortable. When Owen paused, Justice Morland commented that it was indeed "a heart-rending story" and apologised for stopping while, in a traditional gesture to new QCs, he formally welcomed the five barristers who had become Queen's Counsel to the court that day. That brief formality and its untimely insertion into the reading of the diary showed all observers — the case lawyers, the public, the journalists and the families — just how involved and tragic was the story of hGH contamination. A short intrusion by a group of well-dressed lawyers and their families had seemed almost indecent.

Over the next six weeks, 11 expert witnesses and about a dozen witnesses of fact gave evidence. Several interesting points emerged. They included that the legality of the harvesting of glands was "repeatedly questioned" with the MRC and DHSS "but never resolved," according to Owen. The only expert witness called by the government who was also a treating doctor was Dr John Buckler, former director of the Leeds Growth Centre and an honorary consultant paediatrician at the Leeds General Infirmary between 1970 and 1995. He treated 110 hGH-deficient children throughout the Yorkshire area and confirmed that one person diagnosed with probable CJD that week — the eighteenth case in a British recipient — had been one of his patients.

When Robert Owen broke off his questioning to announce that a nineteenth case had also emerged, Isobel Smith and Maureen Newman, mothers of Stuart Smith and Terrence Newman — knowing the anguish in store for the families of the newly diagnosed — immediately broke down in tears. Tam Fry, head of the Child Growth Foundation to which some of the parents of growth-retarded children belonged, and father of an hGH recipient himself, left the court to comfort them. It was the most graphic illustration possible in the austere surrounds of a court of the tragedy not just for the CJD victims, but for those who loved them. There was hardly a dry eye among the 20 lawyers, family members or spectators.

On his return to the courtroom, Tam Fry was furious after hearing part of Dr Buckler's evidence. The evidence was that, in hindsight, if glands from all demented people had been excluded and there was no prospect of synthetic hGH becoming available, he would have been in favour of continuing the HGHP in 1977. This was at the time when the risk of CJD had been made known to the MRC by Dickinson but not communicated to the treating clinicians dispensing hGH. Buckler speculated that even if CJD deaths had started earlier,

I would only then have contemplated this treatment in the unequivocally good responding cases, but the benefit would be so enormous that it might well have been considered worth the risk, even accepting the fatal outcome of CJD … Clearly if the indications had been such that the chance of contracting CJD rose from 1% to 10% or higher, then even the enormous benefits of the treatment to those for whom it was appropriate would probably have been inadequate to justify it.[1]

For those listening to Buckler's evidence it took a short time for the message to sink in. Even if there had been a definite, even growing, risk of CJD contraction in hGH recipients, for those patients who were growing he would have recommended continuing the injections. After the court adjourned that day, the usual calm of the tall, bearded Tam Fry had vanished. "Parents rely on clinicians because they don't know any-thing," he said angrily. "No parent would continue with a treatment that had a risk of killing their child."[2] Ashraf Khan, who did not qualify for legal aid, railed outside the court during an adjournment one day, frus-trated at not being part of the case but unable to fund the consequences if he joined in and lost. "I have lost my son," he said, tears forming in his eyes, "should I lose my house too?"[3]

One of the plaintiffs' expert witnesses gave evidence that even the judge eventually found was more helpful to the government's case than the plaintiffs'. Lawyers describe the phenomenon as their witness "going bad in the [witness] box". Thirteen days into the trial, the portly and snowy-haired Olav Trygstad, head of the department of paediatric endocrinology at the Rijkshospital in Oslo, took the stand. As one of the 11 expert witnesses for the plaintiffs, Trygstad provided valuable sci-entific information about commercial manufacturers of hGH and extraction methods used in European countries. With his refinement of the Roos method of hGH, developed in the early 1960s, he had gone on to personally treat about 300 children in Norway. He also acted as a consultant to Nordisk, which used his extraction method in its com-mercial preparation, Nanormon, from 1972 onwards.

Trygstad, who also extracted hPG for Norwegian gynaecologists, revealed he had not stopped using or prescribing hGH after the CJD cat-astrophe of mid-1985. Nor had Nordisk. Both had continued using pitu-itary-derived hGH until 1987, when first generation synthetic growth hormone had been refined to produce fewer antibodies. Under cross-examination by Fenwick, Trygstad admitted he had discussed the pos-sibility of slow virus infection with Maurice Raben, the American growth hormone pioneer, when he visited Boston in 1969. However, Raben had dismissed it because of the harsh treatment the glands were subjected to in his extraction method. On his return home in 1970, Trygstad had raised the subject with a professor of virology on the remote chance that glands collected from among the population of four million in Norway might be contaminated. "The thought was so far away, so we almost forgot it," Trygstad recalled of the professor's dismissal of the risk.

When he first heard of the CJD deaths in hGH recipients in April 1985, Trygstad erroneously thought one patient had been from Papua New Guinea and had probably died of kuru. He also knew the British had initially thought that Alison Lay's CJD had resulted from her neurosurgery as a child.

Fenwick: "Even then, you felt that the risk was such on the one hand and the benefit to these children on the other hand was such that you should continue?"

Trygstad: "Yes, of course, because we relied on our growth hormone product ... I did not think it was a risk. Therefore we did continue the treatment."

Trygstad said he did not tell his patients about the risk of CJD. If the parents asked about it he told them there was "no risk ... because we had a pure growth hormone". He thought that, in the rare event of a gland from one of the approximately four CJD deaths each year in Norway finding its way into his batches, his method would remove the infectivity. And while Sephadex gel filtration had been used from 1961 on hGH made in Norway, Trygstad admitted that it was not used on hPG extracted first, before the hGH, and ampouled for use by gynaecologists until 1972 or 1973.

Trygstad's cross-examination concluded with his agreement that no-one could have anticipated the tragedy of CJD in hGH recipients. The fact that there had been no deaths or few deaths from hGH prepared from frozen glands was, he agreed, "good fortune" rather than the fault of others who did things differently.

As the court adjourned for the day Fenwick could barely keep the smile off his face. Trygstad's evidence, although expert and fact-based and supposed to favour neither side in a court case, had been of more help to the government than the plaintiffs.

The plaintiff team sat stony-faced in their seats. Behind, in the public gallery and seated near Noel Baldwin, Maureen Newman and Barham Khan's parents, was the four-man Australian plaintiff legal team preparing for APQ's nervous shock case to be heard in Melbourne the following year. All four lawyers mentally struck Trygstad off their list of potential expert witnesses. Across the other side of the court, the Australian Government solicitor, Geoff McDonald, had been watching the case from the back stalls of the British Government legal team's area for three of the trial's six weeks. In Trygstad he noted a surprising new possibility for his defendant witnesses in APQ's case.

When the court adjourned, the Australian plaintiff lawyers, barristers Jack Rush, QC, and David Beach, and solicitors from the firm Rennick Briggs, Michael Glen and Sean Millard, trooped across the road to El Vino's wine bar. The bar, a historic piece of London on Fleet Street and once the hub of English journalism, was a favourite of countless reporters and columnists fond of a long lunch. On this chilly afternoon, Jack Rush bought a bottle of good red and leaned on the old wooden bar as it was passed around to fill four glasses. Michael Glen proposed a toast. "Here's to the Resurrection," he said as the glasses clinked in unison, "because that's what they're going to need to win this case."

Expert evidence continued from virologists, endocrinologists, neurologists, epidemiologists, neuropathologists, experts in drug manufacturing regulation, scrapie and mortuary practices. Much of the technical detail was complex but well grasped by the barristers on both sides. They treated each other and the court with such sustained politeness that the Australian observers from both sides, unused to such deference even in a civil trial, were astonished. There was not one objection to anything from either side in the six-week trial. Neither Dickinson, whose role was obvious from documentation, nor Anne Stockell Hartree, the biochemist who made the hGH implicated in all British hGH deaths to date, gave evidence at the trial. In fact Hartree, who now lives in America, refused to co-operate with either side in the case, despite a request from the judge that she be called as a witness.

At the close of evidence three last-minute writs were issued. One had been filed on behalf of Heather Caulton, treated with hGH between early 1977 and 1981, a new mother and the eighteenth person in Britain to contract CJD. A second was for Donald Spear, then 33, treated between 1971 and 1981, and the seventeenth victim to be diagnosed with CJD. The last writ issued was for David Tipping, 25, of Swindon, who had left three young daughters when he died of CJD in April 1995.

Two months later on July 19, 1996, it was standing room only in the same courtroom as the red-robed figure of Justice Morland faced the opposing parties in the CJD litigation once more. Family members and journalists lined the walls once the few seats were taken. By now the families of Stuart Smith, Barham Khan, Ronald Cockburn, John Struthers, James Bettinson and Brian Copland had joined the case, bringing the total to 18 litigants. The late inclusions were allowed, as the case was technically still running and able to be joined until final judgment, when provision was to be made for future cases. The unusual nature of the case allowed for the inclusion, at that stage, of any case in which CJD had developed.

A partial Resurrection had indeed occurred for the plaintiffs since Trygstad's testimony. Some observers described the judgment as a well reasoned bet each way. Justice Morland absolved Hartree from any blame, despite her refusal to co-operate. And he found there had certainly been negligence on the part of the government. It had occurred through mistakes and omissions made by the staff of the MRC and the DHSS or by members of the administrative committees which ran the HGHP, or through acts or omissions of the committees themselves. The negligence was dated, though. The judge found that these acts and omissions had followed the oral warning to the MRC of possible CJD contamination by the scrapie expert, Alan Dickinson, in October 1976 and his follow-up letter in February 1977.

As soon as the written warning of possible CJD contamination of pituitary glands was received from Dickinson, four months after his oral warning, "it called for action stations", Justice Morland found. Just because no action was taken anywhere outside Britain did not mean that those responsible were excused. No other country had received such a specific warning. It had become the crux of the case.

Delays in setting up Dickinson's experiment on the hGH extraction protocol and in taking more than 12 months to seek expert advice from Professors Wildy and Mims — who both advised excluding demented patients from gland collection — were negligent, according to the judge. The main steering committee overseeing the program did not inform the committee of endocrinologists overseeing the treating clinicians of the risk of CJD, which was known by late 1977 from Dickinson, Wildy and Mims, the judge found. It was worth noting that once that same committee was told about Alison Lay's death in 1985, the HGHP was immediately stopped.

During the case, Professor Charles Brook, a treating clinician called by the plaintiffs, had said he had sighted, only the week before he appeared in court in 1996, the powerful letters of Mims, warning that demented patients should be excluded from gland collection and Wildy, warning of the "gruesome possibilities and imponderable probabilities" that treating doctors should be immediately warned about. Had Brook seen Wildy's letter in 1977, he said its impact would have been "shattering". A meeting would certainly have been held to decide whether hGH should be suspended pending Dickinson's protocol test results or continued in the light of only theoretical risk.

Justice Morland also found that the failure to introduce a dementia and CJD exclusion criterion until 1980 — three years after several expert warnings to do so — was negligent. An emergency meeting of both the steering committee and the treating doctors' committee should have been called as soon as the Wildy and Mims advice had been received in late 1977.

Taking into account a reasonable time period after Dickinson's follow-up letter of 1977, the judge found that no new patients, apart from hypoglycaemic patients, should have been treated after July 1, 1977 — the date the DHSS had taken responsibility for the therapy from the MRC. The government, he ruled, had been negligent in taking on new patients and this negligence had caused their CJD. The families of these patients alone were eligible for compensation.

This meant that two patients, both of whom had completed their hGH injections by July 1, 1977, were not eligible for compensation at all. They were Alison Lay, the 22-year-old Winchester typist who died first, and Brian Copland, 31, a farm labourer who died in May 1992 in the small Scottish village of Dunblane. Admitting it was a hard decision, the judge, however, ruled out as candidates for compensation any of the CJD victims whose treatment had straddled July 1, 1977. This group comprised the majority of those who had sued, including Terrence Newman, whose family had initiated the legal action.

Excluding hindsight and sympathy, the judge was not satisfied, had an emergency meeting been called in late 1977 to discuss the Mims and Wildy and Dickinson advice, that a recommendation to suspend hGH treatment for existing patients would have been made. And "such a view could not reasonably be categorised as negligent". The judgment did not deal directly with several interesting issues brought up in the trial, including the illegality of harvesting glands from bodies without express permission of the donor or next of kin.

The clear winners in the case included the families of Patrick

Baldwin, 30, whose young daughters Zara and Nichola were left father-less, Bahram Khan, 27, James Bettinson, 25, of Worcester, Kevin Morrison, 25, the father of two toddler boys, and David Tipping. All five were treated with Hartree/Wilhelmi-prepared hGH.

Inevitably, argument followed from families whose child had been a pre-existing patient and was omitted from the terms of judgment. Some said, long before the court case began, that had they been told of the CJD risk in 1977 they would have chosen to stop hGH therapy. The so-called "straddlers" of July 1, 1977, included Terrence Newman, Saul Hefferon-Waldon, Mark Smith of Glasgow (who died at 20 in March 1990), Carol Ann Taylor of Peterborough (who died at 20 exactly four months later), John Struthers, 28, from the Lake District in northern England, Stuart Smith of Northamptom, Ronald Cockburn of Scotland, Donald Spear, Heather Caulton and Maureen (Millie) Turrell. Turrell, of Petersfield in Hampshire, was 34 and left a husband, Michael and a three-year-old daughter, Sarah, when she died on April 5, 1995 — the same day as Barham Khan. All 10 straddlers to then were treated with Hartree-prepared hGH.

Meanwhile, despite years of parents being told that their children were lucky to be treated with hGH because the drug was so scarce, the trial had been told that a staggering 25 kilograms of dried glands were left over when Hartree handed over production of hGH to the Centre for Applied Microbiological Research (CAMR) in 1980. And when the program was stopped after the first four deaths from hGH in May 1985, another 30,000-odd unprocessed glands were kept in storage. Their disposal, or distribution for research, according to a spokeswoman for the Department of Health in 1996,[4] awaits the eventual outcome of the undoubtedly long-running CJD litigation.

Across the world in New Zealand, the CJD toll had climbed alarmingly. On January 19, 1996, almost nine years after Deborah McKenzie's untimely death, a 42-year-old man died of CJD. Having been treated between 1967 and 1969, his minimum incubation period was about 26 years. This was roughly in the ballpark of an American man who had received hGH manufactured in a university laboratory, but outside the NHPP auspices, between 1956 and 1966. He had died aged 41 in 1990 — 25 years after his last hGH treatment and 35 years after his first injection.[5]

Then less than three weeks after the first New Zealand man's death, another strikingly similar case followed. A second male, also aged 42, had received hundreds of hGH injections between 1965 and 1972. He died of CJD on February 4, 1996. His minimum incubation period was 23 years.

These deaths were followed by a fresh scare in May of that year, after local blood transfusion services quarantined more than 4500 of 8916 bottles of plasma and other blood products that included a donation from a woman who died earlier in the year of CJD.[6] At least 47 haemophiliacs had received Factor VIII from the donor pool. In mid-May, quarantining of products was announced again when it was discovered that the sister of a regular blood donor had died of CJD in the 1980s. The second quarantining followed the protocol established in Canada, the US and Australia that anyone with a family history of any TSE be excluded from blood donation.

The fuss over potentially contaminated blood had barely died down when another man, a long-ago recipient of Wilhelmi-prepared hGH, died after an agonising deterioration from CJD. He was 46, and also had a 23-year minimum incubation period for the disease. He was treated, like the second man, between 1965 and 1972. All three had been among 49 New Zealanders that government records show received Wilhelmi-prepared hGH from America. Once the New Zealand program began in 1978 a further 116 children were treated with hGH prepared under the local Chapman method, with some receiving the hormone from another source as well.

In addition, due to shortages, 21 New Zealanders were given hGH between 1976 and 1978 that had been manufactured by Australia's CSL.[7]

From figures compiled by the New Zealand Ministry of Health, incomplete but existing records show that at least 143 women and 10 men also received the fertility drug, hPG, in the 20-odd years to 1985. It is estimated that about 38 of the hPG recipients received injections prepared by Dr James Brown in Melbourne and about another 30-odd received the drug imported from Wilhelmi at Emory University in the 1960s and early 1970s. Another 13 received hPG from CSL while the remaining 71 received the local Chapman-manufactured drug. It appears that no other cadaver-derived drugs were used in New Zealand. Nor were any central records kept of the numbers of multiple births resulting from hPG.

Staff at Auckland Hospital initially began tracking human hormone recipients when the bad news about CJD burst forth in 1985. But 10 years later, the task was taken over by the Ministry of Health. By mid-1997 it had found and counselled 95 per cent of the 153 hGH and 143 hPG recipients in this tiny two-island nation, plus a few recipients of human hormone drugs from other countries who have since migrated to New Zealand. It was only in 1996, after the new hGH deaths became public, that recipient support groups were formed.

The real horror came with the fourth death. A former Wilhelmi-manufactured hGH recipient was only 41 when he died on September 5, 1996. He had been treated between 1964 and 1966. It meant his incubation period was at least 30 years.

On October 31, 1996, one week after *Nature* published the first direct scientific link between BSE and the new variant CJD found in the molecular marker in monkeys, Heather Caultan died. She was a very unlucky straddler in that her treatment began on June 22, 1977, one week before Justice Morland's deemed negligence period began. She was the eighteenth former hGH recipient to succumb to CJD and left a husband, Mark Woods and a daughter, Chelsea, who was only eight months old. Donald Spear, the man proud to carry the tattoo "Immortal So Far" for the 13 months before his death, died earlier the same week, leaving his heartbroken young wife behind. Three more hormone recipients were also dying of CJD at this time.

By the end of the year nvCJD deaths linked to British beef products rose to 14 UK cases and one in France. A second French case, in a 52-year-old woman, was originally published as a possible nvCJD case. However, it was later reclassified as a dura mater-linked case (she died 11 years after the grafting) after chemical analysis of the PrP in her brain was carried out. She became the world's twenty-sixth known CJD victim following a dura mater implant.[8]

On Thursday, December 19, 1996, the plaintiffs in the CJD litigation, led by Robert Owen, QC, faced the defendants, led by Justin Fenwick, QC, once again, this time in the Crown Court in the Welsh capital, Cardiff, where Justice Morland was on circuit. While argument was made for costs and whether the judge would be prepared to widen the ambit of his July 1996 judgment to include the straddlers whose hGH treatment had predated July 1, 1977, the judge had disturbing news.

Not only did he confirm his ruling that compensation should be paid only to those who were new patients after July 1, 1977, but he restricted it even further to apply to any new patient after 1977 who had been treated with the Hartree acetone-stored method of hGH extraction. If any of the CJD victims who had been treated after July 1, 1977, had received exclusively hGH manufactured from frozen pituitaries via the Lowry method, or from either frozen glands or acetone-stored glands manufactured from 1979 onwards at CAMR at Porton Down, then they would be ineligible for compensation.

By then 20 hGH recipients were dead — all of them treated with Hartree hGH alone. It remained to be seen in any future victims whether cases would arise from a combination of Hartree and Lowry or Hartree, Lowry and CAMR-produced hGH.

In February 1997 the plaintiff legal team appealed the judge's exclusion of the straddlers and a few weeks later the government appealed the entire judgment of Justice Morland. The band of Celts looked with interest Down Under, to see what sort of precedent would be set by the test case in which APQ was suing on behalf of Australia's equivalent of the "well-but-worried" human hormone recipients.

APQ was not very well and still very worried. For more than three years, scientific consultants to the Melbourne firm Rennick Briggs had pored over truckloads of documents relating to the AHPHP and CSL to establish state of knowledge on CJD — a key plank in APQ's case. The firm, which had undergone both a name change and a dramatic down-sizing from 1993 when it had issued writs on behalf of the families of the four women who had died of CJD, remained confident that APQ had by far the best case. She was treated late in AHPHP, well after the 1982 destruction of glands at CSL that contained a probable CJD-infected gland. An alternative fertility drug, hMG, used extensively around the world, had been available at the time, although it had been expensive because it was not government-sponsored like hPG.

No CJD-related deaths have resulted from hMG.

APQ also clearly demonstrated the requisite psychiatric injury necessary to mount a case. As an adult at the time of treatment, APQ may have refused to take hPG if she had been told the known risks of CJD, or other diseases being transmitted by the hormone, or even that it was a human biological product. APQ's anxiety was palpable and unrelenting and she still needed either weekly or fortnightly counselling. Her hair was so thin she had bought a turban to wear in court.

Her claim for legal aid was finally denied by the Commonwealth Attorney-General's Department on December 20, 1996 — 18 months after she had first applied for it. An appeal and lobbying by Rennick Briggs for reconsideration by the Commonwealth Government — the main defendant in the case, which had already indemnified the second defendant, the now-privatised CSL Ltd — were turned down.

By this time, too, the length of the trial had blown out to almost four months, chiefly due to the number of witnesses expected to be called by the Commonwealth — at least 25. Some of these experts were to be flown in from overseas, while others had been members of HPAC, which oversaw the running of the AHPHP.

Rennick Briggs was in a grim position. A sole practitioner, Michael Glen owned the firm, and Sean Millard, as the senior solicitor, had conduct of the APQ case. The decision not to legally aid APQ was made in a climate of massive cuts to Commonwealth legal aid funding, introduced by the new Federal Government of Liberal Prime Minister, John Howard, and his Treasurer, Peter Costello. It spelt the end of her test case. There was nowhere to move. Guidelines to both the Special Circumstances Scheme and the Commonwealth Cases of National Importance Scheme, under which APQ had earlier appeared clearly entitled to funding, were amended after the Howard Government was elected in March 1996. The revamped Public Interest Test Case Scheme specifically excluded funding for negligence actions against the Commonwealth.

Frantically, after the Christmas/New Year break, Millard contacted major product liability firms in Melbourne in the hope that they might help fund the case, which many lawyers believed had a good chance of winning. However the fact that the government had refused to consider any settlement of APQ and had stated that the matter would be fought all the way to the High Court, meant that no other firm would take on the litigation without legal aid. As a last-ditch attempt, Rennick Briggs requested that the group of litigants for which APQ was the test case help fund the escalating trial costs. Eighty-five of the 132 agreed to pay another $750 each, which was in addition to stamp duty each had had to pay. Even so, the $46,000 raised was not enough.

In late March other eleventh-hour manoeuvres aimed at reversing the decision on legal aid included the tabling of questions on the case by two non-government politicians in the Australian Senate. Millard conceded on ABC Radio and in the *Sydney Morning Herald* that without legal aid the trial might be abandoned.[11] The Australian Plaintiff Lawyers' Association also raised the conflict of interest issue of the Commonwealth refusing aid to a plaintiff who was suing it.[12]

All the manoeuvres were futile. A proposal for a group settlement was made to the government. By Easter, when no answer had been received, Sean Millard was desperate enough to pass a letter to the sister of the Federal Health Minister, Michael Wooldridge. Even a plea to lift the daily court trial fees of $273 levied effectively as State Tax Relief, was refused by the trial judge on the basis of APQ's assets — half share in the family house and car. Administrative costs in the case alone — including jury fees of $50,000, witness expenses and accommodation — would cost up to $170,000. Even the plaintiff lawyers had agreed to vastly reduced trial fees. But no bank would lend Rennick Briggs more money to run the case.

The start of the trial had by now been put back to April 7. On Tuesday April 2, the first working day after the Easter break, the government made a formal once-only offer of settlement. It was bitterly disappointing. The government's proposal offered no money at all for APQ's alleged psychiatric injury, sustained since being told of her CJD risk — the very point on which she was suing. Instead, it guaranteed to compensate her family for her loss of earnings, loss of support to her family and pain and suffering should she die of CJD. Medical and other costs would be met from the Human Pituitary Hormones Trust Fund Account set up in the wake of the Allars report. As well, all legal costs to date would be met by the government.

Michael Glen rang APQ that day and asked her to come to his office. "I thought it would be some sort of offer," APQ said of the great secrecy that surrounded her visit the next day to the offices of the firm in Little Collins Street. By 3.30 p.m. on Wednesday, April 3, APQ had agreed to the settlement. "I was resigned to the fact that that was the only way," APQ recalls of that day. Few people, apart from her husband and her fellow hPG-recipient friend, had been told that she was APQ, that she was at risk of CJD, or even that she had taken fertility drugs. She had not told her young children, her parents or other family members. Her absence from home during the trial was to be put down to "a meeting" for anyone who asked.

The solicitors told APQ that the offer was a once-only offer and that the attempts to put a counter proposal had been rejected. In the circumstances, it was the best that could be done. While it was her decision to accept the offer, realistically there appeared no alternative. After meeting with the lawyers, "I had the afternoon to comprehend what was being said to me and to decide. I was very tired. They said this offer, if you accept it, will be the end. The same offer will apply to other litigants regardless. To get an offer out of the government at all was pretty unusual and there would be no other offer. I was so confused at the end of it all. There was no other choice. There was not going to be a case anyway because we could not afford it. Every avenue to fund the trial had been exhausted. I didn't want to end it for everyone but I couldn't see any other way. There was no other way and there isn't one now."[13]

APQ does not regret her decision, although she acknowledges that others in her situation might have rejected the offer. She felt that, just as in May 1985 when she lost her babies, "I had come home with my arms just as empty". For her, as well as scores of others who decided to accept the offer in the weeks that followed, the feeling that their lives had been on hold for years pending the court case gradually lifted. Some slept better than they had in ages. APQ was relieved not to have to endure recalling the distress and emotion of her miscarriage, the fear and anxiety that followed being told of her CJD risk and listening to the technical and scientific expert evidence that would have dominated the case for weeks.

Her conviction that she did the right thing — with no obvious support from other litigants bar one letter from a woman in Adelaide several years before — was also tied to her unshakeable fatalism that she *will* die of CJD. "I was born weighing 2 lb 2 ozs in 1955 and survived, I conceived triplets, and the rare hydatidiform mole, CFS and ear problems. I am quite convinced I will get CJD. If anyone is going to get it, it will be me. I cannot shake off the notion. I think of it daily," she says.

When the news of APQ's settlement was announced in the Victorian Supreme Court on Friday, April 4, 1997, and was immediately welcomed by Wooldridge as "compassionate", it sparked immediate anger and disbelief among the other 132 litigants. Many had been expecting money if the case had been won, or at the least, a chance to "see the doctors [who ran the AHPHP] fry on the stand". Some then contacted other prominent product liability specialist law firms in the hope that they would take on the case, even mount a class action. But the fact remained that there was no money. None of the litigants would be eligible for legal aid after APQ was turned down.

In the two months that followed, the Federal Government exerted pressure on all litigants to settle or bring on their cases immediately — whether they had legal representation or not. By the end of May 1997, the majority of Rennick Briggs' 132 clients had settled their cases. But a grim core of human hormone recipients, including Geraldine Brodrick, by now the CJD Support Group coordinator for the state of Queensland, opted to explore other means of suing.

The government then extended its settlement offer to the end of June 1997. By that time 85 recipients had settled through Rennick Briggs. Five days before the deadline, a Senate inquiry was announced. Its terms of reference included investigating the refusal by the government of APQ's legal aid and the fairness of its settlement offer to her. The settlement deadline was extended and expanded to include anyone treated officially on the AHPHP.

By the end of June 1997 the British tally of CJD in former hGH recipients had leapt by four in a few short months to 25, about half the known CJD deaths in France. At the same time in Australia news spread like wildfire of the initial diagnosis of possible CJD in a woman treated with hPG in 1971. This meant, if the CJD was confirmed after her death, that she had had an incubation period of 26 years, a horrific thought for the world's hPG recipient community. On top of New Zealand's last hGH recipient CJD death, 30 years after his last treatment, this news was all bad and getting worse.

CHAPTER 22

The shocking legacy of cannibalism

FORTY YEARS AFTER the discovery of kuru and more than 70 years after Bertha E catapulted Hans Creutzfeldt into the history books, the triggering cause of transmissible spongiform encephalopathies — prion diseases — remained a mystery.

The notion that a prion, a corrupted or abnormal protein, could transmit disease by itself had moved inch by inch — with nothing contrary to impede its progress — from the heretical to the mainstream by 1997.

The acceptance of prions by the scientific establishment could not have been shown more clearly than by the award of the Nobel Prize in Medicine to Professor Stanley Prusiner in October 1997. "Stanley Prusiner has added prions to the list of well known infectious agents including bacteria, viruses, fungi and parasites," the Karolinska Institute, which awarded the prize, stated. "There are still people who don't believe that a protein can cause these diseases, but we believe it." Prusiner's prions, it went on, provide "important insights that may furnish the basis of understanding the biological mechanisms underlying other types of dementia related illnesses — for example, Alzheimer's disease — and establishes a foundation for drug development and medical treatment strategies."

The award to the self-promoting neurologist, who had driven the bulk of research at the molecular level in TSEs since the early 1980s, was immediately controversial. This was not merely because of the speed of acceptance of his still-contentious theory, which had undergone several changes in its evolution. The latest addition to his hypothesis was "Protein X", in 1995, an additional molecule which might interact with the prion protein in the course of prion replication. In other words Protein X might act as a chaperone or co-factor in the conversion or refolding of normal prion protein into its evil twin, protease-resistant protein (PrP). All major theories on the cause of TSEs — prion, unconventional virus, virino or other — remain to be proved. According to sceptics, the protein-only theory does not adequately explain the existence of different strains of prion diseases. Even John Collinge in London, whose Prion Disease Group is a testament to Prusiner's catchy name for the infectious agent, admitted he thought the prize would come at a later time given, "important unresolved issues".

One outspoken opponent of the prion hypothesis, Dr Robert Rowher, director of the molecular neurovirology unit at the Veterans Affairs Medical Center in Baltimore, decided that the prize may in the end be good for a research field that had for years been plagued by "paroxysms of Nobel-itis". Laura Maneulidis, Yale University professor of neuropathology who maintains a virus will be found responsible for TSEs, hopes Prusiner's accolade will not prevent further inquiry into the puzzle. "That's the problem with Nobel Prizes," she said afterwards. "If people think that everything is decided, you can't possibly risk going against the grain."[1] After the announcement Prusiner broke his decade-long self-imposed media silence to declare: "Awards do not vindicate a piece of science. Only data does that."[2]

Possibly the final chapter on the cause of new variant CJD, what was formerly a suspected link to BSE became, in October 1997, a confirmed link. Two independent studies at different ends of Britain established beyond reasonable doubt that it was caused by the same strain of agent or prion. This meant that the only explanation for nvCJD was human exposure to BSE, most likely before the SBO ban of November 1989 when the most infective parts of cattle were banned from the human food chain.

In one of the studies Moira Bruce and colleagues from the Institute of Animal Health in Edinburgh injected brain samples from nine sporadic CJD and nvCJD patients, as well as BSE-infected cows into mice.[3] The symptoms, presentation and course of the disease in those mice after two years, were identical in BSE and nvCJD. Previous transmission in mice — which had been injected with BSE-infected samples of brain from sheep, a goat, a pig, unrelated cattle, domestic cats, a nyala and a greater kudu — studied by this group of researchers had showed a "BSE signature" — very similar incubation periods and patterns of brain damage. This was important. More than 30 years of scrapie experiments in Britain involving sheep, goats, minks and a mule deer with chronic wasting disease, had never produced the BSE signature.

Professor John Collinge and others from the Prion Disease Group at the Imperial College School of Medicine at St Mary's Hospital in London used a biochemical assay that resulted in the same conclusion via a different method.[4] Using normal and also transgenic mice — those in which the mice prion protein had been replaced with human prion protein — the group produced pathology in the brains of the mice that was indistinguishable between BSE and nvCJD. SEAC members described both studies as "compelling" evidence that nvCJD was human BSE.[5]

New variant CJD patients, all of them unwilling participants in a lottery of death from BSE-infected beef products, were all found to have the same tiny variation (MM at codon 129 on the PRNP gene) in their genetic makeup. At the time of writing, the initial 10 cases of CJD that shook the world in March 1996 had more than doubled to 23 confirmed cases. This had implications for the extent of the human epidemic stemming from BSE. Some experts predicted that the small amount of cases was in direct proportion to the end of the human epidemic, with numbers remaining in the low hundreds. Others describe the doubling of cases in the first 12 months since the announcement as the beginning of an epidemic curve that could climb well into the thousands.

Just how many thousands is far too early to tell. The kuru epidemic began in numbers of only tens and twenties earlier this century and peaked at hundreds a year in the late 1950s. It has taken at least 40 years to measure that epidemic. Many felt that the upper end of Professor Richard Lacey's doomsday prediction of between 500 and 500,000 Britons who may to succumb to nvCJD, to be merely that. The slowly climbing, and some say completely under-reported toll of BSE in other European countries may also alter predictions of nvCJD in years to come. Some observers have estimated that it may take 25 years for the scale of a potential nvCJD epidemic to be judged.

One fact is certain and might help to extrapolate in future: no cases of nvCJD have been identified with an onset of symptoms before 1994.[6] Incubation periods in continuing cases of kuru and pituitary hormone-linked CJD, two other known routes of accidental peripheral CJD infection, will provide future estimates of the extent of the epidemic from their longest incubation periods. Also a factor to be considered will be

the amount of infectious material that has entered the food supply —
something that may never be known.

There are an estimated 44 million head of cattle in the US, of which
about seven million are killed annually for food. American agricultural
and health regulators kept an eagle eye on the BSE crisis in both Britain
and the European Union, as new measures banning the use of cattle
parts in animal feed swung into effect in the US in late 1997. No cases
of BSE have been detected there, despite some claims that downer cows
could be the US version of BSE.

The Australian CJD Registry is on the alert for any nvCJD cases, providing a vital world observation post given the complete absence of
BSE in Australian cattle (as well as no scrapie in sheep).

The British Ministry of Agriculture, Fisheries and Food (MAFF) has
since admitted to the presence of at least five cases of BSE that pre-date
Colin Whitaker's visit to the Kent farm in April 1985. Abnormal conditions in cattle have always been coded by MAFF. In 1986 the symptoms
of one condition stored on hole punch computer cards at the Central
Veterinary Laboratory, together with five preserved brains kept there,
matched the symptoms then becoming apparent in rising numbers of
cattle.[7]

The epidemic itself, having killed hundreds of thousands of cattle —
half of them slaughtered before they succumbed to the disease itself —
is expected to result in the deaths of about 7,000 confirmed BSE-
infected beasts between late 1997 and 2001. By then experts estimate it
will have petered out, although pockets of infection will doubtless
remain. This will be due to a small incidence of vertical transmission
— identified in MAFF experiment results in 1996 — in mothers incubating BSE who deliver calves in the year before they develop symptoms. It is not known why this happens. Horizontal spread between animals in the field may also prevent the disease from dying out completely for decades yet.

In a statement issued in July 1997, Britain's Royal Society acknowledged fears that sheep fed the same contaminated meat and bonemeal
as cattle, may develop BSE — as distinct from scrapie. If that were to
happen, the consumption of those animals would definitely pose a
hazard to humans. Sheep and goat heads were only banned from human
consumption in Britain in September 1996. Other types of potentially
infectious sheep offal include the gut, which is used in sausages, and the

spleen and lymph nodes, which are used in other meat preparations. Ovine spinal cord, more difficult to remove than bovine spinal cord, continues to enter the human food supply in Britain — although France, at the time of writing, had recommended that the above-mentioned sheep offal be prohibited.

Of vast interest around the world for a variety of reasons was the news in August 1997 that a 24-year-old Englishwoman, who had turned vegetarian at the age of 12 because of her love for animals, had become the twenty-second person in Britain to contract nvCJD. She had been engaged to be married when struck down by nvCJD, which was diagnosed more than a year after onset via a new pre-mortem diagnostic tool — a tonsil biopsy — at St Mary's Hospital in London.

Clare Tomkins came from Tonbridge, in Kent, the area where Colin Whitaker identified the first reported case of BSE. Her condition was at first misdiagnosed, and she was treated for severe depression.

The apparently long incubation period in Clare Tomkins' case suggested that the epidemic, whatever its size, had not peaked. It reflected, merely, possible infection from the period before BSE was recognised in cattle — probably dating back to the 1970s. On the contrary, it might indicate that despite her devotion to eating only vegetarian food, she was unwittingly exposed to beef products in store-bought food including baby food. Her father, Roger, told reporters his daughter did eat cheese and milk, which prompted SEAC chairman, John Pattison, to remark that evidence which had previously cleared these two food types from known risk of infection should be reviewed.

In September 1997 the *New Statesman* published an open letter, signed by 16 of the families affected by nvCJD at that stage and several TSE experts including emeritus professor of neurology at the University of Oxford, Bryan Matthews, and Alan Dickinson. In it the families of Stephen Churchill, Michelle Bowen, Anne Richardson, Adrian Hodgkinson, Donna Mellowship, Clare Tomkins, Matthew Parker, Gulcan Hassan, Alison Margaret Williams, Victoria Lowther, Keith Humphries, Christopher Warne, Nina Cadwallader, Janice Stuart, Peter Hall and Barry Baker demanded a full inquisitorial public judicial inquiry. They wanted the reasons for the rise of nvCJD explained so that "no such public health disaster will ever happen again".[8] The majority of those families intended to sue Britain's public health regulators, MAFF and the Department of Health, for negligence.

Echoing the thoughts of many, Henry Carey, the husband of the twenty-first victim of nvCJD, Sue Carey, said this to the *Guardian* newspaper in the months after her death at age 36 in early 1997: "I think it is scandalous that the farmers who have supplied the meat which presumably gave Sue the disease are getting billions of pounds in compensation and we are getting nothing."[9] He also damned the role of politicians and health and agricultural officials: "They told us that beef was safe. God knows they ought to take the responsibility."

In late 1997 carriage of potential nvCJD litigation was in the hands of David Body, the Sheffield-based Irwin Mitchell solicitor who had successfully sued the British Government on behalf of some of the families of hGH recipients.

Pending any announcement of a judicial inquiry, claims were to be filed within the three-year statute of limitations after the date of knowledge (the March 20, 1996 announcement of a link between BSE and nvCJD). The claims would be filed on the basis of the alleged failure of the British Government to properly respond to the public health challenge of BSE and to implement safety procedures to limit BSE in British beef herds.[10]

If they were to go ahead, these potential cases would touch on virgin legal territory. They might help define the parameters of "failure" in the government's responsibility to its citizens for food regulation or ensuring the availability of safe food. Never had a case been tried around a decision, or omission, of the food regulator — the government — that has apparently exposed a substantial proportion of the population to an allegedly avoidable risk.

Meanwhile in America, another potential source of CJD infection — squirrel brains — was raised for discussion again in 1997. University of Kentucky neurologist, Dr Joseph Berger, noted at a university-sponsored conference on emerging infectious diseases the "interesting observation" that all the CJD patients from Kentucky that he and another neurologist had treated were squirrel-brain eaters.[11] Some ate them as dumplings in soup, while others added them to a vegetable stew known as burgoo. While eating squirrel — meat or brains — may turn out to be an unwise dietary practice, the theory of an undetected "mad squirrel disease" could be tested via transmission experiments with laboratory animals, Berger suggested.

Devising methods of treatments for TSEs, particularly given the nvCJD outbreak, has become imperative. Diagnostic tests are paramount and include the tonsil biopsy methods used in Clare Tomkins' case, as well as the relatively accurate pre-mortem 14-3-3 abnormal protein antibody test. NIH researcher Paul Brown identifies strategies for preventing or treating patients with inherited TSEs like GSS and FFI that include selective abortion. Parents could be tested, if at familial risk, for confirmation that they do or do not carry a lethal gene. "New millennium" options, as he terms them because they won't be available until at least then, include genetic engineering or treatment with chemotherapy compounds called sulfated glycosaminoglycans (GAGS). GAGS appear to be able to interfere with the formation of amyloid plaques, the lethal deposits of protein found in CJD, Alzheimer's disease and other chronic inflammatory diseases. Clinical trials for GAGS were not expected before the turn of the century.

In a paper published in *Science* just after the announcement of his Nobel Prize, Prusiner suggested that interfering with the conversion of normal cellular PrP^c to the rogue PrP^{sc} was "the most attractive therapeutic target".[12] Drugs that can enter the central nervous system could be devised to bind themselves to the protein to stop it acting as a template. Other proteins — chaperones such as the alleged Protein X — could also be modified. "Understanding how PrP^c folds and refolds into PrP^{sc} not only has implications for interfering with the pathogenesis of prion disease, but may open new approaches to deciphering the causes of and developing effective therapies for the more common neurodegenerative diseases, including Alzheimer's disease, Parkinson's disease, and amyotrophic lateral sclerosis (ALS)," he said.

A protein abnormality that affects yeast might yet hold answers for prion protein research in mammals. University of Chicago researchers found that when a yeast protein flipped into a different shape, just like rogue prion protein, it appeared to convert normal protein to its own abnormal shape and formed aggregations that looked almost identical to PrP plaques.[13] By tinkering with the production of a chaperone protein, the misshapen protein has reverted to its normal shape in experiments. Translating that result to prion protein, which has a role that remains unknown in mammals, is merely a hope at the time of writing.

Further experiments with transgenic mice in conjunction with molecular modelling may help answer questions such as how TSE infection moves from the point of infection to the brain? How does the TSE agent replicate and infect neighbouring cells? And why does the damage inflicted cause holes rather than some other form of damage?

Around the world, CJD tolls from various causes continue to climb. The World Health Organisation recommended in March 1997 that human dura mater grafts be stopped. This followed the news at a meeting, held to review research on TSEs, that Japan was about to announce a staggering 25 cases of CJD in graft recipients in recent years. In fact, in May 1997 Japan announced that an epidemiological study had found infected dura mater had caused as many as 43 cases of CJD in the previous 10 years.[14]

The WHO recommendation was regarded by some as controversial given that it remains unknown whether CJD transmission occurs with grafts used in places other than the brain, such as dental surgery. Paul Brown, the NIH investigator who attended the Geneva meeting in March 1997, weighed in heavily on the issue. "This is like using an elephant gun on a flea, since a lot of dura may be risk free."[15] The additional Japanese cases brought the toll of human dura mater cases by late 1997 to more than 70 worldwide.

In Queensland, Australia, a woman in her twenties died of CJD after the Japanese announcement of May 1997. In what is one of the world's longest incubation periods for this type of CJD, she died 15 years after she received a dura mater graft during neurosurgery in 1982. This was the same year, and in the same state, that Australia's first CJD case from a dural graft was infected. The woman was the third Australian to die from this form of accidental transmission.

In February 1997 this author contacted Peter Derbes, the New Orleans-based lawyer who had represented Father Richard Nesom, the Catholic priest who had sued the German manufacturer of Lyodura, B Braun Melsungen AG, in March 1988. In a precursor to the APQ case, Fr Nesom had claimed damages for fear and emotional distress over his CJD risk following a graft to repair a dural tear and subsequent cerebro-spinal fluid leakage after a mastoidectomy in March 1987. His appeal was dismissed in 1993.

This was despite arguments based on 36 *Morbidity and Mortality Weekly* reports that CJD incubation could range anywhere from 16 months to 21 years. In a late night conversation with Derbes, I told him that recent research had shown that incubation periods had now stretched to at least 14 years.

Derbes contacted Fr Nesom, by now living in Mississippi, and was shocked to learn, in May 1997 that his former client had been tentatively diagnosed with CJD — 10 years after his dural graft was implanted. The diagnosis, probable rather than possible, based on his symptoms and an abnormal EEG reading, demonstrated another telling indicator of the variability of incubation periods for TSEs from similar origins. The Connecticut woman who received a graft from the same lot number as Fr Nesom succumbed in just 18 months.

On September 12, 1997 Peter Derbes and colleagues filed suit in the Federal Court in New Orleans against B Braun Melsungen AG of Germany, its Canadian-based distributor, Tri Hawk International, and Tri Hawk's insurers, requesting a trial by jury. The writ alleges that Braun and Tri Hawk, despite advice some time between January 29 and April 8, 1987 from the FDA and the Health Protection Branch of Canada, took no steps to inform health care providers who had purchased Lot 2105 Lyodura of the lethal hazard it posed.

If the case proceeded past summary judgment, a trial was not expected to begin until late 1998 at the earliest.

In Britain, the CJD toll from hGH therapy jumped from the 16 cases known at the start of the High Court trial in April 1996 to 26 dead and dying by late 1997. All had been treated with acetone-stored glands produced by Dr Anne Stockell Hartree at Cambridge University between 1963 and 1979, either solely or in combination with extracts from frozen pituitaries. None had been treated exclusively with hGH produced by CAMR at Porton Down from 1980.

In September 1997, the High Court approved damages ranging from £90,000 to £140,000 for the five successful plaintiffs whose hGH treatment had begun negligently after Justice Morland's cut-off date of July 1, 1977. The range reflected the difference between those who died with dependants, like Patrick Baldwin, and those who did not, such as 2nd Lieutenant James Bettinson of the Welsh Guards, who grew to be 1.8 metres tall. Bettinson's death in 1995 aged 27, after he watched his own passing out parade from the stands because he could not walk in a straight line, was found by a coroner — after the Morland judgment — to have resulted from misadventure "in circumstances where there has been a finding of medical negligence".[16]

In November 1997, the Court of Appeal in London unanimously

ruled that a group of "straddlers", hGH recipients whose treatment had straddled the July 1, 1977 cut-off point by a few weeks or months could return to the High Court and argue individual claims for negligence. These cases, which included Stuart Smith and Donald Spear who both missed the cut-off date by about three months, Terrence Newman whose family launched the first negligence case, Saul Hefferon-Waldon, and Heather Caultan who began her treatment a week before July 1, 1977, may total twelve.

Meanwhile in Australia, a fifth woman recipient of the fertility drug, hPG, had negotiated a compensation settlement with the government based on the protocol established in the wake of the APQ settlement.[17] Without having to prove negligence, Mrs Margaret Bansemer's lawyer, Michael Glen from Rennick Briggs in Melbourne, was able to settle a compensation claim on the balance of probabilities that she had CJD. Taken into account were her degenerative symptoms, a tentative diagnosis of the disease by an Adelaide neurologist, and two courses of hPG injections which resulted in the birth of her third child, Jason.

Under this historic agreement — the first outside France for a living and presumed victim of CJD — Mrs Bansemer, unlike those Australian victims before her, was given substantial damages for pain, suffering and loss of income.[18] Despite all the good intentions of the Allars Report, which resulted in the establishment of a $10 million trust fund to provide medical and financial help in the event of further CJD cases, the Federal Department of Health was accused of undue slowness when word filtered back in mid-1997 that 55-year-old Bansemer appeared to have the preliminary signs of CJD. She had been treated in 1970 with two courses of the drug, at least one of them from batch 3 of the CSL-manufactured hPG — a batch not implicated in any of the other five Australian deaths. The government finally approved funds from the trust fund to her family and settled the compensation claim in late October. Alive at the time of writing, should she die of CJD, Margaret Bansemer would be the third woman to succumb who had been treated with hPG at Adelaide's Queen Elizabeth Hospital.

Her tentative diagnosis in May 1997 — after an apparent 27-year incubation period — caused shock waves in Australia's human hormone recipient community. Many recipients were unaware of the 30-year incubation period for the disease in New Zealand and American hGH recipients, which were in any case not linked to CSL-manufactured drugs. The belief by many hPG recipients that they were hopefully out of danger once 16 years had passed since the end of their treatment (the period after which Jan Blight contracted CJD) was shattered. In some, anxiety resurfaced with a vengeance as they waited for autopsy confirmation in the Bansemer case. If confirmed, the Bansemer case would raise the pituitary hormone toll of CJD in Australia to six, including "Stephen", the sole hGH patient.

Meanwhile in September 1997, Stacey C, a former podiatrist, died in Brooklyn, New York, after three years in a vegetative state. A positive Harrington spot test result, her former treatment with hGH and her symptoms before she lapsed into a coma-like state, were all indicative of CJD. Her family hired a New York law firm which issued writs in a multi-defendant action aimed at including all treating centres, manufacturers and distributors of hGH, including Emory University, during the years she received hGH injections. That she survived so long totally incapacitated, curled in a foetal position, her eyes open and unblinking, was due, Paul Brown from the NIH acknowledges, to the superb nursing care she received.

Her family was among several, on both sides of the United States who by early 1997 had filed writs seeking damages for negligence or wrongful death. Statutes of limitation and other legal technicalities were sometimes unbeatable. Cases filed on behalf of the families of 32-year-old Tracia Hagy of Issaquah, Washington, who died aged 32 in November 1992 and Linda Ann Sluder Shipman, who died in Florida in 1995 — both having received years of hGH injections — had failed in their preliminary stages by late 1997.

The families of some of the four New Zealand men who died from CJD in 1996 were contemplating legal proceedings in the United States in late 1997 based on injuries from Wilhelmi-manufactured hGH imported from Emory University.

In France the CJD toll in hGH recipients had climbed from 48 in 1996 to a staggering 58 by late 1997. For a recipient of Pasteur Institute-manufactured hGH this translated to roughly a one in 30 chance of contracting the disease for the 1,700-odd children at risk — shocking odds for such a rare disease. Judicial inquiries continued following the January 1997 media revelations that FF5.5 million (more than US$800,000 or £550,000) was saved when distribution with hGH — untreated by Urea 8 — continued beyond May 1985. Any court case (at least six lawyers had been retained by 20 families[19]) remained a long way off in late 1997.

CJD deaths from pituitary hormone contamination have passed 110 worldwide and continue to rise. The toll doubled in the three years between 1993 and the end of 1996. This indicates that the peak of this mini-epidemic may not yet have been reached. To date not one of these deaths has been attributable to commercial preparations of the drug although one of the French CJD victims was treated with both French-manufactured hGH and Kabi hGH when French stocks ran low.

There remains — as with blood transfusions and bone grafts — no evidence of maternal or vertical transmission of CJD of any type from mother to child. (Nor, it should be stressed, is there evidence or anecdotal reports of transmission through sexual intercourse.)

Women in recent times who were symptomatic with CJD while pregnant number only a handful. They include the Swiss woman, infected via depth electrodes for her epilepsy, whose child was born on September 11, 1976; the Japanese woman who contracted apparent sporadic CJD during her pregnancy and gave birth in the late 1980s; the second American woman to be infected via a dura mater graft whose baby boy was born in February 1991;[20] and two British women. One of those British women, Michelle Bowen, was a nvCJD victim and died soon after giving birth to her son Anthony in November 1995. The second, was Heather Caultan, a former child recipient of hGH who died in 1996, shortly after giving birth.

None of these children, who range in age from toddlers to the now 21-year-old (in late 1997) offspring of the Swiss woman, is known to have contracted CJD. Nor have any of the children born to pregnant or lactating Papua New Guinean Fore kuru sufferers developed kuru.

On February 18, 1997, in the Frederick County Circuit Court in Maryland, 73-year-old Professor Daniel Carleton Gajdusek pleaded guilty to sexually abusing one of his dozens of Micronesian adopted sons. The NIH announced his immediate retirement from his US$123,000 a year post as chief of the Laboratory of Central Nervous System Studies, his pension intact, on the same day.

The plea by the Nobel Prize winner was given front page treatment in the *New York Times* and the *Washington Post*, which reported the following exchanges with Circuit Court Judge G. Edward Dwyer to whom he made his plea. Responding to a question, he said he was taking several medicines, then added, "You want the biochemical names of them?" When the judge ask if he could read and write the English language, Gajdusek replied, "and many others". And finally, asked if he was pleading guilty because he was, in fact, guilty of child abuse, he responded, "Yes, I am".[21]

Under a plea agreement worked out just a week before his trial was due to start, Gajdusek, who faced up to 30 years in jail, would serve only one year after federal and state sexual abuse charges against him were dropped. Despite a lengthy probationary period he was to be allowed to leave the United States after his sentence was served to continue studies into virus-borne diseases. Two months later, in tears and surrounded by his network of friends and family, he made his farewells before going to jail. His release was expected to occur as this book was published. All the children in his household returned to their families in Micronesia and Papua New Guinea.

Forty years after Gajdusek and Zigas worked and worried over the increasing and dramatic toll of kuru cases, a benchmark in kuru history occurred. The last confirmed case of the disease then known, a 63-year-old man from the South Fore region, died on April 11, 1997. Only a few months earlier, in December 1996, two other kuru victims, a man aged about 46 and a woman in her fifties died, thanks to the legacy of one or more cannibal feasts four to six decades earlier.

Kuru is the beginning of this fascinating area of research and may yet provide clues for the end. Its incubation periods provide the end point of estimated incubation periods for all types of accidentally transmitted CJD. Michael Alpers, director of the Papua New Guinea Institute of Medical Research, still hopes to document the last case of kuru. As he pointed out soon after the death of the 63-year-old man: "This is the first time in the history of this disease that we have no confirmed case."

However, since that kuru death in April 1997, four decades after cannibalism was outlawed, two more cases of kuru have since been confirmed. The first was in a 60-year-old woman who died in August 1997 and the second was in a 49-year-old man who had entered the midcourse of the disease at the time of writing in early 1998. Alpers expects one or two cases of kuru to emerge each year well into the new millennium. The incubation period could still be as long, or longer, than the human life span.

And kuru research, although unpublished for years, will continue. In mid-1997 a collaboration on genetic studies was announced between Alpers and John Collinge in London. Original kuru data computerised in PNG and combined with more recent field data dating from the mid-1980s, might reveal previously unappreciated patterns. Or, with no common genetic trait yet visible, the new collaboration might reveal some sort of susceptibility to kuru. Genes other than the PRNP gene may be implicated.

Many lives have changed irrevocably through the accidental transmission of CJD and the taking of the therapeutic products that caused it. Children are motherless, husbands are without spouses, wives are without husbands, parents mourn their children and others live with the frightening knowledge that it could happen to them.

In September 1973 the mother of New Zealand's first set of quintuplets, Shirley Ann Lawson was divorced from her husband, Sam.[22] Nine years later, in February 1982, she was fatally shot in the head by her second husband, Gary Eyton, from whom she was separated, following previous threats to kill her. He then turned the gun on himself, a coroner later found.[23]

Lee Allender, the son of Jane Allender, the first woman to succumb to CJD via hPG fertility treatment, has undergone years of psychological treatment following the death of his mother from a drug she took to create him. His father, Ted, was likely to move to China on a joint venture environmental project after heavy involvement in various groups and councils related to CJD support. He also designed and set up the Australian CJD support web site on the Internet — one of a group visited frequently on the World Wide Web.

Stephen Cummings, who lost his wife Vonda to hPG-related CJD in 1991, has moved with his children back to Western Australia. Noel Halford, whose wife Jenny was diagnosed after the stupendous coincidence of being examined by the same neurologist as had seen Jane Allender, has remarried. Geraldine Brodrick has retired, her last child has left school and she is writing her own book.

Paul Andrews, the British hGH recipient who sat in court for much of the six-week CJD litigation in 1996, is trying to put his fear of CJD in perspective and has found a new career — as a primary school teacher. Previously a Conservative, his disappointment with the Tory Government's refusal to grant an inquiry into CJD contamination of pituitary hormones has changed him. He has joined New Labour and the National Union of Teachers.

As the new millennium approaches, technological and scientific change proceeds faster than ever before. Genetic testing for a variety of diseases is available to potential parents and family members — from specialised clinics — and even through the mail in some countries. Cloning, once in the realms of science fiction, has become a common topic for bioethical debate. This followed the first report of a successful sheep cloning in March 1996, demonstrating that it was possible to clone an adult mammal.[24] Even artificial human chromosomes, made in a laboratory from a blend of natural and synthetic human DNA, held up a future vision of custom-designed genes for people suffering inherited diseases.[25]

The way is also open in the future for xenografts or transplants of animal organs and tissue into humans. In early 1997 the US Government banned the practice, saying the risks needed to be studied. Following the BSE crisis the British Government also announced a moratorium on xenotransplantation due to continuing uncertainty about safety and the obvious dangers of transferring hitherto unknown animal viruses, particularly retroviruses, like HIV, to humans.[26]

But the British moratorium, announced in early 1997, was only temporary. Clinical trials of pig hearts genetically engineered to reduce the risk of rejection in humans were ready to go. Others were in the offing. Safeguards and stringent regulations, capable of being policed by a regulatory body, are paramount for any xenotransplant program. Otherwise, the lessons from the tragic legacy of accidental transmission of TSEs — particularly kuru, pituitary hormone extracts and dura mater grafts — may have to be learned all over again.

Afterword

THE GLOBAL LEGACY of accidental CJD transmission continues. As time passes, so the unruly threads of the disease legacy spread — overshadowed, ominously, by the uncertainty of the extent of the nvCJD threat to the human population.

In late 1997 the horror of the 1974 transmission of CJD via corneal transplants (and two subsequent transmissions, one of them in a German woman 30 years after a transplant[1]), was revisited when Britain's organ donation screening system became the subject of an inquiry. Marion Hamilton, a 53-year-old Scotswoman died of inoperable lung cancer at the Strathcarron Hospice near Stirling in February 1997. Her corneas and the white part of an eye were donated to two men and a woman aged in her eighties. It was not until much later in the year that the cause of Mrs Hamilton's additional neurological problems was confirmed by the CJDSU as sporadic CJD. The recipients of her ocular tissue were traced and told they were potential walking time bombs.[2]

In Australia a similar incident had occurred in the late 1970s but was not reported in medical literature until 1995 after two young doctors completed a research study on CJD. Corneas from a man later found to have died of CJD were transplanted into two women, one 33 years old and the other 65, at a Sydney hospital. The younger patient's graft was removed within 48 hours of revelation of the cause of the donor's death.[3] Both women were lost to follow-up by the treating hospital within five years. In 1997, neither was traceable by the Australian CJD Registry.

In other developments, better surveillance and awareness of CJD resulted in the addition of China, Venezuela and Korea to the world map of reported incidence of the disease. The Netherlands joined Australia and Brazil, each with a single victim of CJD after hGH therapy, this time in a 39-year-old woman who had been treated more than 20 years earlier.[4] The first German, a woman, joined the ranks of unfortunate CJD victims due to contaminated dura mater infections — seven years after the event.[5] And Mike Harrington's new 14-3-3 protein antibody was successful in differentiating for the first time between familial CJD sufferers with the codon 200 mutation and healthy carriers of the mutation, whose spinal fluid carried no trace of it.[6]

Concern over blood products and potential CJD transmission continued. Canada made its first warning to hospitals in March 1997 that up to 100,000 patients in the early 1990s may have received blood products from pooled donations linked to a healthy carrier of a familial CJD mutation. In the Middle East nearly 80 expectant mothers carrying babies conceived through in-vitro fertilisation at clinics in Israel and the Palestinian West Bank, were warned by the Israeli health ministry of a slight CJD risk. Albumin, an essential product in the nurturing of their fertilised eggs, was traced back to an American CJD donor. All the women opted to continue with their pregnancies.

Britain's Department of Health began a search for the blood products made from the donations of three sufferers and another suspected sufferer of nvCJD to head off a potential scare when the cases were aired on a television documentary in late 1997. The chief medical officer, Sir Kenneth Calman, admitted that although no evidence existed of human-to-human transmission of CJD via blood, "we do not know whether the same will apply to new variant CJD".[7] The United Kingdom Haemophilia Centre Directors' Organisation executive committee also warned that the anxiety created in haemophiliacs from the withdrawals involving nvCJD donors should not be underestimated and that counselling was necessary.[8] Later, New Zealand and Irish health authorities began tracing up to 400 people who received imported blood derivatives from a British donor who died of nvCJD.[9]

On the human hormone extract front, a joint-party Senate committee of the Australian Federal Government found that legal aid was not unfairly denied to APQ, the hPG recipient who was forced to settle her test case for nervous shock on the eve of her trial in April 1997. Among the 18 unanimous recommendations of the committee, however, was the key suggestion that recipients of hPG and hGH who could prove psychiatric injury should be compensated. The compensation should be paid on a one-off basis from a fresh injection of funds to a trust account set up in the wake of the damning Allars inquiry findings of 1994. And the minimum suggested was the equivalent cost of defending potential litigation — hundreds of thousands of dollars.[10]

In the wake of APQ's controversial settlement, 85 others at risk of

CJD also settled on the same grounds — that their legal expenses were paid and that they would be guaranteed damages, without having to prove negligence, in the event that they ever contracted CJD. The Senate committee report also recommended that those who had settled their cases should also be eligible for the one-off payment from the trust account, providing they had evidence of psychiatric injury. At the time of writing more than 50 others who had sued but not settled their cases pending the outcome of the Senate inquiry remained in legal limbo, unwilling to decide on future legal action until the response of the Federal Government was known.

In Britain, meanwhile, the APQ equivalents — the "well-but-worried" — scored a significant legal victory on December 18 in the High Court. Justice Morland ruled that pending proof of psychiatric injury, the 40-odd hGH recipients whose treatment with Hartree-manufactured hGH began after July 1, 1977 were eligible to sue for compensation. "A psychiatric injury can be readily induced by an accumulative awareness or drip-feed of information over a prolonged period of time although the court will scrutinise rigorously a claim so based," the judge ruled. He said the MRC and the DHSS had "committed a wrong" on these hGH recipients "by imperilling their lives from a terrible fatal disease … I cannot see in the facts and circumstances of this litigation why public policy including social and economic policy considerations should exclude them from compensation".[11] The government was expected to appeal before a series of individual trials was due to start in April 1998.

Concurrently, and in a re-run of the near-hysteria that followed the March 1996 announcement of the initial link between BSE and nvCJD, in mid-December 1997 the British Government banned the sale of any beef products with bones. In response to advice from SEAC in the wake of new tests which showed a small risk of infectivity in cattle bone marrow and the dorsal root ganglia within cattle spinal columns, the strictly precautionary ban included T-bone steaks, ribs of beef and oxtails. These cuts of beef can no longer be sold in shops and restaurants and have to be de-boned by butchers before sale for either domestic or export sale. The same applies to imported beef. Manufacturers cannot make soup, stock cubes or gelatin using British cattle bones over six months old.

But just like the SBO ban on cattle offal, none but the most deliberately obvious flouting of the ban would be punishable. A bad blow for British farmers that will force many out of business — and just as consumer confidence was returning after the 1996 BSE/CJD scares — the meat-on-the-bone ban killed any hope of an early lifting of the European Commission's embargo on British beef products imposed in 1996.

SEAC committee members Jeffrey Almond and John Collinge on a television program aired concerns that BSE may have already spread from cattle to sheep via ruminant protein supplements fed to sheep after they were banned from cattle feed. The EU then reportedly considered banning meat on the bone from sheep more than six months old exported from Britain and other BSE-affected countries. As the year drew to a close the United States banned all beef and sheep meat imports from any EU country, regardless of whether it had reported cases of BSE or not. A rift with European partners erupted over British regulations from January 1, 1998 banning beef imports that did not conform to its own anti-BSE standards. Swill with pig meat was to be banned from British pig feed after further advice from SEAC recommended that recycling of waste as feed within a species created the potential for a major BSE-like epidemic. And the House of Commons Agriculture Committee estimated the cost of BSE to Britain between 1996 and 2000 — during which the culling of all cattle over 30 months would continue — would be an estimated £3.5 billion. CJD, meanwhile, remained a disease that was not notifiable anywhere in the world.

Just days before Christmas, the New Labour Government of Tony Blair announced a long-awaited independent judicial inquiry into the disastrous ramifications of the BSE epidemic. The Minister for Agriculture, Jack Cunningham, also announced a one-off £85 million BSE aid package to beef and some sheep farmers. Lessons to be learned from the year-long inquiry and on-going research will hopefully ensure that the tragedy of this sort of accidental disease transmission is never repeated — and that the time-honoured taboo against cannibalism is respected.

Hormone production
methods

USA: After Maurice Raben's first published treatment of a pituitary dwarf in 1958, hGH was produced for a time in some academic laboratories from glands collected by the Veterans Administration Pituitary Bank. Distribution of hGH began centrally in 1963 by the National Pituitary Agency and ran for 20 years. Replaced by the National Hormone and Pituitary Program (NHPP) in 1983, about 7,000 American children received hGH under the auspices of both. Another 3,000 children received commercial hGH — Crescormon by KabiVitrum from 1978 and Asellacrin by Ares-Serono from 1980 — either solely or as a supplement to NHPP hGH. A small number of women were treated in the 1960s with hPG.

About 80,000 glands — frozen, stored in acetone or taken from embalmed bodies (the latter only until 1977) — were collected each year by 5,000 pathologists. In the early years patient ages and disease process were "immaterial". By the 1970s exclusion criteria for glands were merely those that were"diseased" but afterwards included glands taken from bodies with hepatitis or from drug addicts.

Between 1963 and 1977, hGH was processed at three main centres:
1   New England Medical Centre in Boston where Dr Maurice Raben used his own technique to extract hGH from about 20,000 acetone-stored glands per year pooled in one huge batch.
2   Emory University in Atlanta where Dr Alfred Wilhelmi processed frozen, acetone-stored and embalmed glands using a salt precipitation technique on batches of at 15,000 each.
3   Cornell University Medical College in New York where Dr Brij Saxena used a modified Raben procedure to extract hGH from batches of 15,000 each.

From 1977 onwards Dr Albert Parlow used a far less crude preparation method on frozen glands exclusively to make hGH at the University of California Research Institute at Harbor General Hospital, Torrance.

Britain: The Human Growth Hormone Program began in 1959 as a Medical Research Council hGH trial. It continued for 17 years and treated 642 children. In 1977 the Department of Health and Social Services (DHSS) took over the program, hGH became an officially endorsed therapy for pituitary dwarves and another 1,243 children were treated until mid-1985. Over the 26 years of the program about 960,000 pituitaries were collected from cadavers at many hospitals and public mortuaries. No specific exclusion criteria ever applied to glands stored in acetone. From 1976, glands to be frozen were excluded only if taken from a body more than 96 hours after death, taken from an embalmed body, or taken from a patient suffering from hepatitis, sepsis, meningitis, encephalitis or multiple sclerosis. Injecting drug users, organ transplant and patients who had been on kidney dialysis were also excluded.

Pituitary glands were processed at three main centres:

1   At the University of Cambridge, biochemist Dr Anne Stockell Hartree made hGH between 1963 and 1980 from acetone-stored glands. From 1968 she devised her own method refined from that of Wilhelmi. As many as 30,000 powdered pituitaries were processed at once.

2   In a laboratory at St Bartholomew's Hospital in London, Dr Philip Lowry refined the extraction method of Swedish biochemist, Paul Roos, by adding an ion-exchange step and an isoelectic precipitation step. He extracted hGH from two batches per month, each of 800 frozen glands between 1975 and 1980.

3   From 1980 to 1985 hGH production switched to the Centre for Applied Microbiological Research (CAMR) at Porton Down where hGH was made from acetone-stored glands, in a further refinement of the Hartree-Wilhelmi process, as well as from frozen glands.

Australia: A group of academic researchers, the Victorian Pituitary Group, produced hGH and hPG from two Melbourne hospitals in the early 1960s. Two of them, Dr James Brown, an original member of the Gonadotrophin Club of Europe and Dr Kevin Catt, extracted both hormones from acetone-stored glands, in their Brown/Catt method. Glands were excluded from infectious diseases cases. Simultaneously, scientists Ken Ferguson and Alan Wallace, while researching the influence of pituitary hormones on wool growth in sheep at the Commonwealth Scientific and Industrial Research Organisation, separated human hPG and hGH for use by doctors. In 1966 Commonwealth Serum Laboratories (CSL), using the Ferguson method, began collecting glands from morgues, at the request of the Federal Government which was to sponsor both hGH and hPG. Glands were excluded any from people who had died of viral infections like hepatitis, malignant disease, septicaemia or obvious disease of the gland. This was later updated to include "pre-senile dementia (CJD)".

From 1967, the official start of the Australian Human Pituitary Hormone Program, until 1985, in the biggest program of its type in the world, more than 1,400 women and 62 men were treated with hPG. More than 700 children received hGH. About 170,000 glands were collected in total, an average of 8,500 annually from public hospitals, repatriation hospitals for returned soldiers and their families, and morgues. New Zealand's Chapman production method was introduced in 1984. Glands mixed with Australian supplies, were also sent from New Zealand and Mauritius, and, apparently Papua New Guinea, for periods during the AHPHP.

Canada: The Medical Research Council of Canada began a therapeutic trial of hGH in 1967. Doctors in Montreal collected pituitaries and sent them to Raben who processed them into hGH. Later glands were sent locally for processing at two main centres:

1   Dr Henry Friesen's laboratory at the University of Manitoba.

2   The laboratory of Dr Michel Chrétien in Montreal.

Pituitary gland collections rose to 15,000 per year in the late 1970s.

France: hGH extracted via the Raben method began in 1959. Production between 1973 and 1975 was carried out in several academic laboratories using refined versions. From 1973 pituitaries were collected through the Association France-Hypophyse and from 1975 hGH was extracted in a laboratory at the Pasteur Institute under a refined Roos method and later via the British Lowry method. Gland collection fell so short of demand that by the early 1980s commercial suppliers Kabi, Nordisk and Serono supplied half the hGH given to French patients. At FF350 per ampoule, it was far more expensive than the locally produced equivalent which cost FF200.

Between 1973 and 1988 almost 200,000 pituitaries were collected for local French production — two-thirds of them in France. Half the glands collected between 1983 and 1988 came from Bulgaria and Hungary where exclusion criteria were said to include patients with hepatitis, meningitis, encephalitis, multiple sclerosis, infectious diseases, malignancies, transplanted organs and injecting drug users. After the CJD deaths in 1985, France opted to continue manufacturing cadaver-derived hGH, as did several other countries. All patients were switched to synthetic hGH in 1988.

New Zealand: In 1964 a national pituitary bank was established which began annual collections of up to 2,000 glands per year from 21 morgues. Dr James Brown in Melbourne processed both hGH and hPG from some of these acetone-stored glands. Simultaneously, under a deal struck between local endocrinologists friendly with Wilhelmi of Emory University, Wilhelmi processed hGH and hPG at no cost from glands airmailed to him from New Zealand. He kept any other hormones that were extracted. His 1975 retirement marked the end of the deal. New Zealand turned to Australia for the production of both miracle drugs as a stop-gap measure until its own hormone production could be established. Between 1976 and 1978, 4,518 New Zealand glands, some of them mixed with Australian batches by CSL, were sent back for use in New Zealand. By this time 90 local children had been treated with Wilhelmi or Brown hGH. From 1978 hGH was extracted from frozen glands using the Chapman method at the New Zealand National Hormone Laboratory at the University of Auckland and was injected into another 94 local children. Between 1964 and 1985 about 150 New Zealanders used hPG made variously at Emory University, by James Brown in Melbourne, by CSL in Australia and locally. A total of about 51,000 glands were collected between 1964 and 1984 with no incentive payments to mortuary attendants.

Israel: In a laboratory at the Tel Aviv University, hGH was made from acetone-stored glands, collected indiscriminately from morgues, and processed via the Raben extraction method. From 1974 to 1992, long after most countries had abandoned human pituitary glands for synthetically-produced hGH, Israel continued with cadaver-derived hGH. After Kabi's Crescormon was withdrawn worldwide in 1985, Israeli endocrinologists continued to use other brands of commercially-prepared hGH until the final switch to the synthetic drug in 1992. Between 1964 and 1992, a total of 199 children were treated with cadaver-derived hGH.

Hong Kong: One of the small Government-sponsored programs in various countries which used commercial hGH exclusively until the switch to synthetic hGH after CJD deaths. Between 1978 and 1985 19 hGH-deficient Chinese children were injected three times weekly with Crescormon, on a program run from Queen Mary Hospital made from glands collected in Hong Kong and sent to Sweden for processing.

Cast of characters

ALLARS, Margaret: Sydney administrative law expert who wrote the 815-page report of the Inquiry into the Use of Pituitary Derived Hormones in Australia and Creutzfeldt-Jakob disease.

ALLENDER Jane: First person in the world to die from CJD after hPG infertility treatment in 1988.

ALPERS, Michael: Australian director of the Papua New Guinea Institute of Medical Research who continues to monitor the last cases of the disastrous kuru epidemic which wiped out more than 3,000 villagers in the eastern highlands.

APQ: Australian hPG recipient test case, whose settlement with the Australian Federal Government on the eve of a $1 million four-month civil trial for nervous shock related to her fear of contracting CJD, led to a Senate inquiry.

BODY, David: Welsh Sheffield-based solicitor who spearheaded Britain's CJD Litigation for hGH recipients.

BRODRICK, Geraldine: Mother of the world's only medically recorded set of nontuplets, born after hPG therapy in Sydney, Australia, June 13, 1971.

BROWN, Paul: Neuroscientist, Francophile, medical director of the laboratory of Central Nervous System Studies at the NIH and one of Gajdusek's closest friends.

CREUTZFELDT, Hans Gerhard: German neuropsychiatrist whose 1920 report on a girl with strange neurological symptoms led to his name, perhaps erroneously, being joined with Jakob's to describe a relentless degenerative disease of the brain and central nervous system characterised by microscopic spongy holes.

DAISY, GEORGETTE & JOANNE: First three chimpanzees who died of kuru, thus proving it was a transmissible disease.

DICKINSON, Alan: British geneticist, scrapie expert and founding director of Edinburgh's Neuropathogenesis Unit.

DRAY, Ferdinand: Head of hGH production at the Pasteur Institute.

GAJDUSEK, Daniel Carleton: Eccentric paediatrician and scientist whose studies on kuru won him the 1976 Nobel Prize in medicine.

GEMZELL, Carl Axel: Swedish gynaecologist who first trialed hPG on non-ovulating women in 1958.

GIBBS, Clarence Joseph: Medical microbiologist and Gajdusek's colleague at the NIH who supervised transmission experiments of kuru and CJD in primates.

HADLOW, William: American veterinary pathologist who first recognised similarities between scrapie and kuru.

HALFORD, Jenny: Third Australian woman who died of CJD in 1990 while living in England. Her condition was linked to her hPG only through a bizarre coincidence.

HINTZ, Raymond: Professor of endocrinology at Stanford University who first linked the death of Joe Rodriguez to his hGH therapy.

IRONSIDE, James: Edinburgh neuropathologist who confirmed that uniform "florid" plaques ringed by spongiform change in the brains of nvCJD victims was a new entity.

JAKOB, Alfons: German neuropsychiatrist who reported the first authentic cases of CJD in 1921, followed by a case of familial CJD in 1923.

JOB, Jean-Claude: President of France-Hypophyse which oversaw the French hGH program.

LAY, Alison: First English victim of CJD in 1985 after childhood hGH injection whose death in 1985 forced the shut down of the Human Grown Hormone Program in Britain.

LAZARUS, Leslie: Chairman of the Human Pituitary Advisory Committee (HPAC) which oversaw the 19-year long Australian Human Pituitary Hormone Program.

LOWRY, Philip: British biochemist who produced hGH from frozen pituitary glands in a London laboratory between 1975 and 1980.

McKENZIE, Deborah: First New Zealand victim of hGH, imported from America, in 1987.

NESOM, Richard: American Catholic priest given a dura mater implant in 1985, who unsuccessfully sued the manufacturer over his fear of CJD contraction and was eventually diagnosed with probable CJD in 1997.

NORROY, Isabelle: Youngest CJD victim in the world, aged 10, and among the first French hGH recipients to die of CJD in 1991.

RABEN, Maurice: Pioneer of hGH production who first successfully trialed hGH on a human patient in 1958.

RODRIGUEZ, Joseph: First victim in the world to die of CJD following hGH therapy in 1984.

ROOS, Paul: Swedish biochemist whose refined method of hormone extraction was adopted and modified by many manufacturers.

STOCKELL HARTREE, Anne: American biochemist who manufactured British hGH from acetone-stored pituitary glands at a University of Cambridge laboratory between 1963 and 1979.

WILL, Robert: Scottish neurologist and head of the CJD Surveillance Unit in Edinburgh. Warned experts of an alarming number of cases of atypical CJD in young people in Britain in 1996.

ZIGAS, Vincent: Australian doctor based in Papua New Guinea who made first official report of kuru.

Chronology

1913	Bertha E examined by Hans Creutzfeldt.
1920	Creutzfeldt's paper on Bertha published.
1921	Alfons Jakob's paper on four cases of "spastic pseudo-sclerosis" published.
1923	Familial CJD first identified by Jakob.
1935	Louping-ill vaccine accident in Scotland.
1936	Josef Gerstmann, Ernst Straüssler and Isaak Scheinker publish case report on patient with GSS.
1940s	Experiments reveal scrapie "agent" not entirely destroyed by heating in an autoclave.
1947	First outbreak of Transmissible Mink Encephalopathy.
1956	Zigas makes first official report to PNG health authorities on kuru.
1958	Maurice Raben publishes report of first successful trial of hGH on human patient. Carl Axel Gemzell reports success of hPG on non-ovulating women in Sweden.
1959	In *Lancet* letter William Hadlow recognises similarities between scrapie and kuru. Britain begins trial of hGH on children and hPG on infertile women.
1960	In *Brain* Sam Nevin presents eight patients with "subacute spongiform encephalopathy".
1965	Lawson quins born in New Zealand and thrive. First monograph on slow virus infections produced by Gajdusek, Gibbs and Alpers.
1966	*Nature* paper describes kuru transmission to primates, proving it is infectious.
1967	*Nature* article by Tikvah Alper asks "does the scrapie agent replicate without nucleic acid?" Official start of Australian Human Pituitary Hormone Program.
1968	*Science* paper on CJD records first transmission of CJD to chimpanzees, proving it is infectious.
1969	*Science* paper reveals CJD can be "passaged" through a number of chimpanzees.
1971	Brodrick nontuplets born in Sydney. None survive. Kabi Pharmacia begins production of commercial hGH called Crescormon.
1974	*New England Journal of Medicine* letter reports first case of CJD transmission via corneal graft. *Journal of Neurosurgery* article by Gajdusek advises on autopsy and biopsy precautions for patients with CJD..
1975	*Journal of Clinical Pathology* republishes Gajdusek's precautions to quell fears of pathologists.
1977	*Lancet* letter reveals two cases of CJD transmission via depth electrodes used on epilepsy patients.

Science publishes Gajdusek's Nobel lecture, which contains warning of CJD via tissue transplantation.

1978   In *New England Journal of Medicine* Gajdusek publishes precautions for caring for and handling of material from patients with CJD.

1979   In *Annals of Neurology* paper, Colin Masters and colleagues review Nevin's cases which reveal a cluster of CJD in three patients operated on by the same neurosurgeon in the same hospital. Australia is also included on map of the known world incidence of CJD.

1980   First report of third animal TSE–chronic wasting disease of mule deer and elk.

1982   In the *Journal of Neurology, Neurosurgery and Psychiatry* Robert Will reveals that the three Nevin patients almost certainly contracted CJD in the 1950s from contaminated neurosurgical instruments.

American neurologist Stanley Prusiner commits biological heresy by proposing that corrupted proteins "prions", and not a virus, cause TSEs.

1984   *American Journal of Medicine* reports cases of CJD in people who eat squirrel brains.

Death of Joe Rodriguez, world's first CJD victim following hGH therapy.

1985   Deaths of two more American hGH recipients and Alison Lay, first British recipient of hGH to die of CJD.

Shut downs of Government-sponsored human hormone drug programs in most countries. Kabi stops production of Crescormon.

America starts tracing hGH recipients.

Kent vet, Colin Whitaker, visits farm to find initial case of strange new disease in cows in Britain.

World's first licence for biosynthetic hGH granted in Britain.

1986   *Veterinary Record* reports on new disease in cattle called Bovine Spongiform Encephalopathy.

New England Journal of Medicine article describes FFI as fourth human TSE.

1987   *Morbidity and Mortality Weekly* issues first warning about dura mater after apparent CJD transmission within 18 months of graft.

1988   Jane Allender becomes first person in the world to die of CJD, 13 years after hPG treatment.

British Medical Journal letter begins decade-long debate warning of threat to human health from BSE.

1989   Jan Blight dies 16 years after failed treatment with hPG.

CJD symptoms appear in two French hGH recipients aged 10 and 11.

Official confirmation through molecular genetics that TSEs are both infectious and inheritable.

Disgraced Canadian sprinter Ben Johnson admits taking hGH in lead up to Seoul Olympics.

1990   Jenny Halford dies in England after treatment in Melbourne 14 years earlier with hPG.

1991   Vonda Cummings dies of CJD following unsuccessful hPG injections 15 years earlier.

Peter Costello raises CJD in Australian Federal Parliament and proposes compensation.

Journal of Neurology, Neurosurgery and Psychiatry report on death of Brian Bowler, British dura mater recipient, prompts lapsing of Britain's 20-year licence to import Lyodura®.

Lancet article by Brown and Gajdusek warns against burying BSE cattle without first incinerating remains after experiment with scrapie brain solution shows infective agent still lethal to hamsters after burial for three years.

Lancet article by London neurologist, John Collinge, suggestions genetic predisposition to TSEs through PRNP gene mutations.

"Stephen", Australia's only hGH recipient to contract probable CJD, dies in Sydney.

Brazilian hGH recipient death from CJD reported.

1992   *Le Monde* article on Jean-Philippe Mathieu reveals 10 French hGH recipients are dead from CJD.

Today newspaper series on "Timebomb children" reveals similar hGH death toll in Britain.

Lancet letter by Dumble and Klein claims Australian Government keeping hPG-treated women in the dark about CJD risk.

New England Journal of Medicine report indicates a pregnant Japanese woman who died of CJD had infective brain, placenta, umbilical cord and colostrum in animal transmission experiments. Child still well.

1993   Blight and Cummings' CJD deaths revealed by Australian Federal Government.

Margaret Allars appointed to head inquiry into AHPHP and CJD.

Husbands of Australian women who died of CJD launch legal action for compensation while living hPG recipient, APQ, lodges writ for nervous shock over fear of contraction.

French magistrate launches investigation for involuntary homicide on French hGH program chiefs.

1994   Allars report reveals breached ethics, broken guidelines, and bent rules among litany of faults in a damning report on AHPHP.

Granada TV's "World in Action" documents hGH tragedy. It is seen by at least two hGH recipients who diagnose themselves with CJD.

Families of dead Australian women negotiate compensation settlement.

1995   Recalls of blood products in Canada following scares about CJD infection from donors.

First two teenage cases of nvCJD referred to mystified CJDSU.

1996   March 20 announcement that 10 cases of CJD in people under 42 in Britain must be linked to BSE.

EU places worldwide ban on British beef products.

Gajdusek arrested in America on paedophilia charges.

Neurology report reveals seventh FFI family in the world in Queensland, Australia.

CJD Litigation judgement finds negligence by British Government but only after July 1, 1977.

Four more deaths in New Zealanders treated with American-imported hGH, including one with a 30-year incubation period.

1997   APQ settles nervous shock case with Australian Federal Government after legal aid refused.

Gajdusek jailed after pleading guilty to child sexual abuse.

Stanley Prusiner wins Nobel Prize in medicine.

Nature article reveals final proof that scrapie is not solely an inherited sheep disease.

Nature article reveals best evidence that BSE causes nvCJD.

Neurology report reveals eighth FFI family lives in Victoria, Australia.

Australian Federal Government settles damages case with living woman merely suspected of having CJD following hPG treatment in 1971.

Britain bans all cuts of beef on the bone, including steaks.

High Court judge allows British "well but worried" recipients of hGH treated after July 1, 1977, to sue for compensation.

Britain announces independent judicial inquiry into BSE epidemic.

1998   Illegal use of hGH by elite athletes grabs world attention when a female Chinese swimmer is banned from the World Swimming Championships in Perth, Australia, after hGH found by chance in her luggage in a customs check.

Endnotes

Chapter 1
Kuru: The shivering sickness

1 D. Gajdusek & J. Farquhar (eds), *Kuru: Early Letters and Field-notes from the Collection of D Carleton Gajdusek*, Raven Press, New York, 1976, p. 54.
2 Gajdusek & Farquhar (eds), *Kuru*, p. 57.
3 These types of diseases, triggered by an infection or a genetic abnormality, progress by the action of the body's own immune system attacking itself.
4 V. Zigas, *Laughing Death — the Untold Story of Kuru*, Humana Press, 1990, p. 227.
5 Zigas, *Laughing Death*, p. 226.
6 Gajdusek & Farquhar (eds), *Kuru*, Introduction xxii.
7 Zigas, *Laughing Death*, Foreword vi.
8 D. Gajdusek (ed.), *Correspondence on the Discovery and Original Investigations on Kuru, Smadel-Gajdusek Correspondence, 1955–1958*, NIH, Bethesda, Maryland, 1975, p. 50.
9 Australia granted PNG independence in 1975.
10 Gajdusek & Farquhar (eds), *Kuru*, p. 41.
11 Gajdusek & Farquhar (eds), *Kuru*, p. 41.
12 Gajdusek & Farquhar (eds), *Kuru*, p. 42.
13 Gajdusek & Farquhar (eds), *Kuru*, p. 31.
14 Gajdusek (ed.), *Smadel-Gajdusek correspondence*, p. 88.
15 In Gajdusek's archival cinefilm footage of kuru victims, available at the National Library of Medicine on the campus of the National Institutes of Health in Bethesda, Maryland, kuru victims are a tragic sight seen smiling at first broadly, then hesitantly while trying vainly to balance on one foot. One male cannot bring a cigarette to his lips properly. Inability to perform these simple tasks indicates a neurological problem.
16 M. Alpers, Interview with author, December 1996.
17 D. Gajdusek, "Unconventional viruses and the origin and disappearance of kuru", *Science*, 1977, vol. 197: pp. 943–960.
18 S. Prusiner, D. Gajdusek, M. Alpers, "Kuru with incubation periods exceeding two decades", *Annals of Neurology*, 1982, vol. 12, pp. 1–9.
19 M. Alpers, Interview with author, December 1996.
20 Zigas, *Laughing Death*, p. 251.
21 Zigas, *Laughing Death*, p. 253.
22 I. Klatzo, D. Gajdusek, V. Zigas, *Pathology of Kuru*, Laboratory Investigation, 1959, vol. 8, pp. 799–847.
23 Klatzo, Gajdusek, Zigas, *Pathology of Kuru*, pp. 799–847.
24 M. Alpers, Interview with author, December 1996.
25 S. Lindenbaum, *Kuru Sorcery: Disease and Danger in the New Guinea Highlands*, Mayfield Publishing Company, 1979, p. 20.

26 Lindenbaum, *Kuru Sorcery,* p. 19.
27 M. Alpers, Interview with author, December 1996.
28 Anon., "'Concentration Camp' Attempt to Combat N. G. Disease", *Sydney Morning Herald*, May 23, 1960.
29 M. Alpers, Interview with author, December 1996.
30 D. Gajdusek, C. Gibbs, M. Alpers, "Slow, latent and temperate virus infections", *National Institute of Neurological Diseases and Blindness Monograph,* 1965, vol. 2, pp. 65–82.
31 M. Alpers, "Kuru: implications of its transmissibility for the interpretation of its changing epidemiological pattern, The Central Nervous System, Some Experimental Models of Neurological Disease", *International Academy of Pathology monograph no 9,* Proceedings of the fifty-sixth annual meeting of the International Academy of Pathology, Washington DC, March 12–15, 1967, Williams and Wilkins, Baltimore, 1968, pp. 234–251.
32 M. Alpers, "Reflections and Highlights: A Life with Kuru", *Prion Diseases of Humans and Animals,* Ellis Horwood, New York, 1992, pp. 66-75.
33 D. Gajdusek, "Unconventional viruses and the origin and disappearance of kuru", *Science,* 1977, vol. 197, pp. 943–960.
34 R. Klitzman, M. Alpers, D. Gajdusek, "The natural incubation period of kuru and the episodes of transmission in three clusters of patients", *Neuroepidemiology,* 1984, vol. 3, pp. 3–20.
35 Names were abbreviated for publication in the Klitzman paper.
36 Klitzman, Alpers, Gajdusek, "The natural incubation period of kuru and the episodes of transmission in three clusters of patients", pp. 3–20.
37 S. Prusiner, D. Gajdusek, M. Alpers, "Kuru with incubation periods exceeding two decades", *Annals of Neurology,* 1982, vol. 12, pp. 1–9.

Chapter 2
Creutzfeldt and Jakob: German pathfinders

1 H. Creutzfeldt, "On a particular focal disease of the central nervous system (preliminary communication)", *Zeitschrift fur die gesamte Neurologie und Psychiatrie,* 1920, vol. 57, pp. 1–18. Translated by E. P. Richardson Jr.
2 Creutzfeldt, "On a particular focal disease of the central nervous system (preliminary communication)", p. 1.
3 A. Jakob, "Concerning a disorder of the central nervous system clinically resembling multiple sclerosis with remarkable anatomic findings (spastic pseudosclerosis)", report of a fourth case, *Medizinische Klinik,* 1921, vol. 17, pp. 372–376. Translated by E.P. Richardson Jr.
4 C. Masters, D. Gajdusek, "The spectrum of Creutzfeldt-Jakob disease and the virus-induced subacute spongiform encephalopathies", in *Recent Advances in Neuropathology,* W. Thomas Smith & J. Cavanagh (eds) No. 2, Churchill Livingstone, New York, 1982, Ch. 6, pp 139–163.
5 S. Nevin, W. NcMenemey, S. Behrman, D. Jones, "Subacute spongiform encephalopathy — a subacute form of encephalopathy attributable to vascular dysfunction (spongiform cerebral atrophy)", *Brain,* 1960, vol. 83, part 4, pp. 519–563.

6   A. Jakob, "Spasticshe Psuedosklerosis", in *Monographien aus dem Geramtgebiere der Neurolgie und Psychiatrie 37*, O. Foerster, K. Wilmhans (eds). Julius Springer, Berlin, 1923, p 215.

7   P. Brown, "The brave new world of transmissible spongiform encephalopathy (infectious cerebral amyloidosis)", *Molecular Neurobiology,* 1994, vol. 8, pp. 79–87.

Chapter 3
Scrapie: The trouble with sheep
1   H. Parry, "Scrapie disease in sheep", in *Historical, Clinical, Epidemiological, Pathological and Practical Aspects of the Natural Disease,* D. Oppenheimer (ed.), Academic Press, 1983, vol. 44, p. 169.

2   A. Brash, "Scrapie in imported sheep in New Zealand", *New Zealand Veterinary Journal,* 1952, vol. 1, pp. 27–30.

3   Parry, "Scrapie disease in sheep", p. 51.

4   L. Bull, D. Murnane, "An outbreak of scrapie in British sheep imported into Victoria", *Australian Veterinary Journal,* 1958, vol. 34, pp. 213–215.

5   N. Hunter, "Genotyping and susceptibility of sheep to scrapie", in *Methods in Molecular Medicine Series: Prion Diseases,* H. Bailey, R. Ridley (eds), Humana Press, 1996, p. 211.

6   H. Fraser, Report for CJD litigation held in the High Court, London. April–May 1996.

7   Fraser, Report for CJD litigation, 1996.

8   G. Hartsough, D. Burger, "Encephalopathy of mink: epizootiologic and clinical observations", *Journal of Infectious Diseases,* 1965, vol. 115, pp. 387–392.

9   Hartsough, Burger, "Encephalopathy of mink", pp. 387–392.

10   Hartsough, Burger, "Encephalopathy of mink", pp. 387–392.

11   J. Swanson, *Bovine Spongiform Encephalopathy: Special Reference Briefs,* Animal Welfare Information Center, United State Department of Agriculture, 1990.

12   K. Mulvaney, "Mad cows and the colonies", *The Environmental Magazine,* 1995.

13   Parry, "Scrapie disease in sheep", pp. 43, 56.

14   Formaldehyde is a chemical disinfectant that renders proteins useless. A decent whiff of its acrid small can make your eyes water, and a large dose can cause lung collapse.

15   N. Hunter, D. Cairns, J. Foster, Smith G, W. Goldmann, K. Donnelly, "Is scrapie solely a genetic disease?", *Nature,* 1997, vol. 86, p. 137.

16   E. Williams, S. Young, "Chronic wasting disease of captive mule deer: a spongiform encephalopathy", *Journal of Wildlife Diseases,* 1980, vol. 16, pp. 89–98.

17   A. Dickinson, G. Outram, D. Taylor, J. Foster, "Further evidence that scrapie agent has an independent genome", in *Proceedings of 1986 Paris Symposium: Unconventional Virus Diseases of the Central Nervous System,* L. Court et al. (eds), Atelier d'Arts Graphiques, Abbaye de Melleray, France, 1988.

Chapter 4
Kuru and scrapie: The breakthrough

1   W. Hadlow, "Historical reflections—The scrapie-kuru connection: recollections of how it came about", in *Prion Diseases of Animals and Humans,* S. Prusiner, J. Collinge, J. Powell, B. Anderton, (eds), E. Horwood (publ.), 1992, pp. 40–46.
2   Hadlow, "Historical reflections—The scrapie-kuru connection", pp. 40–46.
3   W. Hadlow, "Scrapie and kuru", *Lancet,* September 5, 1959, pp. 289–290.
4   Hadlow, "Scrapie and kuru", pp. 289–290.
5   Letter from Gajdusek to Hadlow, August 6, 1959, in *Prion Diseases of Animals and Humans,* S. Prusiner, J. Collinge, J. Powell, B. Anderton, (eds), E. Horwood (publ.), 1992, p. 52.
6   I. Klatzo, D. Gajdusek, V. Zigas, *Pathology of Kuru,* Laboratory Investigation, 1959, vol. 8, pp. 799–847.
7   C. Kriss, "Hormone injections help youth grow despite pituitary problem", *Detroit Morning Sun,* New Center News, September 11, 1978.
8   M. Raben, "Treatment of a pituitary dwarf with human growth hormone", *Journal of Clinical Endocrinology and Metabolism,* 1958, vol. 18, pp. 901–903.
9   N. Pfeffer, *The Stork and the Syringe. A Political History of Reproductive Medicine,* Polity Press, 1993, pp. 144–145.
10 Pfeffer, *The Stork and the Syringe,* pp. 144–145.
11 Pfeffer, *The Stork and the Syringe,* pp. 146.
12 M. Allars, *Report of the Inquiry into the Use of Pituitary Derived Hormones in Australia and Creutzfeldt-Jakob Disease,* Australian Government Publishing Service, 1994, p. 154.
13 C. Li, H. Papkoff, "Preparation and properties of growth hormone from human and monkey pituitary glands", *Science,* 1956, vol. 124, pp. 1293–1294.
14 A. Stockell Hartree, "Preparation and properties of human growth hormone", in *Human Growth Hormone,* A Mason (ed.), William Heinemann Medical Books Limited, 1972.
15 P. Roos, Report for CJD litigation, High Court, London, 1996.
16 L. Lazarus, The results of growth hormone therapy in Australia, Patient Management Symposium, Garvan Institute of Medical Research, St Vincent's Hospital, Sydney, 1979, pp. 20–23.
17 C. Gemzell, Report for CJD litigation, High Court, London, 1995.
18 C. Gemzell, Report for CJD litigation, 1995.
19 Pfeffer, *The Stork and the Syringe,* pp. 146.
20 K. Hall, Report for CJD litigation. High Court, London, 1996.
21 P. Roos, Report for CJD litigation, 1996.
22 Dr Louis Lo, Interview with author, November 1993.
23 Hall, Report for CJD litigation, 1996.
24 O. Trygstad, Evidence during the CJD litigation, High Court, London, April 1996.
25 O. Trygstad, Evidence during the CJD litigation, April 1996.
26 O. Trygstad, Evidence during the CJD litigation, April 1996.

27 L. Hunt, "GPs asked to help trace 300 women", *Independent,* September
    2, 1993.
    P. Pallot, "'Mad cow' risk facing 300 fertility drug women", *Telegraph,*
    September 2, 1993.
28 P. Pallot, "Fertility treatment 'killed my mother'", *Daily Telegraph,*
    September 4, 1993.
29 Anon., "Another set of quins: mothers had hormones", *Sydney Morning
    Herald,* July 30, 1965.
30 G. Liggins, H. Ibbertson, "A successful quintuplet pregnancy following
    treatment with human pituitary gonadotrophin", *Lancet,* January 15,
    1966, pp. 114–117.
31 A. Dupree, "Quin scene: triplets next", *Woman's Day,* August 23, 1965,
    pp. 4–5.
32 Anon., "Quins born to New Zealand woman, doctors say all well",
    Sydney Morning Herald, July 28, 1965.
33 Liggins, Ibbertson, "A successful quintuplet pregnancy following
    treatment with human pituitary gonadotrophin", pp. 114–117.
34 Anon., "Mother was hormone test 'guinea-pig'", *Daily Telegraph,* July
    30, 1965.
35 Allars, *Report of the inquiry into the Use of Pituitary Derived Hormones,*
    p. 162.
36 J. Moore, "Fertility test shock", *Australian Associated Press,* July 30,
    1965.
37 P. Brown, M. Preece, R. Will, "'Friendly fire' in medicine: hormone,
    homografts and Creutzfeldt-Jakob disease", *Lancet,* 1992, vol. 340, pp.
    24–27.
38 Allars, *Report of the Inquiry into the Use of Pituitary Derived Hormones,*
    p. 167.
39 Pfeffer. *The Stork and the Syringe,* pp. 147.
40 Anon., "Group asks for use of pituitary glands'. *Seattle Times,* September
    25, 1975.
41 Allars, *Report of the Inquiry into the Use of Pituitary Derived Hormones,*
    p. 74.
42 O. Trygstad, Personal communication, December 1997.
43 M. Alpers, Interview with author, December 1996.
44 D. Gajdusek, C. Gibbs, M. Alpers (eds), "Slow, latent and temperate
    virus infections", *National Institute of Neurological Diseases and
    Blindness Monograph No. 2,* Washington DC, US Government Printing
    Office, 1965, vol. 2, pp. 65–82.
45 D. Gajdusek, C. Gibbs, M. Alpers, "Experimental transmission of a kuru-
    like syndrome to chimpanzees", *Nature,* 1966, vol. 209, pp. 794–796.
46 M. Alpers, Interview with author, December 1996.
47 C. Gibbs, "Historical reflections—Spongiform encephalopathies — Slow,
    latent, and temperate virus infections — in retrospect", in *Prion Diseases
    of Humans and Animals,* S. Prusiner, J. Collinge, J. Powell, B. Anderton,
    (eds), E. Horwood (publ.), 1992, pp. 53–62.
48 M. Alpers, Interview with author, December 1996.
49 M. Alpers, Interview with author, December 1996.
50 C. Gibbs, "Historical reflections—Spongiform encephalopathies", pp.
    53–62.

51 Gajdusek, Gibbs, Alpers, "Experimental transmission of a kuru-like syndrome to chimpanzees", pp. 794–796.
52 M. Alpers, Interview with author, December 1996.
53 Gajdusek, Gibbs, Alpers, "Experimental transmission of a kuru-like syndrome to chimpanzees", pp. 794–796.
54 Gajdusek, Gibbs, Alpers, "Experimental transmission of a kuru-like syndrome to chimpanzees", pp. 794–796.
55 E. Beck, P. Daniel, M. Alpers, D. Gajdusek, C. Gibbs, Preliminary communication, "Experimental 'kuru' in chimpanzees. A pathological Report", *Lancet,* 1966, vol. 2, pp. 1056–1059.
56 P. Brown, Interview with author, June 1996.
57 W. Matthews, Report of Creutzfeldt-Jakob disease in recipients of human growth hormone, Incorporated into transcript of CJD litigation, London High Court, April–May 1996.
58 C. Gibbs, D. Gajdusek, D. Asher, M. Alpers, E. Beck, P. Daniel, W. Matthews, "Creutzfeldt-Jakob disease (spongiform encephalopathies): transmission to the chimpanzee", *Science,* 1968, vol. 161, p. 388.
59 C. Gibbs, D.Gajdusek, "Infection as the etiology of spongiform encephalopathy (Creutzfeldt-Jakob disease)", *Science,* 1969, vol. 165, pp. 1023–1025.
60 M. Alpers, Personal correspondence, April 1997.
61 P. Brown, Interview with author, June 1996.
62 D. Gajdusek, "Unconventional viruses causing subacute spongiform encephalopathies", in *Virology,* B. Fields (ed.) Raven Press, New York, 1990, pp. 2289–2324.
63 Gajdusek, "Unconventional viruses causing subacute spongiform encephalopathies", pp. 2289–2324.

Chapter 5
And then there were nine

1   G. Brodrick, Interview with author, August 1994.
2   Letter of Professor H. Carey to G. Brodrick, January 15, 1971.
3   Brodrick, Interview with author, August 1994.
4   Brodrick, Interview with author, February 1997.
5   Channel 7 interview with Len Brodrick, June 11, 1971.
6   Brodrick, Interview with author, February 1997.
7   Channel 7 News footage of press conference, June 13, 1971.
8   Anon., "Doctors fear for three more babies", *Daily Telegraph,* June 15, 1971.
9   Brodrick, Interview with author, February 1997.
10 J. Parsons, "The Brodrick story. 'I felt it wasn't only our loss.'", *Woman's Day,* August 30, 1971.
11 G. Brodrick, Interview with author, August 1994.
12 Anon., "Drug reaction causes worry", *Daily Telegraph,* June 15, 1971.
13 M. Allars, *Report of the Inquiry into the Use of Pituitary Derived Hormones in Australia and Creutzfeldt-Jakob Disease,* Australian Government Publishing Service, June 1994, p. 210.
14 Allars, *Report of the Inquiry into the Use of Pituitary Derived Hormones,* June 1994, p. 211.

15 Allars, *Report of the Inquiry into the Use of Pituitary Derived Hormones,* June 1994, p. 211.
16 H. Carey, "Induction of ovulation resulting in nontuplet pregnancy", *Australian and New Zealand Journal of Obstetrics and Gynaecology,* 1976, vol. 16, p. 200.
17 Allars, *Report of the Inquiry into the Use of Pituitary Derived Hormones,* June 1994, p. 211.
18 Allars, *Report of the Inquiry into the Use of Pituitary Derived Hormones,* June 1994, p. 208.
19 P. Durisch, "Pill doctor hits out at red tape", *Sunday Telegraph,* August 29, 1971.
20 Allars, *Report of the Inquiry into the Use of Pituitary Derived Hormones,* June 1994, p. 209.
21 Brodrick, Interview with author, August 1994.
22 I. Fraser, "Secondary amenorrhoea", *Medical Journal of Australia,* 1977, vol. 2, pp. 415–416.

Chapter 6
Lethal gifts from medical science

1   P. Duffy, J. Wolf, G. Collins, A. DeVoe, B. Streeten, D. Cowen, "Possible person-to-person transmission of Creutzfeldt-Jakob disease", *New England Journal of Medicine,* 1974, vol. 299, 692–693.
2   P. Liberski, R. Yanagihara, C. Gibbs, D. Gajdusek, "Spread of Creutzfeldt-Jakob disease virus along visual pathways after intraocular inoculation", *Archives of Virology,* 1990, pp. 111, 141–147.
3   M. McKimmie, "Need for baby led to death", *West Australian,* May 19, 1993.
4   M. Allars, *Report of the Inquiry into the Use of Pituitary Derived Hormones in Australia and Creutzfeldt-Jakob Disease,* Australian Government Publishing Service, 1994, p. 153.
5   Allars, *Report of the Inquiry into the Use of Pituitary Derived Hormones,* June 1994, p. 187.
6   Allars, *Report of the Inquiry into the Use of Pituitary Derived Hormones,* June 1994, p. 201–202.
7   Allars, *Report of the Inquiry into the Use of Pituitary Derived Hormones,* June 1994, p. 202–203.
8   Allars, *Report of the Inquiry into the Use of Pituitary Derived Hormones,* June 1994, p. 203.
9   J. Cooke, "Woman confirmed as fourth CJD victim", *Sydney Morning Herald,* May 1, 1993.
10 P. Tuohy, Letters, *Sydney Morning Herald,* February 11, 1993.
11 R. Traub, D. Gajdusek, C. Gibbs, "Precautions in conducting biopsies and autopsies on patients with presenile dementia", technical note, *Journal of Neurosurgery,* 1974, vol. 41, pp. 394–395.
12 W. Schoene, C. Masters, C. Gibbs, D. Gajdusek, H. Tyler, F. Moore, G. Dammin, "Transmissible spongiform encephalopathy (Creutzfeldt-Jakob disease). Atypical clinical and pathological findings", *Archives of Neurology,* 1981, vol. 38, pp. 473–477.
13 R. Traub, D. Gajdusek, C. Gibbs, "Precautions in autopsies on Creutzfeldt-Jakob disease", *American Journal of Clinical Pathology,* 1975, vol. 64, p. 287.

14 E. Allender, Interview with author, June 1993.

15 Human Pituitary Advisory Committee, "Ovulation induction by human FSH — the results of the Australian program", *Australian and New Zealand Journal of Obstetrics and Gynaecology,* 1976, vol. 16, pp. 106–110.

16 Human Pituitary Advisory Committee, "Ovulation induction by human FSH", pp. 106–110.

17 S. Cummings, Interview with author, June 1993.

18 A. Dickinson, Interview with author, February 1997.

19 A. Dickinson, Interview with author, May 1996.

20 P. Martin, "Anthropology or paedophilia", *Observer,* February 16, 1997, Review Section.

21 R. Williams, "Medicine's Indiana Jones", *Australian Way,* 1988, pp. 35–36.

22 A. Dickinson, Letter to Dr S. Ramaswamy at MRC, The possibility of scrapie-like infective agents withstanding hGH preparative techniques, February 22, 1977.

23 Minutes of MRC steering committee for human pituitary collection, March 11, 1977.

24 C. Bernoulli, J. Siegfried, G. Baumgartner, "Danger of accidental person-to-person transmission of Creutzfeldt-Jakob disease by surgery", *Lancet,* 1977, vol. 1, pp. 478–479.

25 D. Gajdusek, "Unconventional viruses and the origin and disappearance of kuru", *Science,* 1977, vol. 197, pp. 943–960.

26 C. Mims, Letter to Dr S. Ramaswamy at MRC, November 29, 1977.

27 Mims, Letter to Dr S. Ramaswamy at MRC, November 29, 1977.

28 Synopsis of plaintiffs' opening address, CJD Litigation, High Court, London, April 1996, p. 12.

29 Minutes of MRC steering committee for human pituitary collection, December 16, 1977.

30 R. Milner, Witness statement, CJD Litigation, High Court, London, September 1995, p. 15.

31 D. Gajdusek, et al., "Precautions in the medical care of, and in handling materials from, patients with transmissible virus dementia (Creutzfeldt-Jakob disease)", *New England Journal of Medicine,* 1977, vol. 297, pp. 1253–1258.

32 *Code of practice for the prevention of infection in clinical laboratories and post-mortem rooms,* Her Majesty's Stationery Office, London, 1978, p. 3.

33 Synopsis of plaintiffs' opening address, CJD Litigation, High Court, London, April 1996, p. 13.

34 S. Ramaswamy, Letter from MRC to Dr Carleton Gajdusek, April 28, 1978.

35 Reply from Dr Colin Masters at Gajdusek's NIH laboratory to Dr Saroja Ramaswamy at the MRC, May 8, 1978.

36 Synopsis of plaintiffs' opening address, p. 12.

37 Synopsis of plaintiffs' opening address, p. 11.

38 D. Tyrrell, Letter to Dr Barbara Rashbass at the MRC, January 7, 1974.

Chapter 7
What's in a name?
1   S. Stroud, M. Hoog, E. Bieler, "A simple method for the extraction and
    purification of human growth hormone and its assay by paper
    chromatography", *Journal of Clinical Endocrinology and Metabolism,*
    1973, vol. 37, pp. 860–866.
2   W. Katz, Interview with author, April 1996.
3   L. Smith, Interview with author, April 1996.
4   E. Hitchings, Interview with author, April 1996.
5   Katz, Interview with author, April 1996.
6   Smith, Interview with author, April 1996.
7   Hitchings, Interview with author, April 1996.
8   F. Bonnici, Interview with author. April 1997.
9   A. Dickinson, Interview with author, May 1996.
10 M. Allars, *Report of the Inquiry into the Use of Pituitary Derived
    Hormones in Australia and Creutzfeldt-Jakob Disease,* Australian
    Government Publishing Service, June 1994, 1994, pp. 334, 335, 352.
11 Allars, *Report of the Inquiry into the Use of Pituitary Derived Hormones,*
    1994, pp. 352, 334.
12 Allars, *Report of the Inquiry into the Use of Pituitary Derived Hormones,*
    1994, p. 357.
13 R. Rischbieth, "A case of Creutzfeldt-Jakob disease", *Proceedings of the
    Australian Association of Neurology,* 1965, pp. 3, 11.
14 Allars, *Report of the Inquiry into the Use of Pituitary Derived Hormones,*
    1994, pp. 356–357.
15 Allars, *Report of the Inquiry into the Use of Pituitary Derived Hormones,*
    1994, pp. 358–359.
16 Allars, *Report of the Inquiry into the Use of Pituitary Derived Hormones,*
    1994, pp. 352, 356.
17 D. Gajdusek, "Unconventional viruses and the origin and disappearance
    of kuru", *Science,* 1977, vol. 197, pp. 943–960.
18 C. Masters, J. Harris, D. Gajdusek, C.Gibbs, C. Bernouilli, D. Asher,
    "Creutzfeldt-Jakob Disease: patterns of worldwide occurrence and the
    significance of familial and sporadic clustering", *Annals of Neurology,*
    1979, vol. 5, pp. 177–188.
19 Allars, *Report of the Inquiry into the Use of Pituitary Derived Hormones,*
    1994, p. 364.
20 Allars, *Report of the Inquiry into the Use of Pituitary Derived Hormones,*
    1994, p. 350. (quoted in)
21 P. Brown, F. Cathala, "Creutzfeldt-Jakob disease in France: I,
    Retrospective study of the Paris area during the 10-year period
    1968–1977", *Annals of Neurology,* 1979, vol. 5, pp. 189–192.
22 P. Brown, F. Cathala, D. Sadowsky, D. Gajdusek. "Creutzfeldt-Jakob
    disease in France: II, Clinical characteristics of 124 consecutive verified
    cases during the decade 1968–1977", *Annals of Neurology,* 1979, vol. 6,
    pp. 430–437.
23 P. Brown, F. Cathala, D. Gajdusek. "Creutzfeldt-Jakob disease in France:
    III, Epidemiology study of 170 patients dying during the decade
    1968–1977", *Annals of Neurology,* 1979, vol. 6, pp. 438–446.

24 R. Rappaport, Letter to Professor David Milner, January 28, 1980. Cited in opening address of the CJD Litigation, High Court, London, April 1996.

25 Pathologist, Interview with author, March 1997.

26 Allars, *Report of the Inquiry into the Use of Pituitary Derived Hormones,* 1994, p. 367.

27 Allars, *Report of the Inquiry into the Use of Pituitary Derived Hormones,* 1994, p. 63.

28 Allars, *Report of the Inquiry into the Use of Pituitary Derived Hormones,* 1994, pp. 365–366.

29 Gajdusek, "Unconventional viruses and the origin and disappearance of kuru", pp. 943–960.

30 Gajdusek, "Unconventional viruses and the origin and disappearance of kuru", pp. 943–960.

31 T. Alper, W. Cramp, D. Haig, M. Clarke, "Does the agent of scrapie replicate without nucleic acid?", *Nature,* 1967, vol. 214, pp. 764–766.

32 Gajdusek, "Unconventional viruses and the origin and disappearance of kuru", pp. 943–960.

33 A. Dickinson, G. Outram, "The scrapie replication hypothesis and its implications for pathogenesis", in *Slow Transmissable Diseases of the Nervous System,* S. Prusiner, W. Hadlow (eds) 1979, vol. 2, pp. 29–30.

34 L. Court, F. Cathala, "Virus non conventionnels et affections du systeme nerveux central", *Masson,* 1983, pp. 3–16.

35 A. Dickinson, Personal communication, February 1997.

36 G. Taubes, "The game of the name if fame. But is it science?", *Discover,* December 1986, pp. 28–52.

37 S. Prusiner, "Novel proteinaceous infectious particles cause scrapie", *Science,* 1982, vol. 216, pp. 135–144.

38 J. Lanchester, "A new kind of contagion", *New Yorker,* December 2, 1996, pp. 70–81.

39 R. Kimberlin, "Scrapie agent: prions or virinos?", *Nature,* 1982, vol. 297, pp. 107–8.

40 Editorial, "Scrapie: strategies, stalemates and successes", *Lancet,* 1982, vol I, pp. 1221–1223.

41 G. Kolata, "Viruses or prions: An old medical debate still rages", *New York Times,* October 4, 1994.

42 S. Dearmond, S. Prusiner, "Prion diseases", in *Greenfield's neuropathology,* D. Graham, P. Lantos (eds), London, Edward Arnold, 1997, vol. 2, 235–280.

43 M. Kamin, B. Patten, "Creutzfeldt-Jakob disease. Possible transmission to humans by consumption of wild animal brains", *American Journal of Medicine,* 1984, vol. 76, pp. 143–145.

Chapter 8
Hormones: The first victims

1 P. Brown, "Human growth hormone therapy and Creutzfeldt-Jakob disease: a drama in three acts", *Pediatrics,* 1988, vol. 81, pp. 85–92.

2 Anon., "Fatal degenerative neurologic disease in patients who received pituitary-derived human growth hormone", *Journal of the American Medical Association,* 1985, vol. 254, pp. 475–6.

3   R. Hintz, "A prismatic case. The prismatic case of Creutzfeldt-Jakob disease associated with pituitary growth hormone treatment", *Journal of Clinical Endocrinology and Metabolism,* 1995, vol. 80, pp. 2209–2301.

4   T. Koch, B. Berg, S. De Armond, R. Gravina, "Creutzfeldt-Jakob disease in a young adult with idiopathic hypopituitarism. Possible relation to the administration of cadaveric human growth hormone", *New England Journal of Medicine,* 1985, vol. 313, pp. 731–733.

5   Hintz, "A prismatic case", pp. 2209–2301.

6   Koch, "Creutzfeldt-Jakob disease in a young adult with idiopathic hypopituitarism", pp. 731–733.

7   C. Gibbs, A. Joy, D. Reid Heffner, M. Franko, M. Miyazaki, D. Asher, J. Parish, P. Brown, D. Gajdusek, "Clinical and pathological features and laboratory confirmation of Creutzfeldt-Jakob disease in a recipient of pituitary-derived human growth hormone", *New England Journal of Medicine,* 1985, vol. 313, No. 12, pp. 734–738.

8   Gibbs et al, "Clinical and pathological features and laboratory confirmation of Creutzfeldt-Jakob disease in a recipient of pituitary-derived human growth hormone", pp. 734–738.

9   Brown, "Human growth hormone therapy and Creutzfeldt-Jakob disease: a drama in three acts", *Pediatrics,* pp. 85–92.

10 J. Tatlock, Letter to Dr Robert Blizzard, Chairman, Children's Medical Center, University of Virginia, Charlottesville, June 25, 1985.

11 J. Powell-Jackson, R. Weller, P. Kennedy, M. Preece, E. Whitcombe, J. Newsom-Davis, Preliminary communication, "Creutzfeldt-Jakob disease after administration of human growth hormone", *Lancet,* 1985, vol. 2, pp. 244–246.

12 M. Lay, Excerpt from statement read during opening address of CJD litigation, High Court, London, April 1996.

13 M. Lay, Excerpt from statement read during opening address of CJD litigation, High Court, London, April 1996.

14 World in Action, "The cure that killed", BBC television, October 10, 1994.

15 R. Weller, P. Steart, J. Powell-Jackson, "Pathology of Creutzfeldt-Jakob disease associated with pituitary-derived human growth hormone administration", *Neuropathology and Applied Neurobiology,* 1986, vol. 12, pp. 117–129.

16 Weller, et al., "Pathology of Creutzfeldt-Jakob disease associated with pituitary-derived human growth hormone administration", pp. 117–129.

17 Anon., "Fury of victims' parents", *Today,* July 5, 1994.

18 P. Brown, Interview with author, June 1996.

19 Brown, Interview with author, June 1996.

20 G. Northam (presenter), Panorama, "The great British beef fiasco", BBC 1 television, June 17, 1996.

Chapter 9
Tracking the CJD culprit

1   R. Hintz, "A prismatic case. The prismatic case of Creutzfeldt-Jakob disease associated with pituitary growth hormone treatment", *Journal of Clinical Endocrinology and Metabolism,* 1995, vol. 80, pp. 2298–2301.

2   M. Allars, *Report of the Inquiry into the Use of Pituitary Derived Hormones in Australia and Creutzfeldt-Jakob Disease,* Australian Government Publishing Service, 1994, p. 369.

3   Hintz, "A prismatic case", p. 2298.

4   P. Brown, "Human growth hormone therapy and Creutzfeldt-Jakob disease: a drama in three acts", *Pediatrics,* 1988, vol. 81, pp. 85–92.

5   G. Degerman, *Creutzfeldt-Jakob Disease and Pituitary hGH. A Report on Facts, Scientific Background, Assessments and Conclusions as of the date 13 May, 1985,* KabiVitrum/Peptide Hormones.

6   O. Trygstad, Evidence during the CJD Litigation, High Court, London, April 1996.

7   F. Bonnici, Interview with author, April 1997.

8   Allars, *Report of the Inquiry into the Use of Pituitary Derived Hormones,* 1994, pp. 559–560.

9   L. Lazarus, "Suspension of the Australian human pituitary hormone programme", *Medical Journal of Australia,* 1985, vol. 143, pp. 57–59.

10 P. Brown, "Causes of human spongiform encephalopathy", in *Methods in Molecular Medicine Series: Prion Diseases,* H. Bailey, R. Ridley (eds), Humana Press, 1996, p. 142.

11 P. Brown, M. Preece, R. Will, "'Friendly fire' in medicine: hormones, homografts and Creutzfeldt-Jakob disease", *Lancet,* 1992, vol. 340, pp. 24–27.

12 Trygstad, Evidence during the CJD Litigation, April 1996.

13 Z. Josefsberg, O. Aran, Z. Laron, "Safety of pituitary-growth hormone extracted with acetone/acetic acid", *Lancet,* 1994, vol. 344, p. 613.

14 F. Bonnici, Interview with author, February 1997.

15 Brown, "Human growth hormone therapy and Creutzfeldt-Jakob disease: a drama in three acts", pp. 85–92.

16 A. Dickinson, Personal communication, February 1997.

17 J. Sloggem, Witness statement to the CJD litigation, p. 7.

18 C. Gibbs, D. Asher, P. Brown, J. Fradkin, D. Gajdusek, "Creutzfeldt-Jakob disease infectivity of growth hormone derived from human pituitary glands", *New England Journal of Medicine,* 1993, vol. 328, pp. 358–359.

19 Allars, *Report of the Inquiry into the Use of Pituitary Derived Hormones,* 1994, p. 578.

20 C. Masters, Interview with author, April 1997.

21 R. Tintner, Copy of letter to the Reverend and Mrs Lloyd Tatlock, June 11, 1985.

22 Brown, Interview with author, June 1996.

23 R. Tintner, P. Brown, E. Hedley-Whyte, E. Rappaport, C. Piccardo, D. Gajdusek, "Neuropathologic verification of Creutzfeldt-Jakob disease in the exhumed American recipient of human pituitary growth hormone: Epidemiologic and pathogenetic implications", *Neurology,* 1986, vol. 36, pp. 932–936.

24 P. Brown, Iatrogenic Creutzfeldt-Jakob disease from human growth hormone therapy, World Congress of Neurology, September 2–8, 1985. Hamburg, Germany.

25 M. Croxon, P. Brown, B. Synek, M. Harrington, G. Clover, J. Wilson, D. Gajdusek, "A new case of Creutzfeldt-Jakob Disease associated with human growth hormone therapy in New Zealand", *Neurology,* 1988, vol. 38, pp. 1128–1130.

26 Croxon, et al., "A new case of Creutzfeldt-Jakob Disease associated with human growth hormone therapy in New Zealand", pp. 1128–1130.

27 P. Brown, "The decline and fall of Creutzfeldt-Jakob disease associated with human growth hormone therapy", editorial, *Neurology,* 1988, vol. 38, pp. 1135–1137.

28 Brown, "Human growth hormone therapy and Creutzfeldt-Jakob disease: a drama in three acts", pp. 85–92.

29 M. New, P. Brown, J. Temeck, C. Owens, E. Hedley-Whyte, E. Richardson, "Preclinical Creutzfeldt-Jakob disease discovered at autopsy in a human growth hormone recipient", *Neurology,* 1988, vol. 38, pp. 1133–1134.

30 New, et al., "Preclinical Creutzfeldt-Jakob disease discovered at autopsy in a human growth hormone recipient", pp. 1133–1134.

31 D. Marzewski, J. Towfighi, M. Harrington, C. Merril, P. Brown, "Creutzfeldt-Jakob disease following pituitary-derived human growth hormone therapy: A new American case", *Neurology,* 1988, vol. 38, pp. 1131–1133.

32 P. Brown, "Transmissible human spongiform encephalopathy (infectious cerebral amyloidosis): Creutzfeldt-Jakob disease, Gerstmann-Sträussler-Scheinker syndrome, and kuru", in *Neurodegenerative diseases,* D. Calne (ed.), WB Saunders Company, Philadelphia, 1994.

33 M. Harrington, Correspondence with author, October 1996.

34 M. Harrington, C. Merril, D. Asher, D. Gajdusek, "Abnormal proteins in the cerebrospinal fluid of patients with Creutzfeldt-Jakob disease", *New England Journal of Medicine,* 1986, vol. 315, pp. 279–283.

35 Brown, "The decline and fall of Creutzfeldt-Jakob disease associated with human growth hormone therapy", pp. 1135–1137.

36 R. Donald, chairman of clinical subcommittee of the National Hormone Committee in a letter to Dr R. Riseley, Medicines and Benefits, New Zealand Department of Health, December 21, 1988.

37 Letter from members of clinical subcommittee of the National Hormone Committee to the Director-General of Health, May 3, 1988.

Chapter 10
Jane Allender: The price of infertility

1   L. Allender, Interview with author, September 1993.

2   P. Mayo, Interview with author, September 1993.

3   M. Cant, Interview with author, September 1993.

4   E. Allender, Interview with author, September 1993.

5   Diary notations of Jane Allender, 1975.

6   K. Allender, Interview with author, September 1993.

7   P. Mayo, Interview with author, September 1993.

8   L. Allender, Interview with author, September 1993.

9   E. Allender, Interview with author, September 1993.

10 J. Cochius, Interview with author, June 1996.

11 R. Burns, Letter to Dr Brummitt, November 18, 1988.
12 P. Blumbergs, Report on brain of Jane Allender, March 22, 1989.
13 P. Purcell, Letter to Ted Allender, March 31, 1989.
14 D. Sharp, Letter from the *Lancet* to Dr J Cochius, February 28, 1990.
15 M. Allars, *Report of the Inquiry into the Use of Pituitary Derived Hormones in Australia and Creutzfeldt-Jakob Disease,* Australian Government Publishing Service, 1994, p. 589.
16 J. Cochius, R. Burns, P. Blumbergs, K. Mack, C. Alderman, "Creutzfeldt-Jakob disease in a recipient of human pituitary-derived gonadotrophin", *Australian and New Zealand Journal of Medicine,* 1990, vol. 20, pp. 592–594.

Chapter 11
BSE and brains: Transmission spreads

1   T. Holt, J. Phillips, "For debate... Bovine spongiform encephalopathy", *British Medical Journal,* 1988, vol. 296, pp. 1581–1582.
2   Anon., "Comment. Keeping BSE in proportion", *Veterinary Record,* May 21, 1988, vol. 122, p. 1.
3   R. Southwood, *Report of the Working Party on Bovine Spongiform Encephalopathy,* British Department of Health, Ministry of Agriculture, Fisheries and Food, February 1989.
4   G. Wells, A. Scott, C. Johnson, R. Gunning, R. Hancock, M. Jeffrey, M. Dawson, R. Bradley, "Novel progressive spongiform encephalopathy in cattle", *Veterinary Record,* 1987, vol. 121, pp. 419–420.
5   A. Dickinson, Interview with author, April 1996.
6   B. Ford, *BSE the facts. Mad Cow Disease and the Risk to Mankind,* Corgi Books, 1996, pp. 155–157.
7   Holt, Phillips, "For debate... Bovine spongiform encephalopathy", pp. 1581–1582.
8   H. Grant, Interview with author, April 1995.
9   Anon., "German firm denies product link with brain disease", *Reuters News Service,* September 2, 1993.
10 T. Esmonde, C. Lueck, L. Symon, L. Duchen, R. Will, "Creutzfeldt-Jakob disease and lyophilised dura mater grafts: report of two cases", *Journal of Neurology, Neurosurgery and Psychiatry,* 1993, vol. 56, pp. 999–1000.
11 D. Fletcher, "Mad cow disease fears for brain patients", *Daily Telegraph,* August 10, 1991.
12 J. Martinez-Lage, M. Poza, J. Sola, J. Tortosa, P. Brown, L. Cervenáková, J. Esteban, A. Mendoza, "Accidental transmission of Creutzfeldt-Jakob disease by dural cadaveric grafts", *Journal of Neurology, Neurosurgery and Psychiatry,* 1994, vol. 57, pp. 1091–1094.
13 H. Willison, A. Gale, J. McLaughlin, "Creutzfeldt-Jakob disease following cadaveric dura mater graft", *Journal of Neurology, Neurosurgery and Psychiatry,* 1991, vol. 54, p. 940.
14 Willison, et al., "Creutzfeldt-Jakob disease following cadaveric dura mater graft", p. 940.
15 T. Kelsey, "Thousands facing fatal brain disease", *Independent,* September 2, 1993.

16 "Centers for Disease Control. Rapidly progressive dementia in a patient who received a cadaveric dura mater graft", *Morbidity and Mortality Weekly Report,* 1987, vol. 36, pp. 49–50, 55.

17 V. Thadani, P. Penar, J. Partington, R. Kalb, R. Janssen, L. Schonberger, C. Rabkin, J. Pritchard, "Creutzfeldt-Jakob disease probably acquired from a cadaveric dura mater graft", *Journal of Neurosurgery,* 1988, vol. 69, p. 766–769.

18 Editorial, *Communicable Diseases Intelligence,* bulletin, 1989, p. 5.

19 Judgement, Richard M. Nesom vs Tri Hawk International, United States Court of Appeals, Fifth Circuit, March 8, 1993.

20 G. Johnson, FDA import alert #84 – 03 on Lyodura, June 6, 1987.

21 Judgement. Richard M. Nesom vs Tri Hawk International, 1993.

22 T. Nisbert, I. MacDonaldson, S. Bishara, "Creutzfeldt-Jakob disease in a second patient who received a cadaveric dura mater graft", *Journal of the American Medical Association,* 1989, vol. 261, p. 1118.

23 Anon., "Update: Creutzfeldt-Jakob Disease in a second patient who received a cadaveric dura mater graft", *Communicable Diseases Intelligence,* bulletin, 1989, p. 5.

24 C. Masullo, M. Pocchari, G. Macchi, G. Alema, Piazza G, M. Panzera, "Transmission of Creutzfeldt-Jakob disease by dural cadaveric graft", *Journal of Neurosurgery,* 1989, vol. 71, pp. 954–955.

25 J. Martinez-Lage, J. Sola, M. Poza, J. Esteban, "Pediatric Creutzfeldt-Jakob disease: probable transmission by a dural graft", *Childs Nervous System,* 1993, vol. 9, pp. 239–242.

26 D. Simpson, C. Masters, G. Ohlich, G. Purdie, G. Stuart, A. Tannenberg, "Iatrogenic Creutzfeldt-Jakob disease and its neurosurgical implications' *Journal of Clinical Neuroscience,* 1996, vol. 3, pp. 118–123.

27 K. Miyashita, T. Inuzuka, H. Kondo, "Creutzfeldt-Jakob disease following a cadaver dura mater graft", *Neurology,* 1991, vol. 41, pp. 940–941.

28 Willison, et al., "Creutzfeldt-Jakob disease following cadaveric dura mater graft", p. 940.

29 T. Kelsey, "Thousands facing fatal brain disease", *Independent,* Reuters News Service, September 2, 1993.

30 J. Laurance, "12,000 at risk from brain disease may never be traced", *The Times,* September 3, 1993.

31 D. Fletcher, "Mad cow disease fears for brain patients", *Daily Telegraph,* August 10, 1991.

32 P. Pallot, "Cross-infection fears over human mad cow disease", *Daily Telegraph,* September 3, 1993.

33 Martinez-Lage, et al., "Pediatric Creutzfeldt-Jakob disease", pp. 239–242.

34 K. Lane, P. Brown, D. Howell, B. Crain, C. Hulette, P. Burger, S. DeArmond, "Creutzfeldt-Jakob disease in a pregnant woman with an implanted dura mater graft", *Neurosurgery,* 1994, vol. 34, pp. 733–740.

35 M. Thomas, "Mad cow disease kills brain patient", *Sunday Star Times,* July 10, 1994.

36 T. Weber, H. Tumani, B. Holdorff, J. Collinge, M. Palmer, H. Kretzschmar, K. Felgenhauer, "Transmission of Creutzfeldt-Jakob disease by handling of dura mater", *Lancet,* 1993, vol. 34, pp. 123–124.

37 Esmonde, et al., "Creutzfeldt-Jakob disease and lyophilised dura mater grafts", pp. 999–1000.

38 M. Pocchiari, C. Masullo, M. Salvatore, M. Genuardt, S. Galgani, "Creutzfeldt-Jakob disease after non-commercial dura mater graft", *Lancet,* 1992, vol. 340, p. 501.

39 K. Foster, Medical Devices Alert No. 104, Bureau of Radiation and Medical Devices, Health Protection Branch, Ottawa.

40 M. Clavel, P. Clavel, "Creutzfeldt-Jakob disease transmitted by dura mater graft", *European Neurology,* vol. 36, pp. 239–240.

41 Clavel, Clavel, "Creutzfeldt-Jakob disease transmitted by dura mater graft", pp. 239–240.

42 M. McKimmie, "Need for baby led to death", *West Australian,* May 13, 1993.

43 M. Allars, *Report of the Inquiry into the Use of Pituitary Derived Hormones in Australia and Creutzfeldt-Jakob Disease,* Australian Government Publishing Service, 1994, p. 584.

44 T. Billette De Villemeur, P. Beauvais, M. Gourmelen, J. Richardet, "Creutzfeldt-Jakob disease in children treated with growth hormone", *Lancet,* 1991, vol. 337, pp. 864–865.

45 T. Billette De Villemeur, P. Beauvais, M. Gourmelen, J. Richardet, "Maladie de Creutzfeldt-Jakob chez quatre enfants traités par hormone de croissance", *Revue de Neurologie,* 1992, vol. 148, pp. 328–334.

46 F. Renault, P. Richard, "Early electroretinogram alterations in Creutzfeldt-Jakob disease after growth hormone treatment", *Lancet,* 1991, vol. 338, p. 191.

47 Billette De Villemeur, et al., "Maladie de Creutzfeldt-Jakob chez quatre enfants traités par hormone de croissance", pp. 328–334.

Chapter 12
Jenny Halford: A pattern emerges

1   M. Knight, Personal correspondence with author, June 1994.
2   N. Halford, Interview with author, August 18, 1993.
3   Knight, Personal correspondence with author, June 1994.
4   J. Cochius, N. Hyman, M. Esiri, "Creutzfeldt-Jakob disease in a recipient of human pituitary-derived gonadotrophin: a second case", *Journal of Neurology, Neurosurgery and Psychiatry,* 1992, vol. 55, pp. 1094–1095.
5   N. Hyman, Personal correspondence with author, May 1996.
6   Halford, Interview with author, August 18, 1993.
7   Hyman, Personal correspondence with author, May 1996.
8   Knight, Personal correspondence with author, June 1994.
9   Hyman, Personal correspondence with author, May 1996.
10 J. Cochius. Interview with author, June 1996.
11 Cochius. Interview with author, June 1996.
12 Halford, Interview with author, August 18, 1993.
13 Halford, Interview with author, August 18, 1993.
14 Halford, Interview with author, August 18, 1993.
15 M. Allars, *Report of the Inquiry into the Use of Pituitary Derived Hormones in Australia and Creutzfeldt-Jakob Disease,* Australian Government Publishing Service, 1994, p. 650.
16 Halford, Interview with author, August 18, 1993.

17 Knight, Personal correspondence with author, June 1994.
18 Knight, Personal correspondence with author, June 1994.
19 Knight, Personal correspondence, June 1994.
20 Knight, Interview with author, June 1994.
21 S. Heath, "Fertility treatments, virus linked after 20 years", *Age,* October 31, 1990.
22 J. Cochius J, R. Burns, P. Blumbergs, K. Mack, C. Alderman, "Creutzfeldt-Jakob disease in a recipient of human pituitary–derived gonadotrophin", *Australian and New Zealand Journal of Medicine,* 1990, vol. 20, pp. 592–593.
23 R. Hunt, Interview with author, April 1995.

Chapter 13
"Forget the cows, what about the kids?"

1   J. Erlichman, "Are fears about BSE mass hysteria or deep mistrust of Government assurances?", *Guardian,* May 15, 1990.
2   A. Watkins, "Scandal of timebomb children", *Today,* May 14, 1991.
3   A. Watkins, "Doomed: no-one said a word", *Today,* May 13, 1991.
4   D. Body, Interview with author, June 1996.
5   S. Cummings, Interview with author, June 1993.
6   Cummings, Interview with author, June 1993.
7   N. Hakof, Chief executive officer, Queen Elizabeth Hospital, answers to questions from "A Current Affair" television program, February 19, 1993.
8   M. Allars, *Report of the Inquiry into the Use of Pituitary Derived Hormones in Australia and Creutzfeldt-Jakob Disease,* Australian Government Publishing Service, 1994, p. 584.
9   M. Macario, M. Vaisman, A. Buescu, "Pituitary growth hormone and Creutzfeldt-Jakob disease", *British Medical Journal,* 1991, vol. 302, p. 1149.
10 Furbisher J, Fowler R. "Programmed to die — by an NHS blunder", *Sunday Times,* May 17, 1992.
11 Andrews P. Interview with author, May 1996.

Chapter 14
Australia confronts its CJD risk

1   P. Costello, House of Representatives,Hansard, Commonwealth Serum Laboratories, November 27, 1991, pp. 3488–3489.
2   H. Carter, "Compo call on deaths", *Herald-Sun,* November 29, 1991.
3   M. McMurtrie, Personal communication, April 1996.
4   M. Allars, *Report of the Inquiry into the Use of Pituitary Derived Hormones in Australia and Creutzfeldt-Jakob Disease,* Australian Government Publishing Service, 1994, p. 600.
5   J. Mills, J. Fradkin, L. Schonberger, et al., "Status report on the US human growth hormone recipient follow-up study", *Hormone Research,* 1990, vol. 33, pp. 116–120.
6   Allars, *Report of the Inquiry into the Use of Pituitary Derived Hormones,* 1994, p. 670–671.
7   Allars, *Report of the Inquiry into the Use of Pituitary Derived Hormones,* 1994, p. 672.

8   L. Dumble, R. Klein, "Creutzfeldt-Jakob legacy for Australian women treated with human pituitary hormone for infertility", *Lancet,* 1992, vol. 340, pp. 847–848.

9   L. Rogers, "Women at risk of timebomb of 'mad cow disease'", *Daily Mail,* October 12, 1992.

10 J. Cooke, "Surgeon fears brain disease epidemic", *Sydney Morning Herald,* November 27, 1992.

11 D. Armstrong, "Shrouded in silence", *Sydney Morning Herald,* November 28, 1992, p. 1.

12 J. Cooke, D. Armstrong, "The 'experiment' that killed", *Sydney Morning Herald,* November 29, 1992.

13 See chapter 6

14 J. Cooke, "Documents may open way for damages", *Sydney Morning Herald,* December 2, 1992.

15 Letter from Noel Halford and Ted Allender to Brian Howe, December 8, 1992.

16 Surgeon Commander Alistair Miller, Evidence to inquest of Patrick Baldwin, Lincoln Crown Court, November 3, 1993.

17 N. Baldwin, Interview with author, May 1996.

18 Baldwin, Interview with author, May 1996.

Chapter 15
The genetic lottery

1   If genes are words, then DNA is all the letters that can make up a word. A number of words (genes) make up a sentence (chromosome). Alterations to which letters (DNA) are included in a word (gene) obviously change the word (gene), and change the meaning or expression of that word (gene). Thus in the case of the PRNP gene, an alteration to the variety of DNA means that the meaning or expression of the gene is different. A tiny change can be enough to radically alter the structure and thus the properties of the prion protein (PRNP) in the brain, leading to defective functioning (like that found in TSE diseases) or sometimes no function at all.

2   F. Owen, M. Poulter, R. Lofthouse, et al., "Insertion in prion protein gene in familial Creutzfeldt-Jakob disease", *Lancet,* 1989, vol. 1, pp. 51–52.

3   K. Hsaio, H. Baker, T. Crow, et al., "Linkage of a prion protein missense variant to Gerstmann-Straüssler-Scheinker syndrome", *Nature,* 1989, vol. 338, pp. 342–345.

4   J. Collinge, A. Harding, F. Owen, et al., "Diagnosis of Gerstmann-Straüssler syndrome in familial dementia with prion protein gene analysis", *Lancet,* 1989, vol. 2, pp. 15–17.

5   J. Collinge, F. Owen , M. Poulter, et al., "Prion dementia without characteristic pathology", *Lancet,* 1990, vol. 336, pp. 7–9.

6   E. Lugaresi, R. Medori, P. Montagna, et al., "Fatal familial insomnia and dysautonomia with selective degeneration of thalamic nuclei", *New England Journal of Medicine,* 1986, vol. 315, pp. 997–1003.

7   R. Medori, H. Tritschler, A. LeBlanc, et al., "Fatal familial insomnia, a prion disease with a mutation at codon 178 of the prion protein gene", *New England Journal of Medicine,* 1992, vol. 326, pp. 444–449.

8   J. Collinge, M. Palmer, K. Sidl, "Transmission of fatal familial insomnia to laboratory animals", *Lancet,* 1995, vol. 346, pp. 560–70.

9   J. Tateishi, P. Brown, T. Kitamoto, et al., "First experimental transmission of fatal familial insomnia", *Nature,* 1995, vol. 376, pp. 434–435.

10 P. Silburn, L. Cervenáková, P. Varghese, A. Tannenberg, P. Brown, R. Boyle, "Fatal familial insomnia: A seventh family", *Neurology,* 1996, vol. 47, pp. 1326–1328.

11 C. McLean, E. Storey, R. Gardner, A. Tannenberg, L. Cervenáková, P. Brown, "The D178N (cis-129M) 'fatal familial insomnia' mutation associated with diverse clinicopathologic phenotypes in an Australian kindred", *Neurology,* 1997, vol. 49, pp. 552–558.

12 C. Masters, J. Harris, D. Gajdusek, C. Gibbs, C. Bernouilli, D. Asher, "Creutzfeldt-Jakob disease: patterns of worldwide occurrence and the significance of familial and sporadic clustering", *Annals of Neurology,* 1979, vol. 5, pp. 177–188.

13 M. Alter, E. Kahana, "Creutzfeldt-Jakob disease among Libyan-born Israelis", *Neurology,* 1976, vol. 29, pp. 225–31.

14 R. Raubertas, P. Brown, F. Cathala, I. Brown, "The question of clustering of Creutzfeldt-Jakob disease", *American Journal of Epidemiology,* 1989, vol. 129, 146–154.

15 L. Goldfarb, A. Korczyn, P. Brown, J. Chapman, D. Gajdusek, "Mutation in codon 200 of scrapie amyloid precursor gene linked to Creutzfeldt-Jakob disease in Sephardic Jews of Libyan and non-Libyan origin", *Lancet,* 1990, vol. 336, p. 637.

16 P. Brown, S. Galvez, L. Goldfarb, et al., "Familial Creutzfeldt-Jakob disease in Chile is associated with the codon 200 mutation of the PRNP amyloid precursor gene on chromosome 20", *Journal of Neurological Sciences,* 1992, vol. 112, pp. 65–57.

17 P. Brown, F. Cathala, R. Raubertas, et al., "The epidemiology of Creutzfeldt-Jakob disease: conclusion of a 15-year investigation in France, and review of the world literature", *Neurology,* 1987, vol. 37, pp. 895–904.

18 Masters, et al., "Creutzfeldt-Jakob disease", pp. 177–188.

19 B. Matthews, Report on Creutzfeldt-Jakob disease in recipients of human growth hormone, The CJD Litigation, High Court, London, April 1996.

20 The procedure is no longer used with the advent of computed tomography (CT) scans, which X-ray layers of the brain.

21 R. Will, W. Matthews, "Evidence for case-to-case transmission of Creutzfeldt-Jakob disease", *Journal of Neurology, Neurosurgery and Psychiatry,* 1982, vol. 45, pp. 235–238.

22 See chapter 2 for review of Nevin's cases.

23 S. Nevin, W. McMenemey, S. Behrman, D. Jones, "Subacute spongiform encephalopathy — a subacute form of encephalopathy attributable to vascular dysfunction (spongiform cerebral atrophy)", *Brain,* 1960, vol. 83, pp. 519–569.

24 S. Nevin, W. McMenemey, S. Behrman, D. Jones, "Subacute spongiform encephalopathy", pp. 519–569.

25 S. Nevin, W. McMenemey, S. Behrman, D. Jones, "Subacute spongiform encephalopathy", pp. 519–569.

26 P. Brown, "Causes of human spongiform encephalopathy", in *Prion diseases. Methods in Molecular Medicine,* H. Baker, R. Ridley (eds), New Jersey, Humana Press, 1996, p. 141.

27 R. Will, W. Matthews, "Evidence for case-to-case transmission of Creutzfeldt-Jakob disease", *Journal of Neurology, Neurosurgery and Psychiatry,* 1982, vol. 45, pp. 235–238.

28 P. Brown, P. Liberski, A. Wolff, D. Gajdusek, "Resistance of scrapie infectivity to steam autoclaving after formaldehyde fixation and limited survival after ashing at 360°C: Practical and theoretical implications", *Journal of Infectious Diseases,* 1990, vol. 161, pp. 467–472.

29 P. Brown, D. Gajdusek, "Survival of scrapie virus after 3 years interment", *Lancet,* 1991, vol. 337, pp. 269–270.

30 Brown, Gajdusek, "Survival of scrapie virus", pp. 269–270.

31 R. de Silva, "Human spongiform encephalopathy. Clinical presentation and diagnostic tests", in *Prion Diseases. Methods in Molecular Medicine,* H. Baker, R. Ridley (eds), New Jersey, Humana Press, 1996, p. 19.

32 P. Brown, F. Jannotta, C. Gibbs, H. Baron, D. Guiroy, D. Gajdusek, "Coexistence of Creutzfeldt-Jakob disease and Alzheimer's disease in the same patient", *Neurology,* 1990, vol. 40, pp. 226–228.

33 W. Schoene, C. Masters, C. Gibbs, et al., "Transmissible spongiform encephalopathy (Creutzfeldt-Jakob disease). Atypical clinical and pathological findings", *Archives of Neurology,* 1981, vol. 38, pp. 473–477.

34 P. Brown, Editorial, "The decline and fall of Creutzfeldt-Jakob disease associated with human growth hormone therapy", *Neurology,* 1988, vol. 38, pp. 1135–1137.

35 F. Bastian (ed.), *Creutzfeldt-Jakob Disease and Other Transmissible Spongiform Encephalopathies,* Mosby-Year Book, Inc., Chicago, 1991, p. 56.

36 J. Collinge, M. Palmer, A. Dryden, "Genetic predisposition to iatrogenic Creutzfeldt-Jakob disease", *Lancet,* 1991, vol. 337, pp. 1441–1442.

37 P. Brown, M. Preece, R. Will, "'Friendly fire' in medicine: hormones, homografts and Creutzfeldt-Jakob disease", Review article, *Lancet,* 1992, vol. 340, pp. 24–27.

38 L. Dumble, Personal communication, 1994.

39 P. Brown, M. Cervenáková, L. Goldfarb , et al., "Iatrogenic Creutzfeldt-Jakob disease: an example of the interplay between ancient genes and modern medicine", *Neurology,* 1994, vol. 44, pp. 291–293.

Chapter 16
Victims fight back

1 G. Brodrick, Interview with author, March 1997.

2 S. Connor, "Farmer's death 'had no BSE link'", *Independent,* March 13, 1993.

3 Connor, "Farmer's death 'had no BSE link'", March 13, 1993.

4 Media Release, Commonwealth Department of Health, Housing, Local Government and Community Services, April 30, 1993.

5 M. Preece, R. Will, Interview with author, May 1995.

6 J. Cooke, "New death triggers hormone inquiry", *Sydney Morning Herald,* May 12, 1993.

7   G. Richardson, Minister for Health, News Release, Inquiry announced into Creutzfeldt-Jakob disease, May 11, 1993.
8   J. Cooke, "Widowers sue Govt, lab over rare disease", *Sydney Morning Herald,* May 13, 1993.
9   P. Gregory, "Men sue serum lab over deaths", *Age,* May 13, 1993.
10 E. Hunter, Judgement, Richard M. Nesom vs Tri Hawk International, No. 92–3461. United States Court of Appeals, Fifth Circuit, April 14, 1993.
11 Personal communication from E. Jamieson acting for the Bowler family.
12 J. Carnes, Judgement, Julia May McKenzie vs Emory University, Civil Action no 1:93-cv-2677-JEC, United States District Court, Northern District of Georgia, Atlanta Division, February 1, 1995.
13 P. Tuohy, Personal communication, September 1997.
14 M. Allars, *Report of the Inquiry into the Use of Pituitary Derived Hormones in Australia and Creutzfeldt-Jakob Disease,* Australian Government Publishing Service, 1994, 1994, p. 588.
15 Allars, *Report of the Inquiry into the Use of Pituitary Derived Hormones,* 1994, p. 589.

Chapter 17
The French catastrophe

1   P. Aldhous, "French officials panic over rare brain disease outbreak", *Science,* 1992, vol. 258, pp. 1571–2.
2   M. Balter, "Human growth hormone. French scientists may face charges over CJD outbreak", *Science,* 1993, vol. 261, p. 543.
3   O. Trygstad, Evidence to the CJD litigation, High Court, London, April 1996.
4   Z. Josefsberg, O. Aran, Z. Laron, "Safety of pituitary growth hormone extracted with acetone/acetic acid", *Lancet,* 1994, vol. 344, p. 130.
5   G. Mor, International victimology diploma thesis presented to Washington University, May 1995.
6   M. Gerson, "Creutzfeldt-Jakob disease and human growth hormone: is this the beginning of another contamination saga?", Reviews, *Prescribe International,* 1993, vol. 2, pp. 170–174.
7   Balter, "Human growth hormone", p. 543.
8   Gerson, "Creutzfeldt-Jakob disease and human growth hormone", pp. 170–174.
9   J. Goujard, M. Entat, F. Maillard, E. Mugnier, R. Rappaport, J. Job, "Human pituitary growth hormone (hGH) and Creutzfeldt-Jakob disease: Results of an epidemiological survey in France, 1986", *International Journal of Epidemiology,* 1988, vol. 17, pp. 423–427.
10 J. Job, F. Maillard, J. Goujard, "Epidemiological survey of patients treated with growth hormone in France in the period 1959–1990: preliminary results", *Hormone Research,* 1992, vol. 38, pp. 35–42.
11 Mor, International victimology diploma thesis, May 1995.
12 Aldhous, "French officials panic over rare brain disease outbreak", *Science,* 1992, vol. 258, pp. 1571–2.
13 Gerson, "Creutzfeldt-Jakob disease and human growth hormone", pp. 170–174.
14 P. Lowry, Witness statement to CJD litigation, September 1995.

15 T. Witcher, R. Highfield, "Death charges over hormone taken from corpses", *Daily Telegraph,* July 22, 1993.
16 Balter, "Human growth hormone", p. 543.
17 T. Patel, "France reels at latest medical scandal", *New Scientist,* July 31, 1993.
18 A. Casteret, "A new medical scandal", *L'Express,* January 9, 1997.
19 Casteret, "A new medical scandal", pp. 37–41.
20 F. Delbrel, *Pour Benedicte,* Éditions Du Rocher, Jean-Paul Bertrand, 1996.
21 Delbrel, *Pour Benedicte,* Jean-Paul Bertrand, 1996.
22 J. Nau, "CJD compensation", *Lancet,* 1993, vol. 342, p. 1169.
23 P. Brown, Interview with author, June 1996.

Chapter 18
An independent inquiry

1 C. Lawrence, Ministerial statement on the Allars report, June 28, 1992.
2 M. Allars, *Report of the Inquiry into the Use of Pituitary Derived Hormones in Australia and Creutzfeldt-Jakob Disease,* Executive Summary, Australian Government Publishing Service, 1994, p. 7–8.
3 Allars, *Report of the Inquiry into the Use of Pituitary Derived Hormones,* p. 461.
4 J. Cooke, "Medical minefield. The shocking truth behind Australia's human hormone program", *Sydney Morning Herald,* July 2, 1994.
5 Allars, *Report of the Inquiry into the Use of Pituitary Derived Hormones,* p. 473.
6 Allars, *Report of the Inquiry into the Use of Pituitary Derived Hormones,* p. 526.
7 Allars, *Report of the Inquiry into the Use of Pituitary Derived Hormones,* p. 526.
8 Allars, *Report of the Inquiry into the Use of Pituitary Derived Hormones,* p. 474.
9 Allars, *Report of the Inquiry into the Use of Pituitary Derived Hormones,* p. 474.
10 Allars, *Report of the Inquiry into the Use of Pituitary Derived Hormones,* p. 464.
11 Allars, *Report of the Inquiry into the Use of Pituitary Derived Hormones,* p. 478.
12 Allars, *Report of the Inquiry into the Use of Pituitary Derived Hormones,* p. 190.
13 Allars, *Report of the Inquiry into the Use of Pituitary Derived Hormones,* pp. 190–191.
14 J. Talbot, M. Dooley, J. Leeton, et al., "Gonadotrophin stimulation for oocyte recovery and in vitro fertilisation in infertile women", *Australian and New Zealand Journal of Obstetrics and Gynaecology,* 1976, vol. 16, pp. 111–117.
15 Allars, *Report of the Inquiry into the Use of Pituitary Derived Hormones,* p. 205
16 Allars, *Report of the Inquiry into the Use of Pituitary Derived Hormones,* p. 194.

17 Allars, *Report of the Inquiry into the Use of Pituitary Derived Hormones,* p. 196.
18 J. Cooke, "Bioethicists urged to act on victimisation of women", *Sydney Morning Herald,* April 23, 1994.
19 B. Fih, "Simon is kept waiting to grow", *Age,* June 11, 1985.
20 Allars, *Report of the Inquiry into the Use of Pituitary Derived Hormones,* Executive Summary; p. 4.
21 Allars, *Report of the Inquiry into the Use of Pituitary Derived Hormones,* p. 180.
22 Allars, *Report of the Inquiry into the Use of Pituitary Derived Hormones,* p. 214.
23 Allars, *Report of the Inquiry into the Use of Pituitary Derived Hormones,* p. 213.
24 Allars, *Report of the Inquiry into the Use of Pituitary Derived Hormones,* p. 213.
25 Allars, *Report of the Inquiry into the Use of Pituitary Derived Hormones,* pp. 214–215.
26 Allars, *Report of the Inquiry into the Use of Pituitary Derived Hormones,* Executive summary, p. 5.
27 Allars, *Report of the Inquiry into the Use of Pituitary Derived Hormones,* Report, pp. 57–65.
28 Allars, *Report of the Inquiry into the Use of Pituitary Derived Hormones,* p. 64.
29 Allars, *Report of the Inquiry into the Use of Pituitary Derived Hormones,* p. 64.
30 M. Kingston, J. Cooke, "Doctors to pay for mistakes", *Sydney Morning Herald,* November 8, 1994.
31 Anon., "$10m an insult, say hormone victims", *Telegraph-Mirror,* November 10, 1994.
32 J. Cooke, "Four settle fertility drug claims", *Sydney Morning Herald,* December 23, 1994.
33 J. Heffey, State Coroner Victoria, Record of investigation into death, Case No 2353/95, February 23, 1996.
34 Anon., Eleventh report of the PHS interagency coordinating committee on human growth hormone and Creutzfeldt-Jakob disease to the assistant secretary for health, December 1991.
35 M. Grossman, R. Blizzard, R. Barth, Progress report and prospectus for the National Pituitary Agency, February 1969.
36 C. Mautalen, R. Smith, "Lipolytic effects of human growth hormone in resistant obesity", *Journal of Clinical Endocrinology,* 1965, vol. 25, pp. 495–498.
37 Anon., Report of the National Pituitary Agency, National Institute of Arthritis, Metabolism and Digestive Diseases, December 31, 1976.
38 Minutes of the meeting of the PHS interagency coordinating committee on human growth hormone and Creutzfeldt-Jakob disease, November 8, 1989.
39 Minutes of meeting of MRC steering committee for human pituitary collection, December 16, 1977.
40 Minutes of meeting of MRC steering committee for human pituitary collection, December 16, 1977.

41 Allars, *Report of the Inquiry into the Use of Pituitary Derived Hormones,* Report, p. 353.
42 Allars, *Report of the Inquiry into the Use of Pituitary Derived Hormones,* Report, p. 354. Quoting letter from Dr Bangham to Dr FT. Perkins, World Health Organisation February 26, 1980.
43 L. Smith, Interview with author, April 1996.
44 F. Bonnici, Personal communication, May 1997.
45 K. Glasbrenner, "Medical news. Technology spurt resolves growth hormone problem, ends shortage", *Journal of the American Medical Association,* 1986, pp. 581–587.
46 H. Dean, H. Friesen, "Growth hormone therapy in Canada: end of one era and beginning of another", *CMAJ,* 1986, vol. 135, pp. 297–301.
47 Allars, *Report of the Inquiry into the Use of Pituitary Derived Hormones,* Report, p. 480.
48 Allars, *Report of the Inquiry into the Use of Pituitary Derived Hormones,* Report, p. 480.
49 S. Haynes, "Growth hormone", Review, *Australian Journal of Science and Medicine in Sport,* 1986, vol. 18, pp. 3–15.
50 J. Cooke, "Steroid link to killer disease CJD", *Sydney Morning Herald,* August 7, 1993.
51 R. Charlesworth, "Don't swallow it", *Inside Sport,* June 1992, pp. 42–46.
52 J. Cart, "Griffith-Joyner denies buying growth hormone", *Los Angeles Times,* part III, September 21, 1989, p. 8.
53 C. Dubin, "Commission of inquiry into the use of drugs and banned practices intended to increase athletic performance", *Positive Test,* pp. 288–291.
54 Dubin, "Commission of inquiry into the use of drugs and banned practices intended to increase athletic performance", p. 120.
55 V. Cowart, "Human growth hormone: The latest ergogenic aid", *Physician and Sports Medicine,* March 1988, vol. 16, pp. 175–185.
56 Anon., Drug misuse. Anabolic steroids and human growth hormone. Report to the chairman, committee on judiciary, US Senate, United States General Accounting Office, August 1989, p. 35.
57 Anon., Drug misuse., p. 36.
58 Drugs in sport, Second (final) report of the senate standing committee on environment, recreation and the arts, Australian Government Publishing Service, May 1990, pp. 332–334.
59 Abstracts, *Journal of the American Medical Association,* 1993, vol. 269, p. 1377.
60 R. Deyssig, H. Frisch, "Self-administration of cadaveric growth hormone in power athletes", *Lancet,* 1993, vol. 341, pp. 768–769.

Chapter 19
Blood: Another route of infection?

1 J.Cooke, "Blood, bone grafts may transmit disease—in theory", *Sydney Morning Herald,* July 3, 1997.
2 P. Brown, "Environmental causes of human spongiform encephalopathy", in *Methods in Molecular Medicine: Prion Diseases,* H. Baker, R. Ridley (eds), Humana Press Inc., New Jersey. 1996, pp. 145–146.

3   E. Manuelidis, J. Kim, J. Mericangas, L. Manuelidis, "Transmission to animals of Creutzfeldt-Jakob disease from human blood", *Lancet,* 1985, vol. 2, pp. 896–897.

4   J. Tateishi, "Transmission of Creutzfeldt-Jakob disease from human blood and urine into mice", *Lancet*, 1985, vol. 2, p. 1074.

5   T. Esmonde, R. Will, J. Slattery, R. Knight, R. Harries-Jones, R. De Silva, W. Matthews, "Creutzfeldt-Jakob disease and blood transfusion", *Lancet,* 1993, vol. 341, pp. 205–207.

6   L. Dumble, R. Klein, "Walls of Silence", Comment, *Medical Observer,* January 22, 1993, pp. 7, 43.

7   L. Dumble, R. Klein, "Transmission of Creutzfeldt-Jakob disease by blood transfusion", *Lancet,* 1993, vol. 341, p. 768.

8   J. Cooke, "Transfusion link to rare disease", *Sydney Morning Herald.* March 20, 1993.

9   N. Heye, S. Hensen, N. Müller, "Creutzfeldt-Jakob disease and blood transfusion", *Lancet,* 1993, vol. 343, p. 298.

10 M. Allars, *Report of the Inquiry into the Use of Pituitary Derived Hormones in Australia and Creutzfeldt-Jakob Disease,* Executive Summary, Australian Government Publishing Service, 1994, p. 657.

11 G. Stachlewski, Statement faxed to media and all members of the House of Representatives, Parliament House, Canberra, March 7, 1995.

12 J. Cooke, "New CJD fear", *Medical Observer,* June 23, 1995, p. 1.

13 N. Kobrinksy, Evidence to the Commission of inquiry on the blood system in Canada, Transcript of Day 161, July 11, 1995.

14 A. Picard, "Blood products being recalled", *Globe and Mail,* Toronto, July 17, 1995.

15 D. McDougall, "Red Cross to throw out blood from donor who has killer virus", *Canadian Press in the Ottawa Citizen,* July 14, 1995.

16 Exhibit 1138, Creutzfeldt-Jakob disease, Chronology for case study, prepared for the Commission of inquiry on the blood system in Canada, November 28, 1995, p. 20.

17 Exhibit 1138, Creutzfeldt-Jakob disease, p. 17.

18 A. Prokopiak, "The Canadian Red Cross Society. Red Cross cautionary withdrawal proceeds smoothly; 25% albumin replacements in by end of week", News Release, July 18, 1995, p. 2.

19 A. Picard, "Blood agencies disorganised. Canadian blood policy lacking", *Globe and Mail,* November 29, 1995.

20 Exhibit 1138, Creutzfeldt-Jakob disease, p. 12.

21 Exhibit 1138, Creutzfeldt-Jakob disease, pp. 29, 33.

22 R. Bragg, "Blood recall 'right thing for wrong reasons'", *Toronto Star,* July 18, 1995.

23 T. Murray, "New blood crisis? Meeting addresses possibility CJD could taint blood supply in Canada", *Medical Post,* June 18, 1996, vol. 32, p. 1.

24 T. Patel, "Placenta donors to be screened for brain disease", *New Scientist,* November 20, 1993.

25 National Health and Medical Research Council, Creutzfeldt-Jakob disease and other human transmissible spongiform encephalopathies, Guidelines on patient management and infection control, December 1995, p. 33.

26 K. Morris, News, "WHO reconsiders risks from Creutzfeldt-Jakob disease", *Lancet,* 1997, vol. 349, p. 1001.

27 J. Cunningham, "Creutzfeldt-Jakob blood riddle", *Calgary Herald,* April 20, 1996.

28 M. Stewart, "Dad's deterioration came swiftly", *Calgary Herald,* April 20, 1996.

29 A. Créange, F. Gray, P. Cesaro, H. Adle-Biassette, C. Duvoux, D. Cherqui, J. Bell, P. Parchi, P. Gambetti, J. Degos, "Creutzfeldt-Jakob disease after liver transplantation", *Annals of Neurology,* 1995, vol. 38, pp. 269–271.

30 E. Operskalski, J. Mosley, "Pooled plasma derivatives and Creutzfeldt-Jakob disease", *Lancet,* 1995, vol. 346, p. 1224.

31 A. Créange, F. Gray, P. Cesaro, "Pooled plasma derivatives and Creutzfeldt-Jakob disease", *Lancet,* 1996, vol. 347, p. 482.

32 T. Patel, "French dismiss transfusion link to brain disease", *New Scientist,* February 25, 1995, p. 5.

33 Y. Tamai, H. Kojima, R. Kitajima, F. Taguchi, Y. Ohtani, T. Kawaguchi, S. Miura, M. Sato, "Demonstration of the Transmissible Agent in Tissue from a Pregnant Woman with Creutzfeldt-Jakob Disease", *New England Journal of Medicine,* 1992, vol. 327, p. 649.

34 M. Ricketts, N. Cashman, E. Stratton, S. Elsaadany, "Is Creutzfeldt-Jakob disease transmitted in blood?", Review, *Emerging Infectious Diseases,* 1997, vol. 3, pp. 155–163.

35 A. Johnson, "Hopes That Died", *Guardian,* February 1, 1995.

36 Johnson, "Hopes That Died", 1995.

37 D. Kennedy, "Young victim of hormone therapy faces death with courage and humour. I regret nothing, says patient dying from growth cure", *The Times,* September 5, 1995.

38 Named patients in this chapter have all been revealed in the media by the families concerned.

39 R. Lacey, "Bovine Spongiform Encephalopathy is being maintained by vertical and horizontal transmission", *British Medical Journal,* 1996, vol. 213, pp. 180–181.

40 N. Hawkes, "Second farmer's death raises fear of 'mad cow' cover-up", *The Times,* August 13, 1993.

41 P. Smith, M. Zeidler, J. Ironside, P. Estiberio, T. Moss, "Creutzfeldt-Jakob disease in a dairy farmer", *Lancet,* 1995, vol. 346, p. 898.

42 N. Delasnerie-Laupretre, S. Poser, M. Pocchiari, D. Wientjens, R. Will, "Creutzfeldt-Jakob disease in Europe", *Lancet,* 1995, vol. 345, p. 898.

43 A. Loudon, "Farmer's wife in new mad cow alert", *Daily Mail,* October 24, 1995.

44 Anon., "Brain deaths", *New Scientist,* October 14, 1995, p. 11.

45 P. Harris, "New Fear Over Mad Cow Link. Secret probe as fourth farmer is hit by brain disease", *Daily Mail,* October 23, 1995.

46 M. Hornsby, "Tighter curb to keep BSE out of food. Prosecution warning to abattoirs", *The Times,* November 10, 1995.

47 D. Bateman, D. Hilton, S. Love, M. Zeidler, J. Beck, J. Collinge, "Sporadic Creutzfeldt-Jakob disease in a 18-year-old in the UK, *Lancet,* 1995, vol. 346, pp. 1155–1156.

48 Bateman, et al., "Sporadic Creutzfeldt-Jakob disease in a 18-year-old in the UK", pp. 1155–1156.
49 T. Britton, S. Al-Sarraj, C. Shaw, T. Campbell, J. Collinge, "Sporadic Creutzfeldt-Jakob disease in a 16-year-old in the UK", *Lancet,* 1995, vol. 346, p. 1155.
50 Britton, et al., "Sporadic Creutzfeldt-Jakob disease in a 16-year-old in the UK", p. 1155.
51 T. Billette de Villemeur, J. Deslys, A. Pradel, C. Soubrie, A. Alpérovitch, M. Tardieu, J. Chaussain, J. Hauw, D. Dormont, M. Ruberg, Y. Agid, "Creutzfeldt-Jakob disease from contaminated growth hormone extracts in France", *Neurology,* 1996, vol. 47, p. 690.
52 I. Shaw, "BSE and farmworkers", *Lancet,* 1995, vol. 346, p. 1365.
53 P. Martin, "The mad cow deceit", *Night and Day Magazine,* December 17, 1995, pp. 21–26.
54 S. Connor, "Closing in on a killer", *Sunday Times,* December 3, 1995.
55 C. Arthur, L. Jury, C. Newman, "Major rejects mad cow link to humans", *Independent,* December 8, 1995.
56 V. Chaudhary, "BSE expert calls for calm", *Guardian,* December 9, 1995.

Chapter 20
A new CJD strain

1   R. Will, Interview with author, May 1996.
2   J. Ironside, Interview with author, June 1996.
3   J. Mills, J. Fradkin, L. Schonberger, et al. "Status report on the US human growth hormone recipient follow-up study", *Hormone Research,* 1990, vol. 33, pp. 116–120.
4   J. Monreal, G. Collins, C. Masters, C. Miller Fisher, R. Kim, C. Gibbs, D. Gajdusek, "Creutzfeldt-Jakob disease in an adolescent", *Journal of the Neurological Sciences,* 1981, vol. 52, pp. 341–350.
5   P. Brown, F. Cathala, R. Labauge, "Epidemiologic implications of Creutzfeldt-Jakob disease in a 19-year-old girl", *European Journal of Epidemiology,* 1985, vol. 469, pp. 42–47.
6   T. Britton, S. Al-Sarraj, C. Shaw, T. Campbell, J. Collinge, "Creutzfeldt-Jakob disease in a 16-year-old in the UK", *Lancet,* 1995, vol. 346, p. 1155.
7   A. Adamson, "Legacy of hope. Scientists will research rare illness after wife's death", *Hull Daily Mail,* January 18, 1996.
8   Ironside, Interview with author, June 1996.
9   J. Collinge, Personal communication, July 1997.
10 Will, Interview with author, May 1996.
11 J. Almond, Interview with author, October 1996.
12 Ironside, Interview with author, June 1996.
13 R. Will, J. Ironside, M. Zeidler, et al., "A new variant of Creutzfeldt-Jakob disease in the UK", *Lancet,* 1996, vol. 347, pp. 921-925.
14 J. Lanchester, "A new kind of contagion", *New Yorker,* December 2, 1996.
15 Anon., "Parents of victim fear link with fast food", *Weekly Telegraph,* April 3–9, 1996.
16 R. Howard, "Creutzfeldt-Jakob disease in a young woman", *Lancet,* 1996, vol. 47, pp. 945–948.

17 Victoria Rimmer died in December 1997, never having woken from her coma.
18 P. Maass, "Colleague defends accused NIH scientist; friend says law enforcement 'setup' led to sexual abuse charges", *Washington Post,* April 8, 1996.
19 P. Pan, K. Vick, "Second youth says he was abused by mad scientist", *Washington Post,* April 18, 1996.
20 J. Gillis, P. Pan, "Scientist described child sexuality. Nobel Prize-winner's journals scrutinised after his abuse arrest", *Pittsburgh Post-Gazette,* April 7, 1996.
21 G. Chazot, E. Broussolle, C. Lapras, T. Blättler, A. Aguzzi, N. Kopp, "New variant of Creutzfeldt-Jakob disease in a 26-year-old French man", *Lancet,* 1996, vol. 347, p. 1181.
22 J. Wise, "Scientists find low level transmission of BSE", *British Medical Journal,* 1996, vol. 313, p. 317. (This preliminary data was confirmed in April 1997 by SEAC, when the experiment, begun in 1989, was finished.)
23 C. Lasmézas, et al., "BSE transmission to macaques", *Nature,* 1996, vol. 381, pp. 743–744.
24 J. Collinge, K. Sidle, J. Meads, J. Ironside, A. Hill. "Molecular analysis of prion strain variation and the aetiology of "new variant' CJD", *Nature,* 1996, vol. 383, pp. 685–690.

Chapter 21
British victims: Their day in court

1 J. Buckler, Witness statement to the CJD litigation, High Court, London, February 1996.
2 T. Fry, Personal communication, April 1996.
3 A. Khan, Personal communication, April 1996.
4 S. Martindale, Personal communication, March 1997.
5 Eleventh report of the PHS interagency coordinating committee on human growth hormone and Creutzfeldt-Jakob disease to the Assistant Secretary for Health, December 1991.
6 P. Smellie, "Bad blood adds CJD to haemophiliac's family fears", *Australian,* May 13, 1996.
7 Answers to author's questions provided by the New Zealand Ministry of Health, June 6, 1997.
8 J. Deslys, C. Lasmézas, N. Streichenberger, et al., "New variant Creutzfeldt-Jakob disease in France", *Lancet,* 1997, vol. 349, pp. 30–31.
9 M. Lees, Question to Senator Newman, Senate Hansard, March 26, 1997, p. 2218.
10 M. Lees, "Australian Pituitary Hormone Program — Government must act now to avoid another 'Voyager'", Media Release, March 26, 1997.
11 J. Cooke, "Denial of legal aid, may stop medical law suit", *Sydney Morning Herald,* March 25, 1997.
12 Cooke, "Denial of legal aid, may stop medical law suit", March 25, 1997.
13 APQ, Interview with author, April 1997.

Chapter 22
The shocking legacy of cannibalism
1   Anon., "The prion hypothesis is finally accepted by the establishment",
    British Medical Journal, News, October 18, 1997, p. 315.
2   J. Knight, N. Boyce, "Nobel splits top brains", *New Scientist,* October
    1997, p. 11.
3   M. Bruce, R. Will, J. Ironside, I. McConnell, et al., "Transmissions to
    mice indicate that 'new variant' CJD is caused by the BSE agent",
    Nature, 1997, vol. 389, pp. 498–501.
4   A. Hill, M. Desbruslais, S. Joiner, K. Sidle, et al., "The same prion strain
    causes vCJD and BSE", *Nature,* 1997, vol. 389, pp. 448–50.
5   J. Wise, "Agents of new variant CJD and BSE are identical", *British
    Medical Journal,* 1997, p. 315.
6   S. Cousens, E. Vynnycky, M. Zeidler, R. Will, P. Smith, "Predicting the
    CJD epidemic in humans", *Nature,* 1997, vol. 385, pp. 197–198.
7   E. Green, "What Clare tells us", *New Statesman,* August 29, 1997, p. 19.
8   Signatories to BSE: an open letter, *New Statesman,* September 12, 1997,
    p. 19.
9   K. Ahmed, "Death from CJD adds to fears of toxic area", *Guardian,*
    August 11, 1997.
10 D. Body, Personal communication, December 1997.
11 J. Warren, "Eating squirrel may be tied to fatal brain disease", *US Knight-
    Ridder Newspapers international,* wire copy, May 1997.
12 S. Prusiner, "Prion disease and the BSE crisis", *Science,* 1997, vol. 278,
    pp. 245–252.
13 A. Coghlan, "Does yeast hold secrets of CJD?", *New Scientist,* May 17,
    1997, p. 16.
14 R. Triendl, "CJD link prompts ban on brain tissue use", *Nature,* 1997,
    vol. 387, p. 5.
15 K. Morris, "WHO reconsiders risks from Creutzfeldt-Jakob disease",
    Lancet, 1997, vol. 349, p. 1001.
16 M. Weaver, "Guards officer died of CJD after growth jabs", *Electronic
    Telegraph,* September 28, 1996.
17 J. Cooke, "First payout for living victim of CJD", *Sydney Morning
    Herald,* December 8, 1997.
18 P. Bansemer, Personal communication with author, October 31, 1997.
19 M. Pelletier, Personal communication, March 1997.
20 Martinez-Lage et al., "Accidental transmission of Creutzfeldt-Jakob
    disease by dural cadaveric grafts", *Journal of Neurology Neurosurgery
    and Psychiatry,* 1994, vol. 57, pp. 1091-1094.
21 J. Gillis, "Nobel winner guilty of abusing boy. Under plea deal, former
    NIH scientist will spend up to a year in jail", *Washington Post,* February
    19, 1997.
22 Anon., "Quins' parents divorced", *Mirror,* September 14, 1973.
23 J. Catt, "Inquest into double killing", *Mirror,* March 24, 1982.
24 K. Campbell, J. McWhir, W. Ritchie, I. Wilmut, "Sheep cloned by
    nuclear transfer from a cultured cell line", *Nature,* 1996, vol. 380, p.
    64–66.

25 R. Weiss, "It's the do-it-yourself chromosome. Gene therapy breakthrough offers hope in fight against disease", *Sydney Morning Herald,* April 2, 1997, p. 1.
26 Anon., "Britain plays it cautions on animal-human transplants", *Nature,* 1997, vol. 385, p. 285.

Afterword
1 J. Heckmann, C. Lang, F. Petruch, A. Druschky, C. Erb, P. Brown, B. Neundorfer, "Transmission of Creutzfeldt-Jakob disease via a corneal transplant", *Journal of Neurology, Neurosurgery and Psychiatry,* 1997, vol. 63, pp. 388–390.
2 B. Christie, "Inquiry ordered after organ donor found to have CJD", *British Medical Journal,* 1997, vol. 315, p. 1485.
3 J. Worthington, S. Stone, "Epidemiology of Jakob-Creutzfeldt disease in Australia 1970 to 1980", *Australian and New Zealand Journal of Medicine,* 1995, vol. 25, pp. 243–244.
4 R. Roos, A. Wintzen, R. Will, J. Ironside, S. van Duinen, "A patient with Creutzfeldt-Jakob disease following treatment with human growth hormone", *Ned Tijdschr Geneeskd,* 1996, vol. 140, pp. 1190–1193.
5 C. Lang, P. Schuler, A. Engelhardt, A. Spring, P. Brown, "Probable Creutzfeldt-Jakob disease after a cadaveric dural graft", *European Journal of Epidemiology,* 1995, vol. 11, pp. 79–81.
6 H. Rosenmann, Z. Meiner, E. Kahana, M. Halimi, E. Lenetsky, O. Abramsky, R. Gabizon, "Detection of 14-3-3 protein in the CSF of genetic Creutzfeldt-Jakob disease", *Neurology,* 1997, vol. 49, pp. 593–595.
7 R. Highfield, "Check on CJD blood donors", *Daily Telegraph,* October 10, 1997.
8 C. Ludlam, "New-variant Creutzfeldt-Jakob disease and treatment of haemophilia", *Lancet,* 1997, vol. 350, p. 1704.
9 Anon., "Nearly 270 people received CJD-contaminated blood", *AFP,* December 14, 1997.
10 Senate Community Affairs References Committee, Report on the CJD settlement offer, Senate Printing Unit, Parliament House, Canberra. October 1997.
11 J. Morland, Judgement, The Creutzfeldt-Jakob disease litigation, Queen's Bench Division, High Court, London. Case 1994 N 05806, December 18, 1997.

Index